2021

ADVANCES IN MOLECULAR PATHOLOGY

EDITOR-IN-CHIEF
Gregory J. Tsongalis, PhD, HCLD

SECTION EDITORS
Ahmad N. Abou Tayoun, PhD, FACMG
Helen Fernandes, PhD
Andrea Ferreira-Gonzalez, PhD, HCLD(ABB), CC(ABB), FACB
Matthew Lebo, PhD, FACMG
Eric Y. Loo, MD
Ann M. Moyer, MD, PhD

ELSEVIER

Publishing Director, Medical Reference: Dolores Meloni
Editor: Lauren Boyle
Developmental Editor: Hannah Almira Lopez

Reprints: For copies of 100 or more of articles in this publication, please contact the Commercial Reprints Department, Elsevier Inc., 360 Park Avenue South, New York, NY 10010-1710. Tel: 212-633-3874; Fax: 212-633-3820; E-mail: reprints@elsevier.com.

Printed in the United States of America.

Editorial Office:
Elsevier, Inc.
1600 John F. Kennedy Blvd,
Suite 1800
Philadelphia, PA 19103-2899

International Standard Serial Number: 2589-4080
International Standard Book Number: 13: 978-0-323-81335-8

ADVANCES IN MOLECULAR PATHOLOGY

ADVANCES IN MOLECULAR PATHOLOGY

CONTRIBUTORS

EDITOR

GREGORY J. TSONGALIS, PhD, HCLD
Professor, Department of Pathology and Laboratory Medicine, The Audrey and Theodore Geisel School of Medicine at Dartmouth, Hanover, NH, USA; Vice Chair for Research and Director, Laboratory for Clinical Genomics and Advanced Technology (CGAT), Department of Pathology and Laboratory Medicine, Dartmouth Hitchcock Medical Center, Lebanon, NH, USA

AUTHORS

MIR B. ALIKHAN, MD
Department of Pathology and Laboratory Medicine, NorthShore University HealthSystem, Evanston, Illinois, USA

RANJANA ARORA, MD
Associate Professor, Department of Pathology and Laboratory Medicine, University of Kentucky, Lexington, Kentucky, USA

DEEPA BHOJWANI, MD
Division of Hematology/Oncology, Children's Hospital Los Angeles, Keck School of Medicine of USC, University of Southern California, Associate Professor, Pediatrics, Keck School of Medicine, University of Southern California, Los Angeles, California, USA

ASHKAN BIGDELI, ALM
Division of Precision and Computational Diagnostics, Department of Pathology and Laboratory Medicine, Lead Bioinformatics Specialist, Hospital of the University of Pennsylvania, Drexel University, School of Biomedical Engineering, Science and Health Systems, Philadelphia, Pennsylvania, USA

JENNIFER A. CAMPBELL, PharmD
Associate Dean of Academic Programs, Manchester University, College of Pharmacy, Natural, and Health Sciences, Fort Wayne, Indiana, USA

MARK A. CERVINSKI, PhD
Associate Professor, Department of Pathology and Laboratory Medicine, Dartmouth-Hitchcock Medical Center, Lebanon, New Hampshire, USA

DEVON CHABOT-RICHARDS, MD
Associate Professor, University of New Mexico Department of Pathology, Albuquerque, New Mexico, USA

BRITTANY B. COFFMAN, MD
Molecular Genetic Pathology Fellow, University of New Mexico Department of Pathology, Albuquerque, New Mexico, USA

YASEMIN COLE, MSc
MD/PhD Student, UNC School of Medicine, The University of North Carolina at Chapel Hill, Chapel Hill, North Carolina, USA

JENSYN K. CONE SULLIVAN, MD
Department of Pathology, Associate Director of Transfusion Medicine and The Neely Cell Therapy Center, Tufts Medical Center, Assistant Professor of Pathology, Tufts University School of Medicine, Boston, Massachusetts, USA

HELEN FERNANDES, PhD
Department of Pathology and Cell Biology, Columbia University Irving Medical Center, New York, NewYork, USA

CAREN GENTILE, MS
Department of Pathology and Laboratory Medicine, Molecular Pathology Laboratory, Hospital of the University of Pennsylvania, Philadelphia, Pennsylvania, USA

NICHOLAS GLEADALL, PhD
Postdoctoral Research Associate, Department of Haematology, University of Cambridge, University of

Cambridge Biomedical Campus, Cambridge, United Kingdom

ROBERT HAMILTON, MD
Department of Pathology and Laboratory Medicine, Dartmouth-Hitchcock Medical Center, Lebanon, New Hampshire, USA

SARAH E. HERLIHY, PhD
Department of Pathology and Laboratory Medicine, Molecular Pathology Laboratory, Hospital of the University of Pennsylvania, Philadelphia, Pennsylvania, USA

CARRIE C. HOEFER, PhD, MBA
Director of Pharmacogenomics, Assistant Professor of Pharmaceutical Sciences, James L Winkle School of Pharmacy and Pharmaceutical Sciences, University of Cincinnati, Cincinnati, Ohio, USA

LEAH K. HOLLON, ND, MPH
CEO, Richmond Natural Medicine, National University of Natural Medicine Residency, Distant Site Supervisor and Board of Directors Member, Richmond, Virginia, USA

JACQUELINE A. HUBBARD, PhD
Assistant Professor, Department of Pathology and Laboratory Medicine, Dartmouth-Hitchcock Medical Center, Lebanon, New Hampshire, USA

NORA JOSEPH, MD
Department of Pathology and Laboratory Medicine, NorthShore University HealthSystem, Evanston, Illinois, USA

KAREN L. KAUL, MD PhD
Department of Pathology and Laboratory Medicine, NorthShore University HealthSystem, Evanston, Illinois, USA

WAHAB A. KHAN, PhD, FACMG
Director, Clinical Cytogenetics, Assistant Director, Molecular Genetics, Department of Pathology and Laboratory Medicine, Assistant Professor, Dartmouth Geisel School of Medicine, Dartmouth College, Dartmouth-Hitchcock Medical Center, Lebanon, New Hampshire, USA

ALEXANDRA E. KOVACH, MD
Division of Hematopathology, Department of Pathology and Laboratory Medicine, Children's Hospital Los Angeles, Associate Professor, Laboratory Medicine, Keck School of Medicine, University of Southern California, Los Angeles, California, USA

WILLIAM J. LANE, MD, PhD
Assistant Medical Director Tissue Typing Lab, Department of Pathology, Brigham and Women's Hospital, Hale Building for Transformative Medicine, Associate Professor, Harvard Medical School, Boston, Massachusetts, USA

ETHAN P.M. LAROCHELLE, PhD
Laboratory of Clinical Genomics and Advanced Technology, Department of Pathology and Laboratory Medicine, Dartmouth Hitchcock Medical Center, Lebanon, New Hampshire, USA; Dartmouth Geisel School of Medicine, Dartmouth College, Hanover, New Hampshire, USA

JOSHUA J. LEVY, PhD
Program in Quantitative Biomedical Sciences, Department of Epidemiology, Dartmouth Geisel School of Medicine, Emerging Diagnostic and Investigative Technologies, Department of Pathology, Dartmouth Hitchcock Medical Center, Lebanon, New Hampshire, USA

M. SHAHEEN S. MALICK, MD
Department of Pathology and Cell Biology, Columbia University Irving Medical Center, New York, New York, USA

KATHY A. MANGOLD, PhD
Department of Pathology and Laboratory Medicine, NorthShore University HealthSystem, Evanston, Illinois, USA

SHANNON M. MCNULTY, PhD
Postdoctoral Research Associate, Department of Genetics, The University of North Carolina at Chapel Hill, Chapel Hill, North Carolina, USA

ROBERT D. NERENZ, PhD
Assistant Professor, Department of Pathology and Laboratory Medicine, Dartmouth-Hitchcock Medical Center, Lebanon, New Hampshire, USA

THOMAS P. OLSON, PhD, FAHA, FACSM
Associate Professor of Medicine, Department of Cardiovascular Medicine, Geneticure, Inc,

Department of Cardiovascular Diseases, Mayo Clinic, Rochester, Minnesota, USA

AMANDA ORAN, PhD
Division of Precision and Computational Diagnostics, Department of Pathology and Laboratory Medicine, Genomic Development Specialist, Hospital of the University of Pennsylvania, Philadelphia, Pennsylvania, USA

ZHIYU PENG, PhD
BGI Genomics, BGI-Shenzhen, Shenzhen, China; College of Life Sciences, University of Chinese Academy of Sciences, Beijing, China

BRADFORD C. POWELL, MD, PhD
Assistant Professor, Department of Genetics, The University of North Carolina at Chapel Hill, Chapel Hill, North Carolina, USA

AYMAN QASRAWI, MD
Assistant Professor, Division of Hematology, Blood and Marrow Transplantation and Cellular Therapy, University of Kentucky, University of Kentucky Markey Cancer Center, Lexington, Kentucky, USA

GORDANA RACA, MD, PhD
Clinical Cytogenomics Laboratory, Center for Personalized Medicine, Children's Hospital Los Angeles, Associate Professor, Laboratory Medicine, Keck School of Medicine, University of Southern California, Los Angeles, California, USA

KALPANA S. REDDY, MD
Department of Pathology and Laboratory Medicine, NorthShore University HealthSystem, Evanston, Illinois, USA

STEFAN RENTAS, PhD
Assistant Professor, Department of Pathology and Laboratory Medicine, The University of North Carolina at Chapel Hill, Chapel Hill, North Carolina, USA

LINDA M. SABATINI, PhD
Department of Pathology and Laboratory Medicine, NorthShore University HealthSystem, Evanston, Illinois, USA

NIKOLETTA SIDIROPOULOS, MD
The Robert Larner, M.D. College of Medicine, The University of Vermont, Genomic Medicine, Department of Pathology and Laboratory Medicine, University of Vermont Medical Center, Burlington, Vermont, USA

LIRON BARNEA SLONIM, MD
Department of Pathology and Laboratory Medicine, NorthShore University HealthSystem, Evanston, Illinois, USA

ERIC M. SNYDER, PhD, FAHA, FACSM
Chief Operating Officer, Geneticure, Inc, Rochester, Minnesota, USA

RYAN SPRISSLER, PhD
Staff Scientist, Manager, Geneticure, Inc, Rochester, Minnesota, USA; Genomics Core Facility, University of Arizona, Tucson, Arizona, USA

SAMANTHA STEPHEN, DO
Department of Pathology and Laboratory Medicine, Dartmouth-Hitchcock Medical Center, Lebanon, New Hampshire, USA

ROBYN SUSSMAN, PhD
Division of Precision and Computational Diagnostics, Department of Pathology and Laboratory Medicine, Molecular Development Assistant Director, Hospital of the University of Pennsylvania, Philadelphia, Pennsylvania, USA

AMOGHA TADIMETY, PhD
Nanopath Inc, Cambridge, Massachusetts, USA

DIANA M. TOLEDO, PhD, MS, CGC
Associate Director, The Broad Institute of MIT and Harvard, Clinical Research Sequencing Platform Laboratory, Cambridge, Massachusetts, USA

LOUIS J. VAICKUS, MD, PhD
Emerging Diagnostic and Investigative Technologies, Department of Pathology, Dartmouth Hitchcock Medical Center, Lebanon, New Hampshire, USA

BRENT L. WOOD, MD, PhD
Division of Hematopathology, Department of Pathology and Laboratory Medicine, Children's Hospital Los Angeles, Professor, Laboratory Medicine, Keck School of Medicine, University of Southern California, Los Angeles, California, USA

JIALE XIANG, MS
BGI Genomics, BGI-Shenzhen, Shenzhen, China; College of Life Sciences, University of Chinese Academy of Sciences, Beijing, China

CONTENTS

VOLUME 4 • 2021

Advances in Molecular Pathology 4 (2021) xv–xvi

ADVANCES IN MOLECULAR PATHOLOGY

Preface

Molecular Pathology: What a Difference a Year Makes

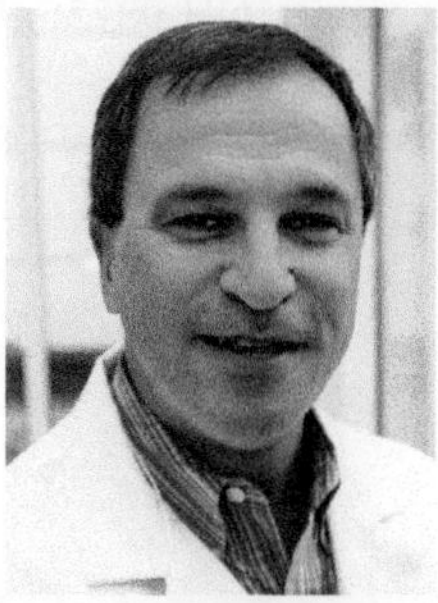

Gregory J. Tsongalis, PhD, HCLD
Editor

This past year brought struggles and challenges to the entire world, including molecular diagnostic laboratories, due to the ongoing severe acute respiratory syndrome coronavirus 2 (SARS-CoV-2) pandemic. Overcoming supply chain issues affecting reagents, other consumables and disposables, along with staffing and equipment issues highlighted the importance of robust laboratory services as well as the ingenuity and creativity of laboratorians to meet those challenges head on. Polymerase chain reaction became a household term and the gold standard for viral detection. The laboratory-developed test in several varieties once again became the go-to assay that saved the day. From diagnostic testing through screening and surveillance testing and ultimately viral sequencing to detect variant strains of SARS-CoV-2, our laboratories delivered on the unmet and uncertain needs of providers and patients globally. At the time of this writing, countries have ramped up efforts to vaccinate individuals with one of several available vaccines, and in the United States, numbers of new cases and deaths due to COVID-19 have significantly subsided. Globally, the virus continues to be a major cause of morbidity and mortality in numerous countries that have had delayed vaccination responses, and the potential resurgence of COVID-19 cases in those younger individuals that have yet to be vaccinated remains a threat. Our hope is that continued vaccination and mitigation strategies will end this pandemic if we remain vigilant and a new sense of "normalcy" will prevail.

In this fourth issue of *Advances in Molecular Pathology*, we include another special section on COVID-19 that highlights experiences from a laboratory perspective, serologic testing, and genomic surveillance of variants. Our colleagues and authors found the time to shed light on some of the more interesting developments in the field of molecular pathology despite the burden that the pandemic has taken on all of us. Clinical genomics is not a passing fad as some had predicted; it is here to stay, and our stewardship of the testing on the analytical and interpretative sides remains critical to patient care. In this issue, we review advances in the field of

https://doi.org/10.1016/j.yamp.2021.06.004
2589-4080/21/

molecular pathology with regards to developments in genetic disease, hematologic disease, infectious disease, pharmacogenomics, solid tumors, and informatics. Several articles present novel technologies, such as optimal genome mapping, point-of-care diagnostics, and artificial intelligence. Operationalizing genomic medicine in a clinical setting and assessing minimal residual disease, cell-free nucleic acids, and tumor mutation burden are discussed as impactful strategies in the management of the patient with cancer. Finally, germline variants, nutrigenomics, and hypertension are presented as new applications of pharmacogenomics.

I am grateful to those friends and colleagues who once again during the most pressing of times agreed to become section editors and authors of the fantastic articles presented here.

Happy reading!

Gregory J. Tsongalis, PhD, HCLD
Department of Pathology and
Laboratory Medicine
Dartmouth Hitchcock Medical Center
1 Medical Center Drive
Lebanon, NH 03756, USA

E-mail address: Gregory.j.tsongalis@hitchcock.org

Genetics

Advances in Molecular Pathology 4 (2021) 1–15
ADVANCES IN MOLECULAR PATHOLOGY

Current Tools, Databases, and Resources for Phenotype and Variant Analysis of Clinical Exome Sequencing

Shannon M. McNulty, PhD[a], Yasemin Cole, MSc[b], Bradford C. Powell, MD, PhD[a], Stefan Rentas, PhD[c,*]
[a]Department of Genetics, University of North Carolina at Chapel Hill, 120 Mason Farm Road, Campus Box: 7264, Chapel Hill, NC 27599, USA; [b]University of North Carolina School of Medicine, University of North Carolina at Chapel Hill, 120 Mason Farm Road, Campus Box: 7264, Chapel Hill, NC 27599, USA; [c]Department of Pathology and Laboratory Medicine, University of North Carolina at Chapel Hill, 111 Mason Farm Road, Campus Box: 7264, Chapel Hill, NC 27599, USA

KEYWORDS
• Exome sequencing • Genomic medicine • Variant prioritization • Phenotype association

KEY POINTS
- The main approaches for incorporating phenotype data in genomic analysis include using manually curated virtual gene panels of high clinical validity, human phenotype ontology database matching, and automated screening of published literature.
- Variant prioritization filters can be based on several American College of Medical Genetics classification criteria to help identify high-impact variants in well-studied and new disease genes.
- Laboratories should keep up-to-date of new disease and gene-focused variant guidelines from ClinGen Clinical Domain Working Groups.
- Phenotype association and variant prioritization methods are both necessary to support a robust genomic analysis workflow. Both data streams are moving toward automation, natural language processing, and machine learning to support rapid primary and reanalysis of genomic data.

INTRODUCTION

Over the last decade, genetic testing has rapidly evolved from single-gene analysis to the feasibility of surveying of a patient's entire genome for disease-causing variants [1–10]. This transformation in molecular diagnostics has been enabled by industry and academic investment in creating and commercializing new technologies like massively parallel multiplex sequencing (otherwise known as next-generation sequencing, NGS), the development of sophisticated statistical and mathematical algorithms to interpret sequence data, and technological improvements in computer processing speed and data storage [11–13]. Consequently, genomic sequencing methods, such as exome sequencing (ES), the targeted sequencing of the protein coding regions of the genome, and whole genome sequencing (GS), are driving a rapid accumulation of human DNA sequence data, which has significantly improved the understanding of genetic variation across ethnically diverse populations [14–16] and propelled exponential growth in the discovery of genes and variants that cause disease [17–20]. The clinical application of genomic sequencing (ie, genomic

*Corresponding author, *E-mail address:* srentas@med.unc.edu

https://doi.org/10.1016/j.yamp.2021.07.001
2589-4080/21/

medicine) [21] has made an especially strong impact on improving the routine care and diagnosis of rare Mendelian diseases [22–24].

The first reported implementation of clinical ES was in 2013 [23], and since then, a growing number of studies have shown trio (mother, father, and proband) ES provides superior diagnostic yield (~36%) compared with standard-of-care chromosomal microarray testing (~10%) in children with suspected genetic disorders [4]. In addition, genomic sequencing impacts clinical management and initiation of therapeutic interventions and can decrease costs to payers and health care systems by reducing unnecessary testing [3,25–33]. Altogether, these studies are adding to a growing consensus that clinical genomic sequencing (ES or GS) should be performed as a first-line test for children with a suspected genetic disorder [2,4,25,28,34,35].

With clinical genomic sequencing poised to become the next standard-of-care test for rare diseases, a growing number of molecular diagnostic laboratories will need to develop clinical ES or GS tests. One of the biggest challenges related to the validation and implementation of a genomic sequencing-based test for rare disease is designing the data analysis workflow [36,37]. The components of a *typical* genomic analysis protocol consist of the following steps: (1) acquiring patient phenotype information, (2) generating sequence data, (3) filtering sequence data for genes with rare and potentially deleterious variants, (4) correlating these impacted genes and their related diseases (if previously established) with the patient's phenotype, (5) classifying variants according to American College of Medical Genetics/Association for Molecular Pathology (ACMG/AMP) guidelines [38], (6) assessing possible ACMG secondary findings [24], and (7) generating reports with pertinent results and case level interpretation. The 2 steps that usually require significant time and effort from a highly trained molecular variant analyst are correlating the patient's phenotype with potentially hundreds of genes (referred to here as phenotype correlation) and determining a variant pathogenicity classification. To help target manual review related to phenotype correlation and variant classification, the last several years have seen an exponential increase in research into algorithms, guidelines, and databases that support these 2 central components of genomic sequencing analysis.

Here, the authors focus on the challenges of developing and implementing robust clinical genomic analysis workflows for rare diseases and pay special attention to the computational tools, databases, and guidelines that are used to contextualize patient phenotype and genotype data. An understanding of how to use these rapidly evolving resources to support analysis procedures is critical to promote excellence and parity in results and in procedures across various clinical ES and GS tests.

PHENOTYPE ASSOCIATION TOOLS AND DATABASES

The use of phenotypic information to identify candidate diagnoses is a common practice in genomic analysis and relies heavily on the Human Phenotype Ontology (HPO), which provides a standardized ontology to describe phenotypic abnormalities. These terms are organized in directed acyclic graphs, which are oriented from general to more specific and allow individual terms to be related to more than 1 parent term. In addition to these terms, the Monarch Initiative maintains disease models to relate collections of human phenotypes to diseases and genes (disease-phenotype annotations and gene-phenotype annotations), effectively defining phenotypic profiles of diseases and/or genes [39–41]. Together, HPO terms and disease models serve as the foundation for 2 main approaches to improve genomic analysis of variants linked to rare Mendelian disease through the inclusion of patient phenotype data: (1) virtual panels to restrict analysis of genes relevant to the patient's phenotype and (2) algorithms to link phenotypes in patients to genes that cause a particular disorder.

Virtual Gene Panels

Patient phenotypes can be used to select one or more virtual gene panels (each representing diagnostic categories) to restrict genetic analysis, narrowing the list of candidate variants for manual gene review. These gene panels can be generated in an ad hoc manner based on gene-phenotype associations in curated databases, including OMIM [42], HGMD [43], Orphanet [44], GeneReviews [45–47], MasterMind [48], and PhenomeCentral [49]. However, selecting genes with sufficient evidence for inclusion on clinical gene panels can be challenging and, until recently, there has been no widely held consensus on how this process should take place. To address this, ongoing efforts, including Genomics England PanelApp [50] and the Clinical Genome Resource (ClinGen) [51], are creating standardized, expert-reviewed gene lists. Regardless of the method used to assemble the gene list, gene panel selection is an iterative process if the original selection is thought to be overly narrow or overly broad. A consequence of using this manual filtration scheme is the potential for limiting the sensitivity of testing by focusing analysis to specific genes: a causative variant may not be identified if the involved gene was not analyzed because of the application of the wrong panel to the case and use of an obsolete version of a phenotype-guided list. Furthermore, the focus on using highly curated genes limits the potential for identifying and reporting new candidate disease genes that may have strong variant and basic science evidence supporting a possible role in causing disease. The main benefit of the virtual panel approach is ensuring that only highly clinically relevant genes undergo analysis and reporting.

Algorithm-Driven Gene Analysis

Numerous computational tools have been developed to aid in the prioritization of genes based on patient phenotype (Table 1). Nearly all tools rely on HPO terms to describe the patient's phenotype, although some tools can accept other ontologies [52,53] or free-text descriptions [54,55]. However, the accurate portrayal of observed phenotypes and identification of phenotypes relevant to disease present a challenge in the correlation of phenotypes to disease in a clinical setting. As a result, the accuracy and precision of patient phenotypes may be affected by noise (inclusion of unrelated phenotypes) and variability in the completeness of the description (some patients may not have had access to specialists or testing needed to identify the precise phenotype). Given that the phenotype or phenotypes observed in a given patient may not be an exact match to the phenotypes defined as part of the known disease/gene phenotypic profile, these tools integrate underlying algorithms to evaluate the similarity between 2 phenotypic terms. Major approaches include measuring semantic similarity [56–58] and using network-based similarity [59,60]. The algorithms then aggregate similarity scores across phenotypes and may also incorporate other information about the associated disease models, including the frequency and age of onset of certain phenotypes, to prioritize candidate genes or diseases. The results are often returned as a ranked list and may also include scores to indicate the strength of the match. These approaches can be independent of the patient's genotype, generating a "personalized gene panel" that can be used for variant filtering, or can integrate genomic data in the form of a list of genes containing variants or the specific variants themselves (see Table 1). Limitations of these approaches include their reliance on concordance of the patient's phenotype to phenotypes described in the HPO database. The HPO database in turn depends on the completeness of descriptions of phenotypes in the medical literature, so the concordance may not be robust to phenotypic expansion. Also, nonspecific phenotypes (like hypotonia and intellectual disability) may pull genes into the ranked list that have either limited clinical validity or a weak association with the observed phenotype (ie, hypotonia could occur rarely in a particular gene-associated disorder). The main benefit of using network-based algorithms for phenotype correlation is eliminating manual effort tied to applying curated gene lists and retaining the possibility of novel gene discovery. When variant information is supplied, these tools typically use a basic filter on genes containing variants that are rare or obviously damaging (eg, nonsense or frameshift variants) and may also integrate inheritance pattern information and include segregation analysis if genotype information from family members is also provided [61,62].

Although most phenotype association tools are strictly based on human disease phenotypes, multiple tools also incorporate model organism data in the identification of gene candidates as a potential method to identify novel candidate gene-disease associations [53,63,64]. Although the extension of the underlying data used in phenotype association from other organisms may be appropriate in a research setting, caution should be used in clinical testing to avoid reporting of genetic variants with an uncertain relationship to human disease.

Capturing Phenotype Information

Multiple methods exist for attaining phenotype data used in virtual gene panel selection or by phenotype association tools. Clinician-selected HPO terms can be captured using annotation aids [65] or dedicated software (eg, PhenoTips [66], MediQuant). PhenoTips [66] and Phenomizer [67] can also provide real-time suggestions of additional terms the clinician can include immediately or should evaluate in the future to further refine the phenotype and differentiate between possible candidate diseases. However, clinician entry of HPO terms can be a time-intensive and redundant task. As an alternative, phenotype terms can be extracted retrospectively from the electronic medical record by manual review or by an automated natural language processing (NLP) method [68–72]. Although NLP of medical text can be challenged by erroneous inclusion of negated phenotypes (features that were specifically noted to be not observed), contradictory information, or phenotypes included as part of family history, phenotypes identified by NLP methods used in downstream

TABLE 1
Summary of Key Features of Phenotype-Driven Prioritization Tools

Tool	Phenotype Input Format	Genotype Input		Variant Pathogenicity Analysis	Output	Access Options	Reference
		Accepted	Format				
AMELIE	HPO	✓	Candidate genes or VCF file (can also include VCF file from parents)	✓	List of candidate genes ranked by phenotypic match score	Web application; API	Birgmeier et al [62], 2020
DeepPVP	HPO or MP (mammalian phenotype ontology)	✓ (required)	VCF file	✓	Prediction score for each variant in the VCF file	Local install	Boudellioua et al [109], 2019
Exomiser (with PhenIX, PHIVE, or hiPHIVE)	HPO	✓ (required)	VCF file (can include multiple family members)	✓	Ranked list of genes with Exomiser score, phenotype score, and variant score	Local install	Smedley et al [61], 2015
eXtasy	HPO	✓ (required)	VCF file	✓	Prioritized variants (global and for each phenotype)	Web application; local install	Sifrim et al [116], 2013
GenIO	HPO and OMIM	✓ (required)	VCF file	✓	Candidate variants associated with phenotype and with secondary findings	Web application	Koile et al [117], 2018
LIRICAL	Phenopacket	✓	VCF file	✓ (via Exomiser)	List of candidate diseases and genes ranked by posttest probability	Local install	Robinson et al [75], 2020
Moon (Diploid/ Invitae)	HPO	✓ (required)	VCF file	✓	Candidate genes, variants, and disease	Web application	NA
Phen2Gene	Phenopacket or list of HPO terms	×		×	Ranked list of candidate genes	Web application; local install; API	Zhao et al [74], 2020

Phen-Gen	Free text	✓ (required)	VCF file	✓	List of candidate genes based on gene scores and variant scores	Local install	Javed et al [55], 2014
Phenolyzer	Free text	✓	Candidate genes or regions	×	Ranked list of candidate genes	Web application; local install	Yang et al [54], 2015
Phenomizer	HPO	×		×	List of candidate diseases and genes ranked by *P* value	Web application	Kohler et al [67], 2009
Phenoxome	HPO	✓	VCF file	✓	List of ranked variants	Web application	Wu et al [59], 2019
Phevor	HPO (or other ontology)	✓ (required)	Candidate genes or VAAST file	×	Ranked list of candidate genes	Web application	Singleton et al [53], 2014
Phrank	HPO (or other ontology)	✓	Candidate genes	×	Ranked list of candidate diseases and genes	Web application; source code	Jagadeesh et al [52], 2019
PubCaseFinder	HPO	✓	Candidate genes	×	Ranked list of candidate diseases and genes and similar publicly available cases	Web application; API	Fujiwara et al [76], 2018

phenotype association tools were demonstrated in a recent study to lead to comparable tool performance relative to manually extracted phenotypes [73]. NLP-guided phenotype extraction was also shown to be faster than manual phenotype extraction, reducing average analysis time by 80% to 99% depending on the NLP method used [69]. There are ongoing efforts to structure phenotypic data in a standardized format after collection as a "Phenopacket" (http://phenopackets.org/), which could also aid in data exchange and streamline analysis, as the standardized file format is the designated input for multiple phenotype-driven prioritization tools [74,75].

The ability to accurately identify candidate genes and variants based on phenotype is limited by the understanding of the phenotypic spectrum associated with a given disease. Although the phenotypes and their associated frequencies in affected individuals are relatively stable for well-characterized diseases, these attributes for recently described or exceptionally rare diseases may be less well characterized or undergoing phenotype expansion. Phenotypes that change throughout the course of the disease and may not have been clinically present at the time of phenotyping can also pose a unique challenge to these tools. Moreover, the rapid pace of novel gene-disease association discovery can lead to delays in the integration of new information into disease knowledge bases. The continued publication of well-phenotyped and -genotyped individuals and the incorporation of this information into HPO disease models are crucial to overcome current limitations of phenotype association tools and provide rich data about phenotype and genotype frequency and age of onset. Multiple recently developed phenotype-driven prioritization tools, including AMELIE [62], DiploidMoon (http://diploid.com), and PubCaseFinder [76], aim to capture recently published information about gene-disease relationships and disease-phenotype associations by including text-mining algorithms that review the literature for new information not yet incorporated into curated databases. For example, PubCaseFinder was used to review annotated titles and abstracts of 1,083,283 case reports and identified 64,794 new disease-phenotype associations not in Orphanet [76]. Such efforts attempt to overcome the limitations of manually curated databases that may lead to the limited coverage of relevant phenotypes. As the understanding of the relationships between genes, diseases, and phenotypes continues to expand, the inclusion of phenotype association will likely prove to be a powerful approach to improve genomic analysis.

VARIANT PATHOGENICITY: EVIDENCE CODES, TOOLS, AND DATABASES

The publication of the standards and guidelines for the interpretation of sequence variants by the ACMG and AMP provided diagnostic laboratories, clinicians, and researchers formalized language and a scoring system to assess the pathogenicity of sequence variants generated from NGS data [38]. The variant classification scheme uses 5 categories: benign, likely benign, variant of uncertain significance (VUS), likely pathogenic, and pathogenic. Variants classified into each category have an increasing likelihood of pathogenicity that fits a quantitative Bayesian formulation with the probability for pathogenicity of a variant classified as benign being less than 0.1%, likely benign 0.1% to 10%, VUS 10% to 90%, likely pathogenic 90% to 99%, and pathogenic greater than 99% [38,77,78]. The criteria used for determining pathogenic variant level classifications are numbered and codified by the strength of the piece of evidence, such as very strong (PVS1), strong (PS1-4), moderate (PM1-6), and supporting (PP1-4). Various combinations of these codes result in the final classification of the variant, for example, a variant with PVS1 (null variant) + PS2 (confirmed de novo) + PM2 (absent from population databases) achieves a pathogenic assertion. In the following section, the authors review several ACMG variant evidence codes and the latest guidelines, tools, and databases that allow for their proper assessment during genomic testing.

PVS1

Very strong evidence of pathogenicity is used when there is as a null variant in a gene whereby loss of function (LOF) is a known mechanism of disease [38]. The types of variants this includes are nonsense, frameshift, canonical ± 1 or 2 splice site, initiation codon, and single- or multi-exon deletion. Further refinement of the PVS1 code was provided by the ClinGen Sequence Variant Interpretation Workgroup [79]. The detailed decision tree from this study incorporates nuances specific to the interpretation LOF variants, such as the variant's location in the gene, the biological significance of the impacted exon, and the possibility of an inframe product. Because the consequence of these nuances may provoke uncertainty that the variant may lead to LOF, the guidelines in this study suggest downgrading the classification to strong or moderate-level evidence depending on this more-granular assessment of the variant. Since the publication of the updated PVS1 guidelines, recent work has shown the branching logic and variables that comprise the PVS1 decision tree can be adopted into an automated classification tool with a graphical user interface (AutoPVS1) [80]. Although this tool or other similar automated approaches may be adopted by clinical laboratories for assessing LOF variants, it is likely that most laboratories will continue using simple bioinformatic filters that bring LOF variants to the forefront for analysis followed by manual review according to the new PVS1 guidelines.

PS1/PM5

The strong evidence code, PS1, is applied when the same amino acid change as a previously established pathogenic variant regardless of nucleotide change has been observed. The moderate strength evidence code, PM5, is used when a novel missense change at an amino acid residue occurs whereby a different missense change has been previously determined to be pathogenic. The most comprehensive databases that support the application of these codes include the Clinical Variant database (ClinVar) [81], Human Gene Mutation Database (HGMD) [43], and Mastermind [82]. ClinVar is maintained by the National Institutes of Health and is a freely available, public archive of human genetic variants and their relationships to diseases. A key strength of ClinVar is that it provides an avenue for large reference laboratories to share their variant-disease interpretations and classifications from patients that received clinical sequencing, thus broadening the number of reported variants with potential clinical significance beyond what is available in the literature. HGMD (Qiagen) is a manually curated database of variant and disease associations reported in the literature, whereas Mastermind (Genomenon) is not curated but functions more as a search engine to identify variant, disease, and phenotype information from millions of full-text scientific articles. HGMD and Mastermind both require a subscription to use and should be used, when possible, in conjunction with ClinVar, to ensure previously reported pathogenic variants are annotated as such during ClinVar analysis.

PS2/PM6

The PS2 code is used when a variant is confirmed to be de novo (both maternity and paternity confirmed) in a gene that matches the patient's disease and has no family history, whereas PM6 can be used if de novo status is assumed but not confirmed. Although this information is acquired by testing parents of an affected proband, new recommendations by ClinGen can allow PS2 to range from supporting to very strong evidence based on the number of affected individuals that have been observed with the same de novo variant [83]. Thus, proper application of this code requires testing parents and evaluation of the literature, evaluation of ClinVar, or access to large internal data sets.

PS3, BS3

The PS3 code can be used when there is evidence of well-established in vitro or in vivo functional studies supportive of the variant's damaging effect on the gene or gene product. A significant amount effort has been put into establishing specific rules that allow for PS3 to range from supporting, moderate, or strong evidence when appropriately controlled and established functional studies have been performed [84]. A careful review of these guidelines when evaluating functional data from the literature is therefore necessary to ensure this code is correctly used. Conversely, if experimental data show a variant has no effect, the BS3 code can be applied. Although experimental studies have historically occurred on a small scale, analyzing a few variants at a time, screening strategies have been recently developed that substitute every amino acid in a protein followed by expression in a mammalian cell line to test the impact on protein function [85,86]. These studies provide predictive information on variants that may not have been encountered in patients and help resolve previously classified VUSs. Data generated from massively parallel reporter assay experiments are typically made available in the MaveDB public repository [87].

PM1

The PM1 code can be applied when a variant is located in a mutational hotspot and/or critical and well-established functional domain (eg, active site of an enzyme) without benign variation. This code is challenging to use for multiple reasons, including mainly that (1) most proteins have not been studied well enough to know the boundaries or full repertoire of functional domains sensitive to pathogenic alterations, and (2) numerous cases are required to establish mutational hotspot signatures, which is difficult to obtain when the implicated gene and disorder are rare. Thus, PM1 is more appropriately used in very well-studied genes and diseases like hypertrophic cardiomyopathy [88], BRCA1/2-related cancer predisposition disorders [89], and collagenopathies [90]. For genes that are not well studied, protein domain analysis can be facilitated by manually reviewing databases like Pfam [91] and UniProt [92].

PM2, BA1, BS1

The PM2 code is among the most frequently applied evidence codes during clinical genomic analysis because it is used when a variant is rare or absent from healthy human populations. Application of this code depends on databases that catalog variant allele frequencies from ES and GS data. The largest repository of human genetic variation that is publicly available for this purpose is the Genome Aggregation Database (gnomAD) [14], with current versions, v2.1.1 and 3.1.1, consisting of more than 125,000 exomes and 70,000 genomes, respectively. Along with providing the frequency of variants in various human populations based on ancestry, the gnomAD data set has provided important insights into gene tolerance for LOF and missense variants and is starting to incorporate frequency information for other types of alterations like copy number and structural variants. Although PM2 was originally considered moderate-level evidence, more recent guidelines suggest rare or absent variants from gnomAD should be downgraded to supporting level evidence because approximately half of all variants in gnomAD are seen once in the entire data set [83,93]. BA1 is standalone evidence for benign assertion and can be used when variants are found in gnomAD with an allele frequency greater than 5%. BS1 can be applied when the allele frequency in a control population is greater than expected for the disorder. Determining disease- and gene-specific allele frequency cutoffs for pathogenic and benign variants is part of a larger effort spearheaded by ClinGen's numerous Clinical Domain Working Groups (CDWG) [94,95]. These expert panels regularly meet to evaluate the clinical validity of gene-disease relationships and pathogenicity of individual genetic variants and compose disease-specific guidelines for the clinical genomics community [94–96]. Examples of gene and disease-focused guidelines include hearing loss [97], *CDH1* [98], and *TP53* [99].

PM3, BP2

Application of the PM3 code occurs when a variant is detected with a second pathogenic or likely pathogenic variant on the other allele in an affected patient in a gene that causes an autosomal recessive disorder. Thus, like the de novo codes (PS2 and PM6), appropriate use of PM3 requires testing biological parents to determine phase or the proximity of both variants needs to be close enough to allow phasing by typical NGS short reads (variants within 100–250 bp of each other). New ClinGen Sequence Variant Interpretation working group recommendations provide an updated scoring system that accounts for each occurrence of the observed variant with a VUS or LP/P variant (confirmed in trans or phase unknown) or in the homozygous state in an affected proband, thus enabling this code to range from supporting to very strong evidence [83]. Alternatively, evidence that a variant is in cis with a pathogenic variant allows for the BP2 code to be used.

PP3, BP4

The PP3 supporting evidence code is applied when computational tools predict a missense or splice site variant is pathogenic by assessing various features of the change, including type of amino acid change (eg, polar to nonpolar) and conservation scores. More recently, these algorithms have become ensemble tools that predict the pathogenicity of missense variants on the basis of scores from several individual tools. A frequently used ensemble tool used for ClinVar analysis is REVEL, which has shown high performance for distinguishing pathogenic from rare neutral variants [100]. Another high-performing missense variant pathogenicity prediction tool with high sensitivity and specificity is ClinPred, which is an ensemble machine learning algorithm that incorporates several in silico prediction tools plus population allele frequency from gnomAD and was trained on variants that were reported as pathogenic in ClinVar [101]. The best-performing computational tool designed to predict splice site gain of function or LOF is SpliceAI [102]. SpliceAI uses a deep neural network that accurately predicts splice junctions from pre-messenger RNA transcript sequence and was validated using RNA sequencing data. REVEL, ClinPred, and SpliceAI data sets are freely available and can be incorporated into genomic analysis pipelines and VCF file outputs. These tools output a score between 0 and 1, which allows for specific pathogenic thresholds to be set by individual laboratories (eg, REVEL score >0.65 supports PP3 assertion, <0.15 supports BP4) or ClinGen CDWGs.

Automating Variant Analysis

The concept of automating variant analysis with tools like AutoPVS1 [80] is enticing for laboratories that wish to increase efficiencies and reduce the number of variants that undergo time-consuming manual review by a molecular variant analyst. Other evidence codes that are amenable to bioinformatic filtering and potential automation include PS2, PM2, PM3, and PP3. The challenge, however, of implementing automation during variant analysis is 2-fold, including (1) ongoing development of gene- and disease-specific classification schemes that negate generalized approaches and (2) most information required to assess a variant is contained in publications, supplementary tables, and databases, which inevitably require manual review and interpretation. Nevertheless, it is likely the future of variant analysis will evolve to include machine learning classifiers that annotate variants within VCF files according to the latest ACMG/AMP criteria. Although the community awaits the development of robust automated classifiers, a simpler strategy that is currently used in genomic laboratories is setting up bioinformatic filtration and prioritization schemes to limit the number of variants for manual interpretation [103,104]. Most of these filtration methods benefit from trio analysis, which allows for inclusion of inheritance status (ie, de novo or cis/trans for multiple variants) along with other features, such as predicted variant impact (nonsense, missense, frameshift, and so forth), classification within ClinVar databases, allele frequency in gnomAD, and predicted impact by in silico tools. If the patient's phenotype is not taken into consideration when developing filtration schemes, the retained variant list will include large numbers of VUSs comprising rare missense variants. Furthermore, such broad analysis can result in identification of variants in genes that are unrelated to the indication for testing. There are statistical and ethical considerations regarding return of such incidental or secondary findings, so the ACMG currently recommends that consideration of return of results in genes not related to the indication for testing be limited to findings that might be considered actionable [105]. Nonetheless, variant prioritization with or without prior filtering of genes that overlap with the patient's phenotype is an important component of creating a robust clinical genomic pipeline [36].

GENOMIC ANALYSIS: CURRENT AND FUTURE AVENUES TO CONSIDER

Although both phenotype association and variant prioritization methods present promising approaches to aid in genomic analysis, neither approach alone is sufficient to ensure rapid and accurate diagnoses. Incompleteness of phenotypes reported in the literature, the pace of new gene discovery, and difficulty accessing these results limit phenotype-driven analysis. Variant first approaches often lead to too many "VUSs" to sift through (such as rare missense variants) or variants in genes that are not related to clinical indication (and therefore not immediately pertinent) or not part of ACMG Secondary Findings 3.0 list [24,105,106] but may confer some risk to disease (leading to a challenging counseling and ethical situation). New analysis strategies may benefit from the use of multiple tools throughout the phenotype collection and association, variant prioritization and interpretation, and reanalysis phases (Fig. 1). For example, implementation of trio analysis, rather than

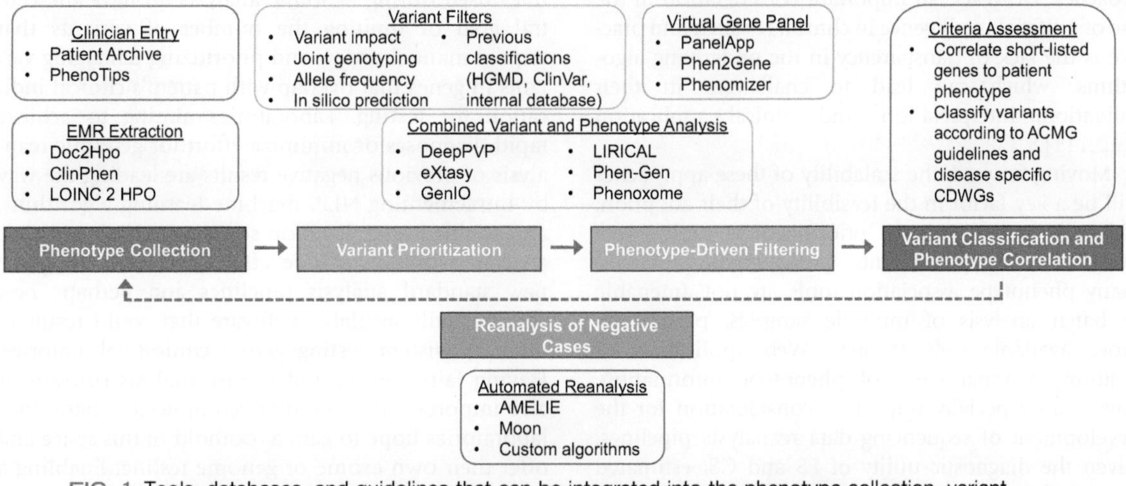

FIG. 1 Tools, databases, and guidelines that can be integrated into the phenotype collection, variant prioritization, filtering, and classification, and reanalysis stages of clinical ES and GS. Tools to aid in phenotype collection can be implemented by clinicians directly entering phenotype information or in automated post hoc extraction of phenotypes from the electronic medical record (EMR). Separate application of variant filters and/or virtual gene panels or use of combined variant and phenotype analysis tools can reduce the number of variants selected for variant classification and phenotype correlation. Negative cases may be monitored by software or custom algorithms to identify cases that may benefit from reanalysis in light of new genetic knowledge or phenotypic information.

proband-only analysis, often provides insight into variant phase and de novo status (PM3, PS2) that can aid in variant prioritization and classification, and at least 2 existing tools are able to integrate genotype information from unaffected family members alongside proband phenotype data [61,62].

Both variant-first and phenotype-driven approaches are tasked with integrating ever-expanding amounts of information about diseases, genes, and variants into robust algorithms. The Bayes statistical framework is a powerful method for combining independent evidence elements and is incorporated into multiple phenotype association and variant prioritization/analysis tools, including Phen-Gen [55], Phrank [52], and MutationTaster [107], to varying degrees. Expansion of the Bayesian framework to predict pathogenicity of variants in light of the given patient's phenotype and genotype (including variant zygosity and, if known, phase) could help bridge the gap between the variant-level interpretation and overall case-level interpretation as it relates to the individual patient [51]. In addition, machine learning and deep learning techniques are increasingly being applied to clinical diagnostics, including variant annotation [108] and phenotype-driven variant prioritization [109], to overcome the hurdle presented by integrating large amounts of available data. These techniques will likely continue to shape future development of phenotype association and variant prioritization approaches. However, an important consideration in the use of artificial intelligence in clinical research and practice is the lack of transparency in the underlying algorithms, which can lead to challenges in their validation, interpretation, and clinical application [110,111].

Moving forward, the scalability of these approaches will be a key factor in the feasibility of their adoption. Although most variant prioritization tools were designed for integration into bioinformatic pipelines, many phenotype association tools are not amenable to batch analysis of multiple samples, particularly those available only through Web application or requiring manual entry of phenotype information. This is an especially important consideration for the development of sequencing data reanalysis pipelines. Given the diagnostic utility of ES and GS, estimated to range from 24% to 41% [4,5,10,112,113], a significant number of nondiagnostic cases may become candidates for future reanalysis. Multiple recent studies that have undertaken bulk reanalysis of ES data noted the need for increased automation of the process to improve the feasibility of its inclusion in routine clinical practice [103,104,114,115]. One such study conducted a reanalysis of ES results for 2250 patients using a semi-automatic pipeline, which incorporated both phenotype matching and variant filtering using 2 levels of stringency [104]. This reanalysis effort led to an increase in the diagnostic rate by 10% to 20%, largely driven by new gene-disease associations and variant reclassification owing to new evidence, also highlighting the need for continual surveillance of the medical literature. In this light, the integration of these tools into reanalysis pipelines, particularly in an automated manner, could potentially be used to prioritize negative cases when genes containing potential variants of interest are newly associated with disease or when the clinician reports new phenotypes identified in the patient. At least 1 recently developed combined phenotype association and variant prioritization tool, AMELIE, supports these efforts via automatic case reanalysis as new papers related to the query phenotypes and/or candidate genes are published [62].

SUMMARY

In this review, the authors discussed the many tools, databases, and guidelines that are used to achieve accurate genetic diagnoses in the phenotypically diverse populations that undergo genomic testing. The various competing "homebrew" bioinformatic pipelines used during genomic analysis all have the central goal of limiting the number of variants that require manual review and prioritizing damaging variants in genes that overlap with patient's clinical indication for testing. Laboratories aiming to achieve rapid diagnoses or minimize effort for genomic reanalysis of previous negative results are leading the way by implementing NLP, machine learning algorithms, and sophisticated filtration schemes to their genomic analysis workflow. These efforts are likely to guide new standard analysis pipelines and perhaps new commercially available software that could result in more consistent testing across clinical laboratories. Having fairly priced and robust analysis software is also important if modestly sized molecular pathology laboratories hope to gain a foothold in this space and offer their own exome or genome testing. Enabling a more equal playing field is in line with efforts from groups like ClinGen who are disseminating free, publicly accessible genomic information for academic and diagnostic purposes. Expanding access worldwide would bring clinical genomic testing into the realm of other routine assays like microarrays and gene panels.

CLINICS CARE POINTS

- Providing molecular diagnostic laboratories with detailed patient phenotypic information using structured terms (e.g., Human Phenotype Ontology), relevant family history, and specimens from family trios (proband and parents) supports greater diagnostic yield for rare diseases.
- Genomic testing falls into the category of non-FDA approved laboratory developed tests; thus, different methods can be used for interpreting genotype and phenotype data. These differences among laboratories can impact which disease-associated variants are analyzed and whether incidental findings and novel candidate disease genes are studied and reported.
- ClinGen is actively developing guidelines for variant classification (general and disease-focused) and new resources that catalogue evidence for gene-disease relationships.
- Continued communication between clinicians and molecular diagnostic laboratories can aid in the accurate interpretation of reported variants, as well as trigger reanalysis of non-diagnostic test results.

DISCLOSURE

The authors have nothing to disclose.

REFERENCES

[1] Green ED, Guyer MS, National Human Genome Research I. Charting a course for genomic medicine from base pairs to bedside. Nature 2011;470(7333):204–13.
[2] Bertoli-Avella AM, Beetz C, Ameziane N, et al. Successful application of genome sequencing in a diagnostic setting: 1007 index cases from a clinically heterogeneous cohort. Eur J Hum Genet 2021;29(1):141–53.
[3] Malinowski J, Miller DT, Demmer L, et al. Systematic evidence-based review: outcomes from exome and genome sequencing for pediatric patients with congenital anomalies or intellectual disability. Genet Med 2020;22(6):986–1004.
[4] Clark MM, Stark Z, Farnaes L, et al. Meta-analysis of the diagnostic and clinical utility of genome and exome sequencing and chromosomal microarray in children with suspected genetic diseases. NPJ Genom Med 2018;3:16.
[5] Taylor JC, Martin HC, Lise S, et al. Factors influencing success of clinical genome sequencing across a broad spectrum of disorders. Nat Genet 2015;47(7):717–26.
[6] Petrikin JE, Cakici JA, Clark MM, et al. The NSIGHT1-randomized controlled trial: rapid whole-genome sequencing for accelerated etiologic diagnosis in critically ill infants. NPJ Genom Med 2018;3:6.
[7] Soden SE, Saunders CJ, Willig LK, et al. Effectiveness of exome and genome sequencing guided by acuity of illness for diagnosis of neurodevelopmental disorders. Sci Transl Med 2014;6(265):265ra168.
[8] Lionel AC, Costain G, Monfared N, et al. Improved diagnostic yield compared with targeted gene sequencing panels suggests a role for whole-genome sequencing as a first-tier genetic test. Genet Med 2018;20(4):435–43.
[9] Bick D, Fraser PC, Gutzeit MF, et al. Successful application of whole genome sequencing in a medical genetics clinic. J Pediatr Genet 2017;6(2):61–76.
[10] Stavropoulos DJ, Merico D, Jobling R, et al. Whole genome sequencing expands diagnostic utility and improves clinical management in pediatric medicine. NPJ Genom Med 2016. https://doi.org/10.1038/npjgenmed.2015.12.
[11] Mardis ER. DNA sequencing technologies: 2006-2016. Nat Protoc 2017;12(2):213–8.
[12] Levy SE, Myers RM. Advancements in next-generation sequencing. Annu Rev Genomics Hum Genet 2016;17:95–115.
[13] Schloss JA, Gibbs RA, Makhijani VB, et al. Cultivating DNA sequencing technology after the Human Genome Project. Annu Rev Genomics Hum Genet 2020;21:117–38.
[14] Karczewski KJ, Francioli LC, Tiao G, et al. The mutational constraint spectrum quantified from variation in 141,456 humans. Nature 2020;581(7809):434–43.
[15] Collins RL, Brand H, Karczewski KJ, et al. A structural variation reference for medical and population genetics. Nature 2020;581(7809):444–51.
[16] Genomes Project C, Abecasis GR, Auton A, et al. An integrated map of genetic variation from 1,092 human genomes. Nature 2012;491(7422):56–65.
[17] Bamshad MJ, Nickerson DA, Chong JX. Mendelian gene discovery: fast and furious with no end in sight. Am J Hum Genet 2019;105(3):448–55.
[18] Chong JX, Buckingham KJ, Jhangiani SN, et al. The genetic basis of Mendelian phenotypes: discoveries, challenges, and opportunities. Am J Hum Genet 2015;97(2):199–215.
[19] Posey JE, O'Donnell-Luria AH, Chong JX, et al. Insights into genetics, human biology and disease gleaned from family based genomic studies. Genet Med 2019;21(4):798–812.
[20] Landrum MJ, Lee JM, Benson M, et al. ClinVar: public archive of interpretations of clinically relevant variants. Nucleic Acids Res 2016;44(D1):D862–8.
[21] Manolio TA, Chisholm RL, Ozenberger B, et al. Implementing genomic medicine in the clinic: the future is here. Genet Med 2013;15(4):258–67.
[22] Retterer K, Juusola J, Cho MT, et al. Clinical application of whole-exome sequencing across clinical indications. Genet Med 2016;18(7):696–704.

[23] Yang Y, Muzny DM, Reid JG, et al. Clinical whole-exome sequencing for the diagnosis of mendelian disorders. N Engl J Med 2013;369(16):1502–11.

[24] Kalia SS, Adelman K, Bale SJ, et al. Recommendations for reporting of secondary findings in clinical exome and genome sequencing, 2016 update (ACMG SF v2.0): a policy statement of the American College of Medical Genetics and Genomics. Genet Med 2017; 19(2):249–55.

[25] Cheema H, Bertoli-Avella AM, Skrahina V, et al. Genomic testing in 1019 individuals from 349 Pakistani families results in high diagnostic yield and clinical utility. NPJ Genom Med 2020;5:44.

[26] Jayasinghe K, Stark Z, Kerr PG, et al. Clinical impact of genomic testing in patients with suspected monogenic kidney disease. Genet Med 2021;23(1):183–91.

[27] Freed AS, Clowes Candadai SV, Sikes MC, et al. The impact of rapid exome sequencing on medical management of critically ill children. J Pediatr 2020. https://doi.org/10.1016/j.jpeds.2020.06.020.

[28] Li C, Vandersluis S, Holubowich C, et al. Cost-effectiveness of genome-wide sequencing for unexplained developmental disabilities and multiple congenital anomalies. Genet Med 2020. https://doi.org/10.1038/s41436-020-01012-w.

[29] Vissers L, van Nimwegen KJM, Schieving JH, et al. A clinical utility study of exome sequencing versus conventional genetic testing in pediatric neurology. Genet Med 2017;19(9):1055–63.

[30] Stark Z, Schofield D, Alam K, et al. Prospective comparison of the cost-effectiveness of clinical whole-exome sequencing with that of usual care overwhelmingly supports early use and reimbursement. Genet Med 2017; 19(8):867–74.

[31] Tan TY, Dillon OJ, Stark Z, et al. Diagnostic impact and cost-effectiveness of whole-exome sequencing for ambulant children with suspected monogenic conditions. JAMA Pediatr 2017;171(9):855–62.

[32] Schofield D, Alam K, Douglas L, et al. Cost-effectiveness of massively parallel sequencing for diagnosis of paediatric muscle diseases. NPJ Genom Med 2017;2doi. https://doi.org/10.1038/s41525-017-0006-7.

[33] Farnaes L, Hildreth A, Sweeney NM, et al. Rapid whole-genome sequencing decreases infant morbidity and cost of hospitalization. NPJ Genom Med 2018;3:10.

[34] Srivastava S, Love-Nichols JA, Dies KA, et al. Meta-analysis and multidisciplinary consensus statement: exome sequencing is a first-tier clinical diagnostic test for individuals with neurodevelopmental disorders. Genet Med 2019;21(11):2413–21.

[35] Kingsmore SF, Cakici JA, Clark MM, et al. A randomized, controlled trial of the analytic and diagnostic performance of singleton and trio, rapid genome and exome sequencing in ill infants. Am J Hum Genet 2019;105(4):719–33.

[36] Hegde M, Santani A, Mao R, et al. Development and validation of clinical whole-exome and whole-genome sequencing for detection of germline variants in inherited disease. Arch Pathol Lab Med 2017;141(6): 798–805.

[37] Roy S, Coldren C, Karunamurthy A, et al. Standards and guidelines for validating next-generation sequencing bioinformatics pipelines: a joint recommendation of the Association for Molecular Pathology and the College of American Pathologists. J Mol Diagn 2018; 20(1):4–27.

[38] Richards S, Aziz N, Bale S, et al. Standards and guidelines for the interpretation of sequence variants: a joint consensus recommendation of the American College of Medical Genetics and Genomics and the Association for Molecular Pathology. Genet Med 2015;17(5): 405–24.

[39] Kohler S, Carmody L, Vasilevsky N, et al. Expansion of the Human Phenotype Ontology (HPO) knowledge base and resources. Nucleic Acids Res 2019;47(D1): D1018–27.

[40] Groza T, Kohler S, Moldenhauer D, et al. The Human Phenotype Ontology: semantic unification of common and rare disease. Am J Hum Genet 2015;97(1):111–24.

[41] Robinson PN, Kohler S, Bauer S, et al. The Human Phenotype Ontology: a tool for annotating and analyzing human hereditary disease. Am J Hum Genet 2008;83(5):610–5.

[42] Amberger JS, Bocchini CA, Schiettecatte F, et al. OMIM.org: Online Mendelian Inheritance in Man (OMIM(R)), an online catalog of human genes and genetic disorders. Nucleic Acids Res 2015;43(Database issue):D789–98.

[43] Stenson PD, Mort M, Ball EV, et al. The Human Gene Mutation Database: towards a comprehensive repository of inherited mutation data for medical research, genetic diagnosis and next-generation sequencing studies. Hum Genet 2017;136(6):665–77.

[44] Ayme S. [Orphanet, an information site on rare diseases]. Soins 2003;(672):46–7, Orphanet, un serveur d'informations sur les maladies rares.

[45] Adam MPDM, A.; Ardinger, H. H.; Pagon, R. A.; Wallace, S. E.; Bean, L. J. H.; Mirzaa, G.; Amemiya, A. GeneReviews. Available at: https://www.ncbi.nlm.nih.gov/books/NBK1116/?partid=1512. Accessed May, 2021.

[46] Fiorini N, Lipman DJ, Lu Z. Towards PubMed 2.0. Elife 2017;6. https://doi.org/10.7554/eLife.28801.

[47] Sayers EW, Barrett T, Benson DA, et al. Database resources of the National Center for Biotechnology Information. Nucleic Acids Res 2011;39(Database issue): D38–51.

[48] Chunn LM, Nefcy DC, Scouten RW, et al. Mastermind: a comprehensive genomic association search engine for empirical evidence curation and genetic variant interpretation. Front Genet 2020;11:577152.

[49] Buske OJ, Girdea M, Dumitriu S, et al. PhenomeCentral: a portal for phenotypic and genotypic matchmaking of patients with rare genetic diseases. Hum Mutat 2015;36(10):931–40.

[50] Martin AR, Williams E, Foulger RE, et al. PanelApp crowdsources expert knowledge to establish consensus diagnostic gene panels. Nat Genet 2019;51(11):1560–5.
[51] Strande NT, Riggs ER, Buchanan AH, et al. Evaluating the clinical validity of gene-disease associations: an evidence-based framework developed by the clinical genome resource. Am J Hum Genet 2017;100(6):895–906.
[52] Jagadeesh KA, Birgmeier J, Guturu H, et al. Phrank measures phenotype sets similarity to greatly improve Mendelian diagnostic disease prioritization. Genet Med 2019;21(2):464–70.
[53] Singleton MV, Guthery SL, Voelkerding KV, et al. Phevor combines multiple biomedical ontologies for accurate identification of disease-causing alleles in single individuals and small nuclear families. Am J Hum Genet 2014;94(4):599–610.
[54] Yang H, Robinson PN, Wang K. Phenolyzer: phenotype-based prioritization of candidate genes for human diseases. Nat Methods 2015;12(9):841–3.
[55] Javed A, Agrawal S, Ng PC. Phen-Gen: combining phenotype and genotype to analyze rare disorders. Nat Methods 2014;11(9):935–7.
[56] Resnik P. Semantic similarity in a taxonomy: an information-based measure and its application to problems of ambiguity in natural language. J Artifial Intelligence Res 1999;11:95–130.
[57] Lin D. An information-theoretic definition of similarity. 1998.
[58] Jiang JJ, Conrath D. Semantic similarity based on corpus statistics and lexical taxonomy. 1997.
[59] Wu C, Devkota B, Evans P, et al. Rapid and accurate interpretation of clinical exomes using Phenoxome: a computational phenotype-driven approach. Eur J Hum Genet 2019;27(4):612–20.
[60] Peng J, Hui W, Shang X. Measuring phenotype-phenotype similarity through the interactome. BMC Bioinformatics 2018;19(Suppl 5):114.
[61] Smedley D, Jacobsen JO, Jager M, et al. Next-generation diagnostics and disease-gene discovery with the Exomiser. Nat Protoc 2015;10(12):2004–15.
[62] Birgmeier J, Haeussler M, Deisseroth CA, et al. AMELIE speeds Mendelian diagnosis by matching patient phenotype and genotype to primary literature. Sci Transl Med 2020;(544):12.
[63] Robinson PN, Kohler S, Oellrich A, et al. Improved exome prioritization of disease genes through cross-species phenotype comparison. Genome Res 2014;24(2):340–8.
[64] Smedley D, Oellrich A, Kohler S, et al. PhenoDigm: analyzing curated annotations to associate animal models with human diseases. Database (Oxford) 2013;2013:bat025.
[65] Hombach D, Schwarz JM, Knierim E, et al. Phenotero: annotate as you write. Clin Genet 2019;95(2):287–92.
[66] Girdea M, Dumitriu S, Fiume M, et al. PhenoTips: patient phenotyping software for clinical and research use. Hum Mutat 2013;34(8):1057–65.
[67] Kohler S, Schulz MH, Krawitz P, et al. Clinical diagnostics in human genetics with semantic similarity searches in ontologies. Am J Hum Genet 2009;85(4):457–64.
[68] Zhang XA, Yates A, Vasilevsky N, et al. Semantic integration of clinical laboratory tests from electronic health records for deep phenotyping and biomarker discovery. NPJ Digit Med 2019;2. https://doi.org/10.1038/s41746-019-0110-4.
[69] Deisseroth CA, Birgmeier J, Bodle EE, et al. ClinPhen extracts and prioritizes patient phenotypes directly from medical records to expedite genetic disease diagnosis. Genet Med 2019;21(7):1585–93.
[70] Liu C, Peres Kury FS, Li Z, et al. Doc2Hpo: a web application for efficient and accurate HPO concept curation. Nucleic Acids Res 2019;47(W1):W566–70.
[71] Savova GK, Masanz JJ, Ogren PV, et al. Mayo clinical Text Analysis and Knowledge Extraction System (cTAKES): architecture, component evaluation and applications. J Am Med Inform Assoc 2010;17(5):507–13.
[72] Aronson AR. Effective mapping of biomedical text to the UMLS Metathesaurus: the MetaMap program. Proc AMIA Symp 2001;17–21.
[73] Son JH, Xie G, Yuan C, et al. Deep phenotyping on electronic health records facilitates genetic diagnosis by clinical exomes. Am J Hum Genet 2018;103(1):58–73.
[74] Zhao M, Havrilla JM, Fang L, et al. Phen2Gene: rapid phenotype-driven gene prioritization for rare diseases. NAR Genom Bioinform 2020;2(2):lqaa032.
[75] Robinson PN, Ravanmehr V, Jacobsen JOB, et al. Interpretable clinical genomics with a likelihood ratio paradigm. Am J Hum Genet 2020;107(3):403–17.
[76] Fujiwara T, Yamamoto Y, Kim JD, et al. PubCaseFinder: A case-report-based, phenotype-driven differential-diagnosis system for rare diseases. Am J Hum Genet 2018;103(3):389–99.
[77] Tavtigian SV, Greenblatt MS, Harrison SM, et al. Modeling the ACMG/AMP variant classification guidelines as a Bayesian classification framework. Genet Med 2018;20(9):1054–60.
[78] Tavtigian SV, Harrison SM, Boucher KM, et al. Fitting a naturally scaled point system to the ACMG/AMP variant classification guidelines. Hum Mutat 2020. https://doi.org/10.1002/humu.24088.
[79] Abou Tayoun AN, Pesaran T, DiStefano MT, et al. Recommendations for interpreting the loss of function PVS1 ACMG/AMP variant criterion. Hum Mutat 2018;39(11):1517–24.
[80] Xiang J, Peng J, Baxter S, et al. AutoPVS1: an automatic classification tool for PVS1 interpretation of null variants. Hum Mutat 2020;41(9):1488–98.
[81] Landrum MJ, Chitipiralla S, Brown GR, et al. ClinVar: improvements to accessing data. Nucleic Acids Res 2020;48(D1):D835–44.
[82] Genomenon. Mastermind genomic search engine. 2021. Available at: https://www.genomenon.com/mastermind. Accessed May, 2021.

[83] Sequence CGR. SVI general recommendations for using ACMG/AMP criteria. 2021. Available at: https://clinicalgenome.org/working-groups/sequence-variant-interpretation/. Accessed May, 2021.
[84] Brnich SE, Abou Tayoun AN, Couch FJ, et al. Recommendations for application of the functional evidence PS3/BS3 criterion using the ACMG/AMP sequence variant interpretation framework. Genome Med 2019;12(1):3.
[85] Findlay GM, Daza RM, Martin B, et al. Accurate classification of BRCA1 variants with saturation genome editing. Nature 2018;562(7726):217–22.
[86] Jia X, Burugula BB, Chen V, et al. Massively parallel functional testing of MSH2 missense variants conferring Lynch syndrome risk. Am J Hum Genet 2021;108(1):163–75.
[87] Esposito D, Weile J, Shendure J, et al. MaveDB: an open-source platform to distribute and interpret data from multiplexed assays of variant effect. Genome Biol 2019;20(1):223.
[88] Waring A, Harper A, Salatino S, et al. Data-driven modelling of mutational hotspots and in silico predictors in hypertrophic cardiomyopathy. J Med Genet 2020. https://doi.org/10.1136/jmedgenet-2020-106922.
[89] Dines JN, Shirts BH, Slavin TP, et al. Systematic misclassification of missense variants in BRCA1 and BRCA2 "coldspots". Genet Med 2020;22(5):825–30.
[90] Savige J, Storey H, Watson E, et al. Consensus statement on standards and guidelines for the molecular diagnostics of Alport syndrome: refining the ACMG criteria. Eur J Hum Genet 2021. https://doi.org/10.1038/s41431-021-00858-1.
[91] Mistry J, Chuguransky S, Williams L, et al. Pfam: the protein families database in 2021. Nucleic Acids Res 2021;49(D1):D412–9.
[92] UniProt C. UniProt: the universal protein knowledgebase in 2021. Nucleic Acids Res 2021;49(D1):D480–9.
[93] Lek M, Karczewski KJ, Minikel EV, et al. Analysis of protein-coding genetic variation in 60,706 humans. Nature 2016;536(7616):285–91.
[94] Rivera-Munoz EA, Milko LV, Harrison SM, et al. ClinGen Variant Curation Expert Panel experiences and standardized processes for disease and gene-level specification of the ACMG/AMP guidelines for sequence variant interpretation. Hum Mutat 2018;39(11):1614–22.
[95] Milko LV, Funke BH, Hershberger RE, et al. Development of clinical domain working groups for the Clinical Genome Resource (ClinGen): lessons learned and plans for the future. Genet Med 2019;21(4):987–93.
[96] Sequence CGR. ClinGen expert panels. 2021. Available at: https://clinicalgenome.org/affiliation/. Accessed May, 2021.
[97] Oza AM, DiStefano MT, Hemphill SE, et al. Expert specification of the ACMG/AMP variant interpretation guidelines for genetic hearing loss. Hum Mutat 2018;39(11):1593–613.
[98] Lee K, Krempely K, Roberts ME, et al. Specifications of the ACMG/AMP variant curation guidelines for the analysis of germline CDH1 sequence variants. Hum Mutat 2018;39(11):1553–68.
[99] Fortuno C, Lee K, Olivier M, et al. Specifications of the ACMG/AMP variant interpretation guidelines for germline TP53 variants. Hum Mutat 2021;42(3):223–36.
[100] Ioannidis NM, Rothstein JH, Pejaver V, et al. REVEL: an ensemble method for predicting the pathogenicity of rare missense variants. Am J Hum Genet 2016;99(4):877–85.
[101] Alirezaie N, Kernohan KD, Hartley T, et al. ClinPred: prediction tool to identify disease-relevant nonsynonymous single-nucleotide variants. Am J Hum Genet 2018;103(4):474–83.
[102] Jaganathan K, Kyriazopoulou Panagiotopoulou S, McRae JF, et al. Predicting splicing from primary sequence with deep learning. Cell 2019;176(3):535–548 e24.
[103] James KN, Clark MM, Camp B, et al. Partially automated whole-genome sequencing reanalysis of previously undiagnosed pediatric patients can efficiently yield new diagnoses. NPJ Genom Med 2020;5:33.
[104] Liu P, Meng L, Normand EA, et al. Reanalysis of clinical exome sequencing data. N Engl J Med 2019;380(25):2478–80.
[105] Miller DT, Lee K, Chung WK, et al. ACMG SF v3.0 list for reporting of secondary findings in clinical exome and genome sequencing: a policy statement of the American College of Medical Genetics and Genomics (ACMG). Genet Med 2021 10.1038/s41436- 021-01172-3.
[106] Green RC, Berg JS, Grody WW, et al. ACMG recommendations for reporting of incidental findings in clinical exome and genome sequencing. Genet Med 2013;15(7):565–74.
[107] Schwarz JM, Cooper DN, Schuelke M, et al. MutationTaster2: mutation prediction for the deep-sequencing age. Nat Methods 2014;11(4):361–2.
[108] Quang D, Chen Y, Xie X. DANN: a deep learning approach for annotating the pathogenicity of genetic variants. Bioinformatics 2015;31(5):761–3.
[109] Boudellioua I, Kulmanov M, Schofield PN, et al. DeepPVP: phenotype-based prioritization of causative variants using deep learning. BMC Bioinformatics 2019;20(1):65.
[110] Price WN. Big data and black-box medical algorithms. Sci Transl Med 2018;10(471). https://doi.org/10.1126/scitranslmed.aao5333.
[111] Bjerring JC, Busch J. Artificial intelligence and patient-centered decision-making. Philosophy & Technology; 2020. https://doi.org/10.1007/s13347-019-00391-6.
[112] Powis Z, Farwell Hagman KD, Speare V, et al. Exome sequencing in neonates: diagnostic rates, characteristics, and time to diagnosis. Genet Med 2018;20(11):1468–71.

[113] Thiffault I, Farrow E, Zellmer L, et al. Clinical genome sequencing in an unbiased pediatric cohort. Genet Med 2019;21(2):303–10.

[114] Baker SW, Murrell JR, Nesbitt AI, et al. Automated clinical exome reanalysis reveals novel diagnoses. J Mol Diagn 2019;21(1):38–48.

[115] Wenger AM, Guturu H, Bernstein JA, et al. Systematic reanalysis of clinical exome data yields additional diagnoses: implications for providers. Genet Med 2017;19(2):209–14.

[116] Sifrim A, Popovic D, Tranchevent LC, et al. eXtasy: variant prioritization by genomic data fusion. Nat Methods 2013;10(11):1083–4.

[117] Koile D, Cordoba M, de Sousa Serro M, et al. GenIO: a phenotype-genotype analysis web server for clinical genomics of rare diseases. BMC Bioinformatics 2018; 19(1):25.

Advances in Molecular Pathology 4 (2021) 17–25
ADVANCES IN MOLECULAR PATHOLOGY

Applications of Noninvasive Prenatal Testing for Subchromosomal Copy Number Variations Using Cell-Free DNA

Jiale Xiang, MS[a,b], Zhiyu Peng, PhD[a,b,*]
[a]BGI Genomics, BGI-Shenzhen, BGI Park, No. 21 Hongan 3rd Street, Yantian District, Shenzhen 518083, China; [b]College of Life Sciences, University of Chinese Academy of Sciences, Beijing 100049, China

KEYWORDS
• Noninvasive prenatal testing • Copy number variation • Subchromosomal abnormalities • Microdeletion • Microduplication • Prenatal screening

KEY POINTS

- Noninvasive prenatal testing (NIPT) is now clinically available for screening fetal subchromosomal copy number variations (CNVs).
- The sensitivity of NIPT for CNVs is challenging to calculate in clinical settings because the number of the missed cases is unknown. This is attributable to the fact that CNV phenotypes can be invisible, mild, or progressive at birth, meaning that some cases require longitudinal follow-up to be identified.
- The positive predictive value (PPV) of NIPT for genome-wide CNVs is 32% to 47%, which is comparable with the PPV for trisomy 13 (43.9%–53%).
- Four critical factors affect the clinical validity of NIPT for detecting subchromosomal CNVs: fetal fraction, sequencing depth, CNV size, and technical variability of the CNV region. Increasing the fetal fraction and sequencing depth improves the NIPT detection rate of subchromosomal CNVs.

INTRODUCTION

In 1997, the detection of male DNA in peripheral blood samples from women bearing male fetuses proved that fetal DNA circulates in maternal plasma and serum [1]. Circulating "fetal" cell-free DNA (cfDNA), which is mainly released from the placenta into maternal circulation, is used in noninvasive prenatal testing (NIPT). Currently, NIPT is primarily used to screen for 3 fetal aneuploidies, trisomy 21, trisomy 18, and trisomy 13, and its performance in detecting these has been well studied in both high-risk and low-risk populations [2]. The high sensitivity, low false-positive rate, and high positive predictive value (PPV) of NIPT have led to its widespread clinical adoption. In recent years, NIPT has revolutionized the prenatal screening landscape and become a routine test in Belgium and the Netherlands [3,4].

Researchers and clinicians have great interest in applying NIPT to screen subchromosomal copy number variations (CNVs) in addition to the 3 traditionally screened aneuploidies. In this review, the authors focus on the current status, development, and challenges of using NIPT to screen fetal subchromosomal CNVs in pregnancies.

Subchromosomal Copy Number Variations

Subchromosomal CNVs are abnormalities in which sections of the genome are deleted (loss) or duplicated (gain). They are relatively common in prenatal

*Corresponding author, *E-mail address:* pengzhiyu@bgi.com

https://doi.org/10.1016/j.yamp.2021.07.002
2589-4080/21/

diagnosis. Wapner and coauthors [5] used chromosomal microarray analysis (CMA) to reveal that 2.5% of samples with normal karyotypes had a microdeletion or microduplication of clinical significance. Based on low-coverage genome sequencing, Wang and colleagues [6] reported that 5.3% of pregnant women undergoing prenatal diagnosis had pathogenic/likely pathogenic CNVs.

Subchromosomal CNVs are associated with severe phenotypes, including structural anomalies, intellectual disability, developmental delay, and autism spectrum disorders [7]. Some presentations, such as structural anomalies, are detectable by ultrasound scans; however, neurologic or neurocognitive features are undetectable via prenatal ultrasound scans. Currently, there are no screening options to identify CNVs at the prenatal stage [8]. To fill this gap, the use of NIPT to screen subchromosomal CNVs is becoming more popular in clinics [4,9,10].

Noninvasive Prenatal Testing for Subchromosomal Copy Number Variations

NIPT can detect aneuploidies through either targeted or random (genome-wide) sequencing, both of which are also technically feasible approaches for detecting subchromosomal CNVs [2]. The targeted approach relies on the amplification of informative single-nucleotide polymorphisms (SNPs) [11]; that is, a targeted SNP-based NIPT is designed to detect a preselected region. In comparison, genome-wide NIPT randomly sequences and analyzes all chromosomes, which has the inherent advantage of detecting CNVs anywhere in the genome instead of only in targeted regions [12].

Selected Copy Number Variations

A handful of selected CNVs with well-defined, severe phenotypes is included in the NIPT screening panel (Table 1), including DiGeorge syndrome (22q11.2 deletion), Prader-Willi and Angelman syndromes (15q11.2-q13 deletion), 1p36 deletion syndrome, Cri-du-chat syndrome (terminal 5p deletion), Jacobsen syndrome (terminal 11q deletion), Wolf-Hirschhorn syndrome (terminal 4p deletion), and Langer-Giedion syndrome (8q24 deletion) [2]. Five of these conditions (DiGeorge syndrome, Prader-Willi/Angelman syndromes, 1p36 deletion syndrome, and Cri-du-chat syndrome) are the best validated and most reported [9,13,14]. The remaining conditions, including Jacobsen syndrome, Wolf-Hirschhorn syndrome, and Langer-Giedion syndrome, are rarely reported [13].

More specifically, Wapner and colleagues [14] validated the use of SNP-based NIPT for CNVs by testing 469 samples (358 plasma samples from pregnant women, 111 artificial plasma mixtures). The results demonstrated that the sensitivity was 97.8% (45/46) for DiGeorge syndrome and 100% for Prader-Willi syndrome (15/15), Angelman syndrome (21/21), 1p36 deletion syndrome (1/1), and Cri-du-chat syndrome (24/24). Later, the same team retrospectively analyzed SNP-based NIPT data (≥3.2 million reads per sample) from 80,449 referrals for DiGeorge syndrome and 42,326 referrals for the other 4 conditions. The PPV was 15.7% (24/153) for DiGeorge syndrome, 0% (0/1) for Prader-Willi syndrome, 1.5% (1/68) for Angelman syndrome, 20% (2/10) for 1p36 deletion syndrome, and 8.9% (4/45) for Cri-du-chat syndrome [15].

Genome-wide NIPT can also be used to identify specific, selected CNVs. Using genome-wide NIPT in 175,393 high-risk pregnancies, Helgeson and colleagues [13] reported the PPV was 100% (23/23) for DiGeorge syndrome, 100% (8/8) for Prader-Willi/Angelman syndromes, 75% (3/4) for 1p36 deletion syndrome, and 66.7% (4/6) for Cri-du-chat syndrome. However, it is worth noting that this study also counted CNVs that were in the maternal genome as true positives; thus, the PPV is likely overestimated. In addition, a prospective study using genome-wide NIPT in 94,085 pregnancies demonstrated that the PPV was 92.9% (13/14) for DiGeorge syndrome, 75% (3/4) for Prader-Willi/Angelman syndromes, 0% (0/2) for 1p36 deletion syndrome, and 50% (3/6) for Cri-du-chat syndrome [9].

Genome-Wide Copy Number Variations

In genome-wide NIPT, all of the chromosomes are randomly sequenced and analyzed, allowing the detection of CNVs in each chromosome [12]. Three studies investigated the analytical validity of genome-wide NIPT for detecting CNVs [16–18]. These studies chose different CNV reporting strategies based on CNV size. In one study, the sensitivity was 97.7% (42/43) for CNVs ≥7 Mb [16], 90.9% (10/11) for CNVs greater than 5 Mb [17], and 14.3% (1/7) for CNVs less than 5 Mb [17]. In another study, sensitivity was 88.9% (24/27) for CNVs greater than 10 Mb [18], and 72.7% (8/11) for CNVs less than 10 Mb [18].

Recently, 3 teams prospectively investigated the PPV of genome-wide NIPT for CNVs in large populations. The first study, reported in 2019, was in the Netherlands, where NIPT is now a routine prenatal test. The researchers recruited 73,239 low-risk pregnancies, accounting for 42% of all pregnancies in the Netherlands at the time. An NIPT with 0.2× genome coverage identified 29 true-positive and 62 false-positive subchromosomal CNVs ranging from 10 to 100 Mb. The overall PPV was 32%. However, the overall

TABLE 1
Characteristics of Selected Subchromosomal Copy Number Variations

No.	Syndrome	Cytoband	Origin	Size	Prevalence	Reference
1	DiGeorge syndrome	22q11.2	90% de novo; 10% inherited	The majority of affected individuals (85%) has a 3-Mb deletion	1/3800–1/6000	[53]
2	Prader-Willi syndrome	15q11-q13	de novo	65%–75% cases have interstitial 5- to 6-Mb deletion	1/10,000–1/30,000	[54]
3	Angelman syndrome	15q11-q13	de novo	65%–75% cases have interstitial 5- to 7-Mb deletion	1/12,000–1/24,000	[55]
4	Cri-du-chat syndrome	5p	~80% de novo; 10% result of a parental translocation; 10% an unusual cytogenetic aberration	Variable, ~5–40 Mb	1/15,000–1/50,000	[56,57]
5	1p36 deletion syndrome	1p36	de novo	Variable, ~1.5 to >10 Mb	1/5000–1/10,000	[57,58]
6	Wolf-Hirschhorn syndrome	4p	55% de novo; 40%–45% inherited from a parent with a balanced rearrangement	Variable, 0.5–2.0 Mb critical region in 4p16.3	1/50,000	[59,60]
7	Jacobsen syndrome	11q23-q25	de novo	Variable, 5–20 Mb	1/100,000	[61]
8	Langer-Giedion syndrome	8q24	de novo	Critical region for the disorder q24.11-q24.13	Unknown	[62]

sensitivity cannot be calculated because data on missed cases are not available [10].

The second study, reported by Liang and colleagues [9] in 2019, recruited 94,085 pregnancies. As a result of maternal age, 40.41% of the participants were high-risk pregnancies, whereas 59.58% were low-risk pregnancies. An NIPT with 10 to 19 million uniquely mapped reads and 36 bp per read (translated to 0.12–0.23× genome coverage) identified 49 true-positive and 71 false-positive subchromosomal CNVs. The overall PPV was 40.8%, including 92.9% for DiGeorge syndrome, 66.7% for 22q duplication syndrome, 50.0% for Cri-du-chat syndrome, 75.0% for Prader-Willi syndrome, 31.9% for CNVs greater than 10 Mb, and 18.8% for CNVs less than 10 Mb. The investigators reported an overall sensitivity of 90.74%.

The final study, reported in 2021, was carried out in Belgium, the first country to implement and fully reimburse NIPT as a first-tier screening test. Van Den Bogaert and colleagues [4] analyzed genome-wide NIPT data from 153,575 pregnancies in the first 2 years (2018–2019) of the national implementation of NIPT. The mean maternal age in 2018 and 2019 was 30.7 years and 30.8 years, respectively. The PPV was calculated to be 47% (43/92). The reported CNV size ranged from 2 to 100 Mb.

To sum up, the sensitivity of NIPT for either selected CNVs or genome-wide CNVs varied between different validation studies [14,16–18]. In clinical settings, however, the sensitivity is challenging to calculate because the number of the missed cases is unknown. This is attributable to the fact that the phenotypes of CNVs could be invisible, mild, or progressive at birth, requiring longitudinal follow-up to identify some cases. The PPV of NIPT for genome-wide CNVs ranges from 32% to 47%, which is comparable with the PPV for trisomy 13 (43.9%–53%), one of the commonly screened chromosome aneuploidies [4,9,10].

Confirmatory Test for Subchromosomal Copy Number Variations

A confirmatory test should be offered when an NIPT identifies a CNV [8]. Karyotyping, fluorescence in situ hybridization (FISH), CMA, and low-coverage genome sequencing can be used to confirm subchromosomal CNVs [19,20]. Briefly, karyotyping is a method using staining procedures to visualize chromosomes in banding patterns with a microscope. Standard banding techniques produce approximately 400 to 500 bands per haploid genome, so karyotyping can normally only detect CNVs larger than 10 Mb. However, a higher-resolution technique achieving approximately 1000 bands per haploid genome can extend the resolution to 3 Mb [20].

FISH is a method for detecting the presence or absence of a particular DNA sequence in situ in a cell. FISH technology relies on DNA probes and provides much higher resolution. A disadvantage of FISH is that it requires prior knowledge of the region of interest in order to design DNA probes [21].

CMA is a method that tests for matches against an array of genomic segments on a microscope slide. Two CMA techniques are used for identifying chromosomal imbalance: comparative genomic hybridization and SNP-based arrays [22]. The resolution of CMA depends on probe density, which varies between CMA platforms. For routine clinical testing, probe spacing on the array provides a resolution of 100 to 250 kb in nontargeted regions and 20 to 50 kb in targeted regions [23]. This resolution is high enough to confirm subchromosomal CNVs that are identified by NIPT.

With the advance of massively parallel sequencing techniques in recent years, low-coverage genome sequencing (~0.25× of the human genome) has been validated to detect genome-wide subchromosomal CNVs greater than 50 kb [24]. In a prenatal diagnosis cohort with 1023 pregnancies, Wang and colleagues [6] compared the performance of low-coverage genome sequencing and CMA. The results demonstrated that low-coverage genome sequencing not only detected all of the pathogenic/likely pathogenic CNVs detected by CMA but also defined 17 additional and clinically relevant pathogenic/likely pathogenic CNVs. These CNVs were missed by CMA because of insufficient probe coverage in the targeted regions.

Opinions of Professional Societies

Although NIPT for subchromosomal CNVs is now clinically available, most professional societies do not recommend its clinical use. In 2020, the American College of Obstetrics and Gynecology recommended that cell-free DNA screening for microdeletion syndromes should not be performed because it has not been validated clinically [25]. In 2016, the American College of Medical Genetics and Genomics recommended informing all pregnant women of the availability of NIPT's expanded use to screen for clinically relevant CNVs when many criteria are met. However, it did not recommend screening for genome-wide CNVs [8]. In 2015, the European Society of Human Genetics and the American Society of Human Genetics did not recommend the expanded use of NIPT for subchromosomal CNVs because of ethical concerns, counseling challenges, and an increase in invasive diagnostic testing [26]. With the availability of prospective studies in large populations in recent years [4,9,10], these recommendations could be reevaluated and discussed further.

FACTORS AFFECTING NONINVASIVE PRENATAL TESTING SCREENING SUBCHROMOSOMAL COPY NUMBER VARIATION

Irrespective of the approach used (targeted or genome-wide), 4 critical factors affect the clinical validity and utility of NIPT for subchromosomal CNVs. These factors are fetal fraction, sequencing depth, CNV size, and biological and technical variability of the CNV region [27].

Fetal Fraction

The ratio of placental to total cfDNA in maternal plasma is known as the "fetal fraction." The average fetal fraction is 10% to 15%, ranging from less than 3% to more than 30% [28]. Using simulated samples, the detection rate of subchromosomal CNVs was shown to increase with fetal fraction [29]. In clinical plasma samples, increased fetal fraction improved the sensitivity for CNVs [30] and reduced maternal background interference [31]. Although NIPT with an increased fetal fraction was reported to have high specificity for CNVs

[30], its impact on the false-positive rate was not systematically compared. It is worth noting that there is controversy about the effect of fetal fraction on the detection of aneuploidies. Hu and colleagues [32] demonstrated that an increase in fetal fraction (from 11.3% to 22.6%) increased the number of false-positive cases from 8 to 10. In contrast, He and colleagues [33] reported that an increase in fetal fraction (from 12.6% to 30.6%) decreased the number of false-positive cases from 11 to 3. Further studies are needed to clarify the impact of increased fetal fraction on NIPT's clinical validity for subchromosomal CNVs.

The fetal fraction can be enriched via different approaches, including **size selection** [34] and **DNA repair** [35]. The enrichment of fetal DNA via size selection relies on the fact that the size profile of fetal and maternal cfDNA is different. In general, fetal cfDNA is shorter than maternal cfDNA [36,37]. To date, magnetic nanoparticles [32,38], E-gel [39,40], and BluePippin [30] have been used for size selection of cfDNA in maternal plasma.

In 2019, Hu and colleagues [32] used magnetic nanoparticles to enrich the fetal fraction. As a result, the fetal fraction increased from 11.3% to 22.6%. In 2020, Zhang and colleagues [38] used 2 types of magnetic nanoparticles (carboxyl-nanoparticles and hydroxyl-nanoparticles) to increase the fetal fraction from 13% to 20%. One caveat was that the enrichment significantly reduced the total amount of cfDNA. The reduction in these 2 studies was 91.76% and 78.41%, respectively [32,38]. This reduction in turn resulted in higher duplicate reads in sequencing and finally a decreased number of unique mapped reads (sequencing depth) for bioinformatic analysis.

Agarose gel electrophoresis is another approach used for size selection in NIPT. Instead of manual gel electrophoresis, which tends to be labor- and time-consuming, there are 2 well-established semiautomatic systems for preparative gel electrophoresis and size selection, the E-gel system and the Pippin serial products.

The E-gel system generally uses precast agarose gels to separate DNA of different sizes and premade holes in the middle of the gel to collect DNA within a specific size range. Since 2018, several studies performed by Wang's group have demonstrated a similar and remarkable increase in fetal fraction by E-gel electrophoresis, which further reduced the "no-call" rate of NIPT for chromosomal aneuploidies in both singleton and twin pregnancies [31,39,40]. For example, Liang and colleagues [31] reported a 2.16-fold increase in fetal fraction and 1.3-fold reduction in maternal background interference in 1004 plasma samples after E-gel–based size selection of 100 to 150 bp. For subjects with high body mass index, E-gel electrophoresis significantly increased the average fetal fraction from 3.4% to 15.48% [40]. Similarly, in 86 plasma samples with dizygotic twin pregnancies, E-gel–based size selection of shorter fragments (107–145 bp) elevated the fetal fraction by around 3.2-fold, strongly enhancing the detection performance of NIPT for chromosomal aneuploidies [39].

Similar to the E-gel system, Pippin series products, including Pippin Prep, BluePippin, and PippinHT, use a precast agarose gel cassette. The systems collect target DNA by switching the channel to Elution Port upon the optical detection of a marker. As early as 2012, Quail and colleagues [34,41] demonstrated that size selection by Pippin Prep was more precise than other methods, capturing a tighter range of DNA size than manual gel electrophoresis or magnetic beads. Recently, Bluepippin was shown to dramatically increase fetal fraction by 2.3-fold in 1264 samples undergoing NIPT, resulting in a 2.2-fold increase in Z scores of positive samples and a substantial gain in sensitivity and specificity for the detection of microdeletions [30]. The analytical sensitivity and specificity were 95.6% and 99.95%, respectively, for the detection of DiGeorge syndrome after size selection [30].

DNA repair

Based on the hypothesis that fetal DNA has more damage than maternal cfDNA, Vong and colleagues [35] used a PreCR repair mix (a commercial DNA repair kit) to repair cfDNA in maternal plasma in pregnant women. The fetal fraction was increased slightly, by 4%, which was attributable to the recovery of a subset of long (>250 bp) cfDNA molecules.

Sequencing Depth

It is clear that a higher sequencing depth is better for accuracy in detecting subchromosomal CNVs. The read depth used for aneuploidies (4–10 million reads per sample) achieved a sensitivity of 83% for CNVs larger than 6 Mb. A higher read depth (up to 120 million reads per sample) increased the sensitivity to 94% [42]. Rampasek and colleagues [43] presented a probabilistic method for detecting fetal CNVs from maternal plasma. With the use of deep sequencing, CNVs greater than 400 kb could be detected with 90% sensitivity and CNVs of 50 to 400 kb with 40% sensitivity if the fetal fraction is sufficiently high (13%). Srinivasan and colleagues [44] estimated that NIPT could detect fetal CNVs as small as 300 kb using one billion reads.

Deeper sequencing improves the resolution and accuracy but substantially increases the cost per test, which precludes its routine use. To balance these factors, studies tend to increase sequencing depth in a limited manner, which has proven to improve the performance of NIPT in detecting subchromosomal CNVs. For example, sensitivity increased from 71.8% to 94.5% for CNVs larger than 1 Mb when the sequencing depth was increased from 3.5 million to 10 million reads [29]. Martin and colleagues [15] increased the sequencing reads from 3.2 million to 6 million for SNP-based NIPT, resulting in an increase in PPV from 15.7% to 44.2% for 22q11.2 and from 5.2% to 31.7% for Prader-Willi/Angelman syndromes, 1p36 deletion syndrome, and Cri-du-chat syndrome. A recent study recommended using 16 to 17 million reads (approximately 0.35× genome coverage) because the detection rate reached a plateau for CNVs larger than 3 Mb at a fetal fraction of 10% [45].

Copy Number Variation Size

In principle, larger CNVs in the fetus are easier to detect against a background of normal maternal DNA. Lo and colleagues [42] reported that NIPT with 4 to 10 million sequence reads and 50 bp per read (approximately 0.07–0.17× coverage) detected 15/18 (83%) samples with pathogenic CNVs greater than 6 Mb but only 2/10 samples with CNVs less than 6 Mb. Similarly, Liao and colleagues [46] used NIPT for common aneuploidies (approximate 0.1× human genome) to detect the CNVs. The detection rate of fetal CNVs greater than 5 Mb and CNVs less than 5 Mb was 90.9% and 14.3%, respectively [17].

Copy Number Variation Region

The CNV region is the fourth factor affecting NIPT detection of subchromosomal CNVs. Biological and technical variability in the CNV region includes GC bias, repetitive elements, and ease of mapping [27], all of which can affect performance.

CHALLENGES

Although the use of NIPT for subchromosomal CNVs has progressed quickly in the past 3 years and become clinically available [4,9,10], many challenges remain in terms of its clinical application, including the selection of CNVs for screening, the presence of maternal CNVs, and the need for counseling. CNVs selected for screening should have severe and well-defined phenotypes with high penetrance. A low penetrance CNV alone does not seem to contribute to developmental, intellectual, and structural anomalies in a prenatal setting [47]. However, screening for such CNVs, for example, 22q11.2 duplication syndrome with a low penetrance of 21.9% [48], was reported [9,49]. This could cause considerable anxiety to couples, especially when the fetus has no ultrasound anomalies. The screening of genome-wide CNVs presents even more challenges. One critical step is to interpret the clinical relevance when CNVs are identified. This cannot be an easy task given the lack, limited, or conflicting phenotypic associations in prenatal setting. Although technical standards for the interpretation and reporting of CNVs were recently published [50], interpretation in the prenatal setting still poses several challenges given the lack of prenatal genotype-phenotype databases, and the penetrance issues described above.

The presence of maternal CNVs is another emerging challenge for screening fetal CNVs. Theoretically, maternal CNVs are easier to identify because around 90% of the cfDNA mixture is maternal in origin [28]. Statistically, maternal CNVs are not as rare as expected. Girirajan and colleagues [51] investigated the inheritance of CNVs using parental data that were available for 653 affected probands. Of 66 CNVs, there were 18 that were exclusively de novo; that is, the majority (48/66) were inherited. Another example is the report by Helgeson and coauthors [13] that identified 55 microdeletions from a randomly selected population of 175,393 pregnancies via NIPT, 25 of which had a maternal contribution. Technically, NIPT can identify maternal CNVs but cannot distinguish whether a CNV is a maternal-only or a maternal-and-fetal abnormality. Prenatal diagnosis is required to determine the status of the fetus when a maternal CNV is suspected, which leads to more invasive testing. However, with knowledge of the fetal fraction and a higher read depth, it is technically possible to determine whether the fetus has inherited the CNVs or not [42]. Further studies are thus warranted.

The last challenge is counseling. Counseling about CNVs is confounded by issues around penetrance [48], variable expressivity [51], CNV size being screened, and genes in the detected CNV [2]. Counseling should be personalized and should provide sufficient information. This is to ensure that patients make autonomous decisions with a full understanding of the benefits and limitations of the test [52]. However, counselors who can discuss prenatal testing options are not always accessible. More importantly, some critical test metrics are currently unavailable for NIPT in CNVs detection. For example, it is challenging to determine the number of missed CNVs in large-scale population studies [10] because subchromosomal CNVs may have variable expressivity, which cannot be identified by a physical check at birth. Long-term follow-up of negative cases has not been done and may not be feasible. As a result, sensitivity and negative predictive value cannot be calculated. When a positive screening result is confirmed, appropriate counseling is important for informed decision making, especially for those with novel CNVs. The American College of Medical Genetics and Genomics recommends providing accurate, balanced, up-to-date information at an appropriate literacy level when a fetus is diagnosed with a CNV [8].

SUMMARY

The application of NIPT for subchromosomal CNVs has been clinically available for several years. Although the sensitivity is unknown in clinical settings, the PPV for genome-wide CNV is clear. It ranges from 32% to 47%, which is comparable with the PPV for trisomy 13 (43.9%–53%), one of the commonly screened chromosome aneuploidies [4,9,10]. Four key factors affect the clinical validity of NIPT for subchromosomal CNVs: fetal fraction, sequencing depth, CNV size, and CNV region. Increasing the fetal fraction and sequencing depth can substantially improve the detection rate of subchromosomal CNVs. However, clinical application of NIPT for CNVs still presents several challenges, including the selection of CNVs for screening, the interpretation of genome-wide CNVs, false positives from maternal CNVs, and the need for appropriate counseling.

DISCLOSURE

J. Xiang and Z. Peng were employed at BGI Genomics at the time of submission.

REFERENCES

[1] Lo YM, Corbetta N, Chamberlain PF, et al. Presence of fetal DNA in maternal plasma and serum. Lancet 1997;350(9076):485–7.

[2] Bianchi DW, Chiu RWK. Sequencing of circulating cell-free DNA during pregnancy. N Engl J Med 2018;379(5):464–73.

[3] Gadsboll K, Petersen OB, Gatinois V, et al. Current use of noninvasive prenatal testing in Europe, Australia and the USA: a graphical presentation. Acta Obstet Gynecol Scand 2020;99(6):722–30.

[4] Van Den Bogaert K, Lannoo L, Brison N, et al. Outcome of publicly funded nationwide first-tier noninvasive prenatal screening. Genet Med 2021;23(6):1137–42.

[5] Wapner RJ, Martin CL, Levy B, et al. Chromosomal microarray versus karyotyping for prenatal diagnosis. N Engl J Med 2012;367(23):2175–84.

[6] Wang H, Dong Z, Zhang R, et al. Low-pass genome sequencing versus chromosomal microarray analysis: implementation in prenatal diagnosis. Genet Med 2020;22(3):500–10.

[7] Capalbo A, Rienzi L, Ubaldi FM. Diagnosis and clinical management of duplications and deletions. Fertil Steril 2017;107(1):12–8.

[8] Gregg AR, Skotko BG, Benkendorf JL, et al. Noninvasive prenatal screening for fetal aneuploidy, 2016 update: a position statement of the American College of Medical Genetics and Genomics. Genet Med 2016;18(10):1056–65.

[9] Liang D, Cram DS, Tan H, et al. Clinical utility of noninvasive prenatal screening for expanded chromosome disease syndromes. Genet Med 2019;21(9):1998–2006.

[10] van der Meij KRM, Sistermans EA, Macville MVE, et al. TRIDENT-2: national implementation of genome-wide non-invasive prenatal testing as a first-tier screening test in the Netherlands. Am J Hum Genet 2019;105(6):1091–101.

[11] Liao GJ, Chan KC, Jiang P, et al. Noninvasive prenatal diagnosis of fetal trisomy 21 by allelic ratio analysis using targeted massively parallel sequencing of maternal plasma DNA. PLoS One 2012;7(5):e38154.

[12] Chiu RW, Chan KC, Gao Y, et al. Noninvasive prenatal diagnosis of fetal chromosomal aneuploidy by massively parallel genomic sequencing of DNA in maternal plasma. Proc Natl Acad Sci U S A 2008;105(51):20458–63.

[13] Helgeson J, Wardrop J, Boomer T, et al. Clinical outcome of subchromosomal events detected by whole-genome noninvasive prenatal testing. Prenat Diagn 2015;35(10):999–1004.

[14] Wapner RJ, Babiarz JE, Levy B, et al. Expanding the scope of noninvasive prenatal testing: detection of fetal microdeletion syndromes. Am J Obstet Gynecol 2015;212(3):332 e1–9.

[15] Martin K, Iyengar S, Kalyan A, et al. Clinical experience with a single-nucleotide polymorphism-based non-invasive prenatal test for five clinically significant microdeletions. Clin Genet 2018;93(2):293–300.

[16] Lefkowitz RB, Tynan JA, Liu T, et al. Clinical validation of a noninvasive prenatal test for genomewide detection of fetal copy number variants. Am J Obstet Gynecol 2016;215(2):227.e1–16.

[17] Li R, Wan J, Zhang Y, et al. Detection of fetal copy number variants by non-invasive prenatal testing for common aneuploidies. Ultrasound Obstet Gynecol 2016;47(1):53–7.

[18] Liu H, Gao Y, Hu Z, et al. Performance evaluation of NIPT in detection of chromosomal copy number variants

using low-coverage whole-genome sequencing of plasma DNA. PLoS One 2016;11(7):e0159233.
[19] Dong Z, Yan J, Xu F, et al. Genome sequencing explores complexity of chromosomal abnormalities in recurrent miscarriage. Am J Hum Genet 2019;105(6):1102–11.
[20] Shaffer LG, Bejjani BA. A cytogeneticist's perspective on genomic microarrays. Hum Reprod Update 2004;10(3): 221–6.
[21] Huber D, Voith von Voithenberg L, Kaigala GV. Fluorescence in situ hybridization (FISH): history, limitations and what to expect from micro-scale FISH? Micro Nano Eng 2018;1:15–24.
[22] Levy B, Burnside RD. Are all chromosome microarrays the same? What clinicians need to know. Prenat Diagn 2019;39(3):157–64.
[23] Miller DT, Adam MP, Aradhya S, et al. Consensus statement: chromosomal microarray is a first-tier clinical diagnostic test for individuals with developmental disabilities or congenital anomalies. Am J Hum Genet 2010;86(5):749–64.
[24] Dong Z, Zhang J, Hu P, et al. Low-pass whole-genome sequencing in clinical cytogenetics: a validated approach. Genet Med 2016;18(9):940–8.
[25] Rose NC, Kaimal AJ, Dugoff L, et al. Screening for fetal chromosomal abnormalities: ACOG Practice Bulletin, Number 226. Obstet Gynecol 2020;136(4):e48–69.
[26] Dondorp W, de Wert G, Bombard Y, et al. Non-invasive prenatal testing for aneuploidy and beyond: challenges of responsible innovation in prenatal screening. Eur J Hum Genet 2015;23(11):1438–50.
[27] Zhao C, Tynan J, Ehrich M, et al. Detection of fetal subchromosomal abnormalities by sequencing circulating cell-free DNA from maternal plasma. Clin Chem 2015; 61(4):608–16.
[28] Canick JA, Palomaki GE, Kloza EM, et al. The impact of maternal plasma DNA fetal fraction on next generation sequencing tests for common fetal aneuploidies. Prenat Diagn 2013;33(7):667–74.
[29] Yin AH, Peng CF, Zhao X, et al. Noninvasive detection of fetal subchromosomal abnormalities by semiconductor sequencing of maternal plasma DNA. Proc Natl Acad Sci U S A 2015;112(47):14670–5.
[30] Welker NC, Lee AK, Kjolby RAS, et al. High-throughput fetal fraction amplification increases analytical performance of noninvasive prenatal screening. Genet Med 2021;23(3):443–50.
[31] Liang B, Li H, He Q, et al. Enrichment of the fetal fraction in non-invasive prenatal screening reduces maternal background interference. Sci Rep 2018;8(1):17675.
[32] Hu P, Liang D, Chen Y, et al. An enrichment method to increase cell-free fetal DNA fraction and significantly reduce false negatives and test failures for non-invasive prenatal screening: a feasibility study. J Transl Med 2019;17(1):124.
[33] He QZ, Wu XJ, He QY, et al. A method for improving the accuracy of non-invasive prenatal screening by cell-free foetal DNA size selection. Br J Biomed Sci 2018;75(3):133–8.
[34] Quail MA, Gu Y, Swerdlow H, et al. Evaluation and optimisation of preparative semi-automated electrophoresis systems for Illumina library preparation. Electrophoresis 2012;33(23):3521–8.
[35] Vong JSL, Jiang P, Cheng SH, et al. Enrichment of fetal and maternal long cell-free DNA fragments from maternal plasma following DNA repair. Prenat Diagn 2019;39(2):88–99.
[36] Lo YM, Chan KC, Sun H, et al. Maternal plasma DNA sequencing reveals the genome-wide genetic and mutational profile of the fetus. Sci Transl Med 2010;2(61): 61ra91.
[37] Fan HC, Blumenfeld YJ, Chitkara U, et al. Analysis of the size distributions of fetal and maternal cell-free DNA by paired-end sequencing. Clin Chem 2010;56(8): 1279–86.
[38] Zhang B, Zhao S, Wan H, et al. High-resolution DNA size enrichment using a magnetic nano-platform and application in non-invasive prenatal testing. Analyst 2020; 145(17):5733–9.
[39] Qiao L, Yu B, Liang Y, et al. Sequencing shorter cfDNA fragments improves the fetal DNA fraction in noninvasive prenatal testing. Am J Obstet Gynecol 2019; 221(4):345.e1–11.
[40] Qiao L, Zhang Q, Liang Y, et al. Sequencing of short cfDNA fragments in NIPT improves fetal fraction with higher maternal BMI and early gestational age. Am J Transl Res 2019;11(7):4450–9.
[41] Quail MA, Swerdlow H, Turner DJ. Improved protocols for the Illumina genome analyzer sequencing system. Curr Protoc Hum Genet 2009 Chapter 18:Unit 18 2.
[42] Lo KK, Karampetsou E, Boustred C, et al. Limited clinical utility of non-invasive prenatal testing for subchromosomal abnormalities. Am J Hum Genet 2016;98(1):34–44.
[43] Rampasek L, Arbabi A, Brudno M. Probabilistic method for detecting copy number variation in a fetal genome using maternal plasma sequencing. Bioinformatics 2014;30(12):i212–8.
[44] Srinivasan A, Bianchi DW, Huang H, et al. Noninvasive detection of fetal subchromosome abnormalities via deep sequencing of maternal plasma. Am J Hum Genet 2013;92(2):167–76.
[45] Kucharik M, Gnip A, Hyblova M, et al. Non-invasive prenatal testing (NIPT) by low coverage genomic sequencing: detection limits of screened chromosomal microdeletions. PLoS One 2020;15(8):e0238245.
[46] Liao C, Yin AH, Peng CF, et al. Noninvasive prenatal diagnosis of common aneuploidies by semiconductor sequencing. Proc Natl Acad Sci U S A 2014;111(20): 7415–20.
[47] Maya I, Sharony R, Yacobson S, et al. When genotype is not predictive of phenotype: implications for genetic counseling based on 21,594 chromosomal microarray analysis examinations. Genet Med 2018;20(1):128–31.
[48] Rosenfeld JA, Coe BP, Eichler EE, et al. Estimates of penetrance for recurrent pathogenic copy-number variations. Genet Med 2013;15(6):478–81.

[49] Hu H, Wang L, Wu J, et al. Noninvasive prenatal testing for chromosome aneuploidies and subchromosomal microdeletions/microduplications in a cohort of 8141 single pregnancies. Hum Genomics 2019; 13(1):14.

[50] Riggs ER, Andersen EF, Cherry AM, et al. Technical standards for the interpretation and reporting of constitutional copy-number variants: a joint consensus recommendation of the American College of Medical Genetics and Genomics (ACMG) and the Clinical Genome Resource (ClinGen). Genet Med 2020;22(2):245–57.

[51] Girirajan S, Rosenfeld JA, Coe BP, et al. Phenotypic heterogeneity of genomic disorders and rare copy-number variants. N Engl J Med 2012;367(14):1321–31.

[52] Sachs A, Blanchard L, Buchanan A, et al. Recommended pre-test counseling points for noninvasive prenatal testing using cell-free DNA: a 2015 perspective. Prenat Diagn 2015;35(10):968–71.

[53] McDonald-McGinn DM, Hain HS, Emanuel BS, et al. 22q11.2 deletion syndrome. In: Adam MP, Ardinger HH, Pagon RA, et al, editors. GeneReviews® [Internet]. Seattle (WA): University of Washington, Seattle; 2020. p. 1993–2021. Available at: https://www.ncbi.nlm.nih.gov/books/NBK1523/.

[54] Driscoll DJ, Miller JL, Schwartz S, et al. Prader-Willi syndrome. In: Adam MP, Ardinger HH, Pagon RA, et al, editors. GeneReviews® [Internet]. Seattle (WA): University of Washington, Seattle; 1998. p. 1993–2021. Available at: https://www.ncbi.nlm.nih.gov/books/NBK1330/.

[55] Dagli AI, Mueller J, CA W. Angelman syndrome. In: Adam MP, Ardinger HH, Pagon RA, et al, editors. GeneReviews® [Internet]. Seattle (WA): University of Washington, Seattle; 1998 1993-2021. Available at: https://www.ncbi.nlm.nih.gov/books/NBK1144/.

[56] Cerruti Mainardi P. Cri du chat syndrome. Orphanet J Rare Dis 2006;1:33.

[57] Firth HV, Richards SM, Bevan AP, et al. DECIPHER: Database of Chromosomal Imbalance and Phenotype in Humans Using Ensembl Resources. Am J Hum Genet 2009; 84(4):524–33.

[58] Jordan VK, Zaveri HP, Scott DA. 1p36 deletion syndrome: an update. Appl Clin Genet 2015;8:189–200.

[59] Battaglia A, Carey JC, ST S. Wolf-Hirschhorn syndrome – RETIRED CHAPTER, FOR HISTORICAL REFERENCE ONLY [Updated 2015 Aug 20]. In: Adam MP, Ardinger HH, Pagon RA, et al, editors. GeneReviews® [Internet]. Seattle (WA): University of Washington, Seattle; 2002 1993-2021. Available at: https://www.ncbi.nlm.nih.gov/books/NBK1183/.

[60] Battaglia A, Carey JC, South ST. Wolf-Hirschhorn syndrome: a review and update. Am J Med Genet C Semin Med Genet 2015;169(3):216–23.

[61] Mattina T, Perrotta CS, Grossfeld P. Jacobsen syndrome. Orphanet J Rare Dis 2009;4:9.

[62] Maas S, Shaw A, Bikker H, et al. Trichorhinophalangeal syndrome. In: Adam MP, Ardinger HH, Pagon RA, et al, editors. GeneReviews® [Internet]. Seattle (WA): University of Washington, Seattle; 2017. p. 1993–2021. Available at: https://www.ncbi.nlm.nih.gov/books/NBK425926/.

Advances in Molecular Pathology 4 (2021) 27–36
ADVANCES IN MOLECULAR PATHOLOGY

Applications of Optical Genome Mapping in Next-Generation Cytogenetics and Genomics

Wahab A. Khan, PhD[a,*], Diana M. Toledo, PhD, MS, CGC[b]

[a]Clinical Cytogenetics, Molecular Genetics, Department of Pathology and Laboratory Medicine, Geisel School of Medicine at Dartmouth College, Dartmouth-Hitchcock Medical Center, Williamson Translational Research Building-4th Floor, 1 Medical Center Drive, Lebanon, NH 03766, USA; [b]The Broad Institute of MIT and Harvard, Clinical Research Sequencing Platform Laboratory, 320 Charles Street, Cambridge, MA 02141, USA

KEYWORDS

- Next-generation cytogenomics • Optical genome mapping • Structural variants • Repeat expansions
- Long-read mapping

KEY POINTS

- Optical genome mapping provides long-range information derived from megabase-size molecules.
- Optical genome mapping detects balanced and unbalanced chromosomal scale variation, submicroscopic copy number alterations, and repeat expansions in a single assay.
- Optical maps provide de novo human genome assemblies with accurate specificity and depth of coverage.
- Paired with long-read sequencing, optical genome mapping has implications in producing individualized high-quality diploid human genomes.

INTRODUCTION

Historically, short-read sequencing has been the preferred method for sequencing targeted gene panels, exomes, and genomes in the clinical laboratory. However, other technologies have begun to show advantages over these traditional sequencing methods. As the name implies, short-read sequencing involves fragmenting (~350 bp) and sequencing the genome in short reads, then tiling those overlapping reads and reconstructing the genome. Although this is a cost-effective and accurate method, there are regions of the genome that will be intractable to being detected using this methodology [1].

Long-read or third-generation sequencing allows for highly accurate sequencing of long stretches of the genome. Two well-known modalities in the long-read sequencing space are Pacific Biosciences (PacBio) with single-molecule, real-time (SMRT) sequencing and Oxford Nanopore Technologies (ONT) with nanopore sequencing. The chemistries used and average read length outputs of these technologies are briefly provided in Table 1. SMRT sequencing is limited by the efficiency and longevity of the polymerase being used and therefore has a shorter average read length than nanopore-based technologies. The sequence reads are able to traverse most repetitive genomic regions with high AT/GC content and tandem repeats. Although this is an advancement over short-read sequencing, accessing highly repetitive regions, such as segmental duplicons, deciphering complex genomic rearrangements, and assembling de novo sequences at the chromosomal level, continue to pose challenges. Often,

*Corresponding author, *E-mail address:* wahab.a.khan@hitchcock.org

https://doi.org/10.1016/j.yamp.2021.07.010
2589-4080/21/

TABLE 1
Comparison of Second- and Third-Generation Sequencing Technologies Relative to Optical Mapping

	Optical Mapping (BioNano)	Pacific Biosciences SMRT	Oxford Nanopore Technologies	Mate Pair Sequencing	Short-Read Sequencing (ex. Illumina)
Average read length	225 kb [2] (molecule length)	10–14 kb [32]	10–30 kb [45]	2–5 kb [46]	150–300 bp
Chemistry	Light microscopy and enzymatic labeling of DNA	Fluorescently labeled nucleotides added to DNA sequence tethered to the bottom of a well in real time	Measures ionic current differences between nucleotides through a nanopore	Biotinylated DNA ends circularized, and cut into smaller fragments, followed by short-read sequencing	Sequencing by synthesis: fluorescently labeled reversible terminator-bound dNTPs
Accuracy, %	98.88	>99	>95	>99	>99
Resolution	>500 bp (large contigs)	Base pair level (continuous long read)	Base pair (ultralong read)	Base pair level	Base pair level (paired-end reads)

consensus calls from multiple long-read technologies are needed to achieve high-quality assemblies in terms of contiguity and completeness [2,3].

Because of these limitations, optical genome mapping (optical mapping) technologies have emerged to bridge the gap between sequencing-based technologies and whole chromosome visualization (ie, karyotyping). Optical mapping uses light microscopy to probe fluorescently labeled sequence motifs (restriction enzyme sites) across the entire genome at a resolution of 500 bp, with an average molecule length of approximately 225 kb [2]. Optical mapping was first described in 1993 in the context of constructing *Saccharomyces cerevisiae* (yeast) chromosomes from ordered restriction maps [4]. In early development, this technology was plagued by low throughput, high error rate, and variability in DNA length and stretching. Since then, advances have been made to resolve many of these early issues by improving the microfluidics, labeling techniques, novel enzymology, and throughput capability [5–7]. Although the current resolution is approximately 500 bp for the Bionano platforms, advancements in algorithms and data analysis software report the capability of a resolution as low as 10 bp [8]. Commercialized efforts have developed multichannel/massively parallel platforms that have increased the application of this technology [9].

Here, the authors highlight applications of optical genome mapping and its utility as a robust benchmark for ushering in next-generation cytogenetics and genomics. This article provides a summary of some of the applications emerging in the area of optical genome mapping. The authors also discuss consideration in bioinformatics support and advantages and disadvantages of this nascent technology.

SIGNIFICANCE

Next-generation optical genome mapping has demonstrated the potential to augment short-read genome sequencing in the near term. This has overarching implications for laboratory diagnostics and can reveal important regions of the human genome implicated in disease (eg, complex structural variants near low copy repeats or intergenic regions, repeat expansions, transposon-mediated pathogenic variants, and balanced cryptic chromosomal rearrangements, among others). The impact would be highest in deciphering structural variation (SV) not amenable to being detected by current short-read technology, such as balanced translocations or inversions. This would further bridge the gap between genomics and cytogenomics. In doing so, optical genome mapping can also aid in a more complete representation of the diploid human genome that complements emerging long-read technologies.

FROM MASSIVELY PARALLEL SEQUENCING TO NEXT-GENERATION KARYO-MAPPING

Illumina-based short-read second-generation sequencing is readily used at scale in clinical and research settings. This technology provides reasonable sequence read depth and base-calling accuracy for small sequence variants discovery and analysis. Despite this, a basic prerequisite of massively parallel short-read sequencing is that the DNA sequence must be aligned to a reference genome. Although this is viewed as the gold standard, the most current reference genome (GRCh38) is not an average of the global population, but rather contains long stretches that are specific to various donors with the majority being sampled from a single donor [10]. Furthermore, SV discovery using short-read sequencing is challenging and can become increasingly complex in areas of the genome with repeat DNA architecture or complex genomic loci, such as the major histocompatibility region.

Optical mapping, using the Bionano Saphyr approach [11], obviates a reference genome. It allows for *de novo* assembly in that it re-creates the genome with no prior knowledge or a reference genome. It also produces long DNA fragments to identify SV with high accuracy (see Table 1). The optical mapping approach, using the Bionano Genomics Irys automated imaging system, was initially described using nanochannel array for SV detection [4,9]. The basic steps start from high-quality genomic DNA extraction and incorporation of fluorescent tags followed by ligation and staining (Fig. 1A). The labeled DNA is loaded onto the nanochannel on the Bionano system and then migrated through the channel by way of electrophoresis (Fig. 1B). This linearizes the DNA molecule, preserving its length and minimizing fragmentation. The fluorescent labels along the length of each linearized kilo- to mega-base pair-sized DNA molecule are then algorithmically processed into an optical sequence motif map [9]. It is also important to note that optical mapping does not generate the physical nucleotide sequence nor does it give a sense of variant allele fraction (VAF). With optical mapping, the nearest labeling site to the copy number interval or structural aberration in question can be visualized.

Briefly, the algorithm generated by the BioNano platform maps the locations of fluorescent labels along the length of each DNA molecule using a proprietary software package (eg, nanoStudio in previous iterations or the latest Access software). The algorithm takes into account sizing errors and differences in length of the optical molecules. The data are transformed using a pairwise comparison of all single-molecule reads using unsupervised clustering. Following this, the individual optical map clusters can be grouped based on signal from the restriction sites, whereas false signals are filtered out, and consensus clusters are joined and mapped to the genome [9]. High-resolution optical mapping using the Bionano system can generate images of molecules with an average N50 contig length of greater than 250 kb pairs. At the time of writing this chapter, this approach currently produces a genome depth of approximately 300× per flow cell with 3 flow cells per chip and 2 chips per instrument [12].

CYTOGENOMIC APPLICATIONS OF OPTICAL MAPPING IN CONSTITUTIONAL DISEASE

Several practical applications that have adopted optical genome mapping are discussed later with respect to structurally complex loci underlying constitutional disease as well as SVs in cancer genomics. Some of these loci can be challenging to resolve by currently available methods, such as karyotyping, chromosomal microarrays (CMA), polymerase chain reaction (PCR)-based tests, and/or short-read next-generation sequencing (NGS). Next-generation cytogenomic mapping of rare, yet recurrent, microdeletion/microduplication syndromes by Bionano Saphyr workflow offers a high-throughput, genome-wide method to interrogate genome structural differences at scale.

Optical Mapping Applied to Genomic Disorders Mediated by Low Copy Repeats

In constitutional disorders, far fewer SVs affect the germline relative to small variants (eg, single nucleotide variants (SNVs), insertion/deletions, or indels). However, collectively, the SVs affect a larger genomic landscape because more base pairs are involved in the rearrangement. Depending on the gene content and size, this arguably can lead to a far greater impact on the patient's phenotype compared with SNVs and indels [13]. Further deep intronic regions of the human genome in which SVs can alter gene expression and regulatory elements are important to capture [14].

Clinically relevant regions investigated by optical mapping often contain genes with paralogs and other complex repetitive structures near centromeres/telomeres [15]. This can complicate the interpretation of data and diagnosis of disease. The Bionano workflow can accurately assemble large contigs (see Table 1) that are able to transverse these regions and has demonstrated the ability to reconstruct segmental duplications with far less read length error rates compared with PacBio SMRT sequencing or ONT [15,16]. In several previously reported microdeletions/microduplications overlapping 7q11.23 (Williams-Beuren syndrome), 15q13.3, and 16p12.2, Bionano optical mapping was

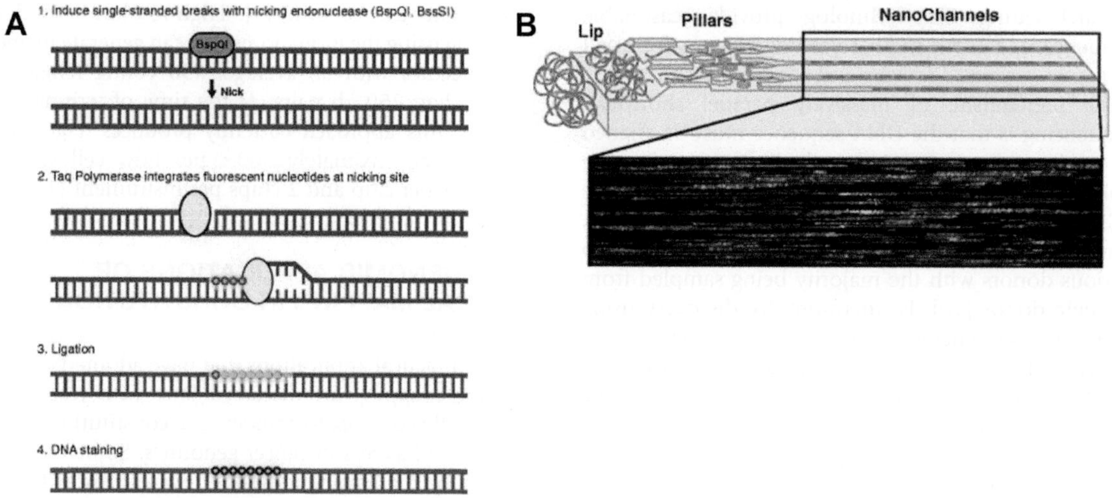

FIG. 1 (**A**) The process of preparing high-molecular-weight DNA for optical mapping is depicted. DNA is nicked with a restriction enzyme (eg, BspQI) in step 1. In step 2, the polymerase integrates fluorescent nucleotides along the length of the DNA. The next process involves a ligation step (step 3) followed by DNA staining (step 4) for downstream processing on the Bionano Irys Saphyr chip. (**B**) As the DNA is loaded onto the chip, a voltage current is applied that concentrates the DNA at the lip (left point in image showing coiled DNA). DNA migrates through the pillars, uncoils, and eventually straightens and migrates into the nanochannels (right point in the image). At the point of contact in the nanochannels, the voltage is removed, and the DNA molecule is stopped and imaged. In zoom view, spectrum blue indicates DNA staining, and spectrum green indicates the interspersed fluorescently labeled nicked sites in the nanochannel structure. (*From* Barseghyan, H., Tang, W., Wang, R.T. et al. Next-generation mapping: a novel approach for detection of pathogenic structural variants with a potential utility in clinical diagnosis. Genome Med 9, 90 (2017); with permission.)

able to localize SVs inaccessible to short-read sequencing [15]. Optical mapping has also demonstrated patterns of SVs across different populations around the world [17]. Optical maps can be implemented to observe SVs and most copy number variants (CNVs) in genomic disorders currently being investigated by CMAs.

Optical Mapping and Single-Gene Disorders: Prototypical Example of Duchene Muscular Dystrophy

In another application, optical mapping was applied to the diagnosis of a single-gene disorder: Duchene muscular dystrophy, typically detected by CMA as well as by multiple-ligation dependent probe amplification (MLPA). Specifically, pathogenic SVs and CNVs were simultaneously detected by optical mapping that spans both single and multiple exons in *DMD* [11]. Of note, optical mapping also picked up a pathogenic 5.1-Mbp balanced inversion disrupting *DMD* that was missed by CMA, MLPA, and clinical exome sequencing [11]. This underscores the ability of optical mapping to identify inversions that are not amenable to detection with CMA or short-read sequencing technologies.

Optical Mapping in Context of Infertility and Prenatal Testing

Balanced reciprocal translocations are chromosomal structural rearrangements occurring in approximately 0.2% of newborns. Most translocations are de novo, whereas others are "private SVs" occurring in family pedigrees. Besides dosage-sensitive genes involved in intellectual disability, chromosomal translocations can perturb critical genes required for normal fertility and reproductive fitness [18]. An NGS technique known as mate-pair sequencing has been used to identify translocation breakpoints [19]; however, this uses sequence reads that can be difficult to accurately map in certain translocation breakpoints traversing repeat regions. Bionano optical mapping, on the other hand, is able to map breakpoints from balanced chromosomal translocations in repetitive DNA. In a recent study, optical mapping was able to correctly identify several genes, *FNDC3A*, *NUP155*, *DPY19L1*, *BAI3*, having known associations with male infertility [18].

Optical mapping has also demonstrated utility in detecting de novo balanced rearrangements occurring prenatally. By Giemsa-banding, these apparently balanced rearrangements can be very difficult to interpret from karyotyping alone. As the gene content and the size of the reciprocally exchanged segments are not revealed by karyotyping, optical mapping can provide a means of assessing whether the balanced translocation interrupts nearby critical disease-specific genes [18,20]. In cases whereby the impacted gene or genes have a dominant phenotype, genetic counseling can be recommended for pregnancy management.

CYTOGENOMIC APPLICATIONS USING OPTICAL MAPPING IN ACQUIRED DISEASE

Up until this point, the authors have highlighted SVs resulting in germline disease. SVs in somatic disease may result from deregulation of DNA repair mechanisms and genomic surveillance. Examples of such SVs have been described in the form of fusion events and a host of other alterations ranging from deletions, duplications, amplifications, and complex chromothripsis. In most cases, optical mapping is able to consolidate current standard-of-care cytogenomics techniques for hematological malignancies, such as chromosomal banding, fluorescence in situ hybridization (FISH), and CMA. Even with short-read genome sequencing, certain cancer rearrangements can be recalcitrant to being detected. Long-read PacBio or ONT sequencing can pose challenges in camouflaged regions of the genome, thus producing sequences with lower base qualities. Therefore, complementary approaches, such as optical mapping, that do not rely on generating a physical sequence would be advantageous in genotyping large genome aberrations.

Optical Mapping in Hematological Malignancies

High-resolution optical genome mapping has been successfully applied to study numerous leukemia samples with simple and complex cytogenetic aberrations [12]. In a recent study, samples previously analyzed using karyotyping, FISH and/or CMAs as part of routine diagnostic testing were assessed using optical mapping. Diagnostically relevant chromosomal aberrations were identified from a combination of myeloid and lymphoid neoplasms (AML, MDS, CML, CLL, ALL, MM, MPN, T-PLL, LYBM) using Bionano optical imaging. This included identification of all previously reported aberrations with a VAF greater than 10% detected by standard of care workflow. Among complex cases with multiple SVs per sample, only 1 case did not exhibit full concordance [12]. Moreover, fusions and SVs affecting novel genes, such as *NOTCH1*, were identified as potentially new findings in a CLL through optical mapping. This approach has also demonstrated potential for "phased" detection of SVs as well as methylation signatures [21].

Optical Mapping in Solid Tumor Genetics

Although large SVs play an important role in intratumoral genetic heterogeneity, optical mapping has, as of yet, not seen widespread application in solid tumor applications. This is in part due to the difficulty of obtaining high-quality, high-molecular-weight DNA from solid tumors. However, analysis using earlier workflow iterations, whereby purified nuclei from tissues are embedded in agarose gel plugs and more recent paramagnetic nanobind disk chemistries to recover nuclei acid material, is improving optical genome map generation [22,23]. Other proof of principle studies showing the importance of optical genome mapping to solid tumor analysis from primary fresh tissue have shown feasibility similar to SV visualization in liquid tumors. For example, optical mapping combined with whole-genome sequencing (WGS) in lung squamous cell carcinoma helped reveal intratumor genetic heterogeneity. Specifically, comparison of SVs from optical mapping and WGS of lung squamous cell carcinoma samples demonstrated nearly a quarter percent of SVs detected by optical mapping overlapped with WGS results. In this study, SVs 5 kb or greater were most amenable to being detected by optical mapping from tumor high-molecular-weight DNA [24]. Overall, the SVs were found to be particularly large in genomic size within the primary tumor and metastasized sections [24]. Additional SV filtering strategies by optical genome mapping have been described across a range of solid tumor tissue types from prostate, ovarian, and kidney to colon and breast [23].

RESOLVING INTRACTABLE REGIONS OF THE HUMAN GENOME: REPEAT EXPANSIONS DISORDERS

Repetitive regions in the genome are challenging to decipher using short-read sequencing technologies. Therefore, repeat expansion disorders are typically identified using technologies that estimate the repeat length, but cannot visualize the context in which these repeats occur and cannot size large intronic expansions (>1000 repeats). Technologies, such as Southern blot and repeat prime PCR, are labor intensive and are difficult to multiplex on a genome scale. Optical mapping can quantify repeat expansion and contraction disorders across the genome. Quantification of repeat numbers by optical mapping is performed by calculating the length of a given repeat unit (eg, triplet repeats or larger intronic repeat). Because optical molecules have embedded within them fluorescently labeled restriction enzyme recognition sites, these sites can be visualized upstream and downstream of the repeat. The labeled restriction sites act as anchor points, and the onboard software deconvolutes the optical image and calculates the distance between the 2 labels. This process is iterated over the length of the exonic or intronic region of interest of a given gene implicated in the repeat expansion disorder to enumerate the repeat units [25]. The enumeration can be performed in both coding and noncoding regions along with SV detection in a single assay using optical mapping. Several examples are presented in later discussion.

Facioscapulohumeral Muscular Dystrophy

Facioscapulohumeral muscular dystrophy (FSHD) presents with muscular weakness involving the facial muscles, scapula stabilizing muscles, and foot dorsiflexor muscles, and this weakness is often progressive and asymmetrical. Rather than an expansion, FSHD1 is caused by the contraction of the D4Z4 repeat region at the subtelomeric end of the long arm of chromosome 4 (4q35). This occurs by activating transcription of a typically dormant gene, *DUX4*, and causes aberrant expression. This region is typically large in a normal allele, with a range of $\geq$12 repeat units, and each repeat unit measures 3.3 kb in length. The pathogenic range of repeat units is $\leq$10 (between 1 and 10 repeat units), with an intermediate zone of 10 to 11 repeat units [26,27].

Optical mapping has been shown to successfully characterize the genetic landscape of the 4q35 region in the context of FSHD molecular diagnostics with Bionano Genomics technology [28]. In addition, other studies have used single-molecule optical mapping as a reliable technique for diagnosing FSHD1 with a workflow that is achievable by most molecular diagnostics laboratories [25]. Taking this a step further, optical mapping has been used toward successful prenatal diagnosis of FSHD1 on cultured amniocytes [29]. This was determined by counting Nb.BssSI restriction enzyme sites in each D4Z4 repeat in the 5′ end of *DUX4* on chromosome 4q35.2. D4Z4 repeat array has only 1 Nb.BssSI restriction site, and there is an additional Nb.BssSI site that is 1.7 kb distal to the last D4Z4 repeat unit. The latter is a marker for the FSHD1 pathogenic haplotype (4qA), whereas the typical haplotype (4qB) does not have this extra site. This allows 2 possible ways to distinguish a wild-type or pathogenic allele using optical mapping [29].

Fragile X Syndrome

Fragile X syndrome is the most common cause of inherited intellectual disability in males and is identified by the expansion of a CGG repeat in the 5′UTR region of the *FMR1* gene on the X chromosome. As with other repeat expansions/contractions, it is largely unknown what the maximum repeat length is for a full mutation because sequencing this region is not possible using short-read technology, but more than 1000 repeats have been estimated (>3000 bp in DNA length). Clinical testing for fragile X is typically done by PCR product sizing using capillary electrophoresis and confirmation in some cases of the full mutation by Southern blotting [30]. Although both of these methods are able to distinguish between normal, intermediate, premutation, or full mutation ranges (>200 repeats), they do not provide a precise CGG length for larger repeats and are only able to infer interruptions within the sequence (eg, AGG). The presence of AGG interruptions within the CGG repeat sequence in a permutation carrier is associated with higher stability and less expansion from generation to generation [31]. Repeat length and AGG triplet interruption can both be necessary pieces of molecular information that genetic counselors and other providers can use in the clinical setting to give more accurate recurrence risk estimates to female premutation carriers [32]. Third-generation sequencing technologies, such as PacBio or ONT, have been used to sequence the *FMR1* 5′UTR region and detect AGG interruptions, albeit at a lower depth of coverage [32]. This has also established precedence in the field to use optical genome maps for high-throughput mapping of this well-known repeat expansion. To this end, the potential to use optical mapping has been considered in a prenatal setting for detecting fragile X expansions in *FMR1* as well as measuring repeat expansion in *DMPK* from patients with type I myotonic dystrophy [33].

Amyotrophic Lateral Sclerosis

Amyotrophic lateral sclerosis (ALS) or frontotemporal dementia (FTD) is a progressive and severe neurodegenerative disorder primarily affecting the motor neurons. About 10% of all ALS/FTD cases may be familial and have a genetic component. Approximately 39% to 45% of all familial and 3% to 7% of simplex cases have a *C9orf72* G_4C_2 hexanucleotide repeat expansion in the pathogenic range. This expansion spans from 61 to greater than 4000 repeats or greater than 24 kb in length [34,35]. Conventional testing methods are able to detect whether an allele is in the pathogenic range, but they cannot definitively determine repeat size and have lower sensitivity in detecting large hexanucleotide expansions (eg, in kilobase range). Recently, investigators used optical mapping to detect a mosaic range of the *C9orf72* G_4C_2 repeat, exhibiting a large expansion of 32 kb or greater than 5000 repeats in length, from a postmortem brain sample of a patient with ALS. Although this repeat expansion was detectable by long-read sequencing, the investigators caution that specificity and sensitivity can be compromised because of polymerase exhaustion using SMRT sequencing and low throughput with ONT [36]. Taken together, the examples presented above lay important groundwork in the field of neurogenetics for using optical genome mapping in complex regions of the human genome.

BIOINFORMATICS WORKFLOW IN OPTICAL GENOME MAPPING

The bioinformatics workflow as it applies to Bionano optical mapping is composed of molecule-map quality control, map alignment, de novo assembly, and scaffolding. Essentially, the file types store similar features to Illumina-based sequencing, such as signal intensity, signal-to-noise ratios, coverage, and call quality (Fig. 2). Specifically, the raw data file generated by the Bionano Saphyr system contains signal intensity and signal-to-noise ratio features in *bnx* format. The *cmap* file in turn contains the assembly sequence and holds information, such as label quality and signal coverage. The alignment file is called *xmap*, and the "structural variation" file is called *smap*. All *xmap* files are generated using a default alignment output through a proprietary RefAligner for *de novo* map assembly on the Bionano system [2]. This, paired with the IrysSolve Scripts package, assists with data analysis of the *smap* SV file. Data visualization and management are then subsequently performed by the Irys

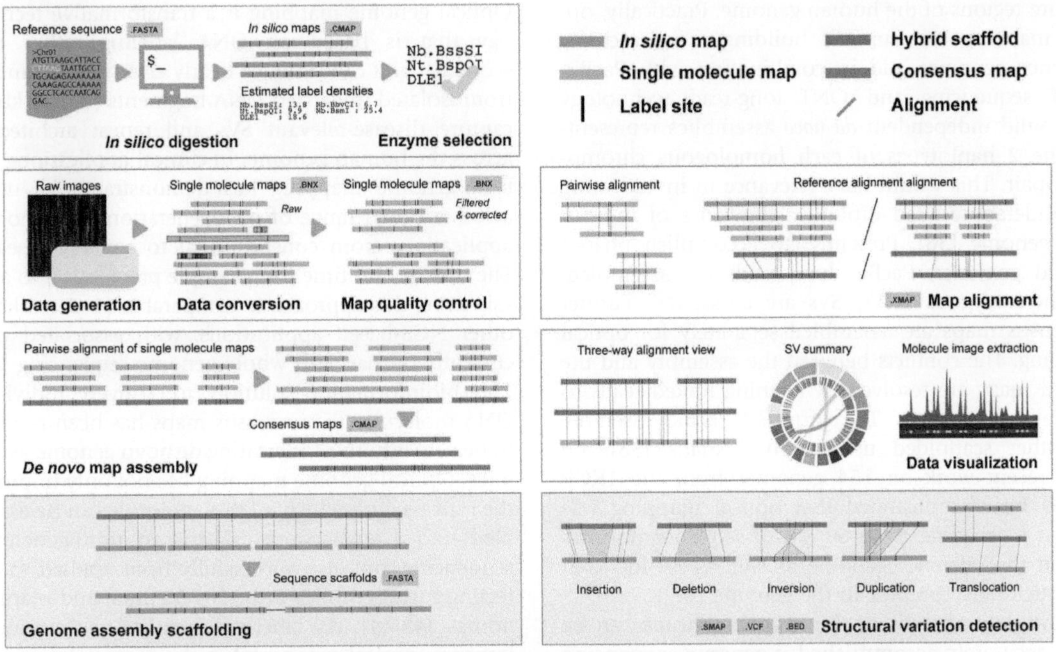

FIG. 2 The optical-mapping bioinformatics pipeline is divided into several major analysis steps. This involves, but is not limited to, molecule-map quality control, map alignment, de novo assembly, and scaffolding. In the bottom right panel, labeled "structural variant (SV) detection," the different scenarios of how the SV data output on the Bionano system postprocessing are shown. Of note, the reference optical map is colored pink, and the patient optical map is blue, indicating insertion, deletion, inversion, duplication, and translocation patterns. (*From* Yuan Y, Chung CY, Chan TF. Advances in optical mapping for genomic research. Comput Struct Biotechnol J. 2020;18:2051-2062. Published 2020 Aug 1. https://doi.org/10.1016/j.csbj.2020.07.018; with permission.)

platform using the IrysView desktop application. Once the *smap* SV file is annotated, optical mapping through the Bionano system can identify deletions and insertions on average greater than 500 bp, duplications greater than 30 kb, inversions on the order of 30 kb, and translocated segments greater than 50 kb [37]. The current state of the bioinformatics, however, has limitations in identifying more complex SV as additional postprocessing steps are needed, but can robustly handle simple SVs as described above.

PRESENT RELEVANCE AND FUTURE AVENUES OF OPTICAL MAPPING IN MEDICAL GENETICS

The survey of the current state of optical genome mapping presented here shows that this technology is ushering in a new era for cytogenetics and genomics. It is permitting identification of previously intractable karyotype-level rearrangements, such as balanced translocations and inversions with high resolution. It is allowing visualization of repeat expansions in the obscure regions of the human genome. Practically, optical mapping can support building more accurate reference genomes and in combination with PacBio SMRT sequencing and ONT long-read technology help build independent *de novo* assemblies representing the 2 haplotypes of each homologous chromosome pair. This would have relevance in investigating the underappreciated diploid architecture of the human genome [38]. Presently, to accomplish phased diploid genomes, PacBio long reads are assembled, and heterozygous SNVs, SVs are annotated. Further consensus maps are assembled separately for optical mapping. The conflicts between the assembly and the optical maps are resolved by aligning linked reads to the PacBio assembly. The corrected PacBio assembly is further scaffolded using optical maps [38]. Of note, recent work on 154 genomes from the 1KGP project has demonstrated that optical mapping was able to localize nearly ~60 Mb of sequence not present in the reference genome as well as 55 loci that are structurally complex in the genome [17].

Complete analysis of the human genome can be more accurately accomplished if genome sequencing is complemented with optical genome mapping. High-quality benchmark data are already leveraging short- and long-read technologies along with optical maps, which will prove invaluable for validation of genomic-scale assays and completing the gaps in the human genome. These complementary approaches can identify SNVs, Indels, CNVs, SVs, and repeat architecture across the human genome [39]. The ability to capture this information might also become part of a novel clinical workflow for unsolved exomes and accurate detection of SVs in cancer cytogenetics and genomics [40].

One important point to reemphasize is that in its current state, optical mapping does not provide nucleotide-level resolution and is therefore not meant for breakpoint discovery [37]. Rather, the physical location of the restriction sites obtained from optical mapping facilitates genome scaffolding and SV calling. However, in the event the restriction sites are incompletely labeled because of various reasons, such as improper uncoiling of the extracted DNA (see Fig. 1B), this can lead to errors in the map itself. However, current estimates suggest this is minimal, and algorithms are being developed to error-correct *Rmap* data for a more contiguous genome scaffold [41].

SUMMARY

Optical genome mapping is a transformative technology that is based on DNA labeling rather than sequencing. It can produce nearly error-free assemblies from isolated linearized DNA fragments (~100 kb) to capture disease-relevant SVs and repeat architecture across the human genome. In clinical applications, optical genome mapping has demonstrated its utility across a broad range of next-generation cytogenomics applications from constitutional to somatic diseases. The turnaround time from sample preparation to analysis using this approach is comparable (1–2 weeks) to other NGS-based applications, with associated costs currently on par with whole genome sequencing [42]. The bioinformatics solution to convert individual DNA molecules to consensus maps has been reported to be very intuitive for creating de novo genome assemblies. Optical genome mapping has not only improved the process with which a DNA molecule can be assembled into a large contig, relative to third-generation sequencing, but also successfully been applied to correcting misassemblies in both vertebrate and plant genomes [43,44]. As labeling chemistries continue to improve, optical mapping has the potential to further empower both genomic- and cytogenomic-based applications.

DISCLOSURE

The authors have nothing to disclose.

REFERENCES

[1] Alkan C, Sajjadian S, Eichler EE. Limitations of next-generation genome sequence assembly. Nat Methods 2011;8(1):61–5.

[2] Yuan Y, Chung CY-L, Chan T-F. Advances in optical mapping for genomic research. Comput Struct Biotechnol J 2020;18:2051–62.

[3] Miga KH, Koren S, Rhie A, et al. Telomere-to-telomere assembly of a complete human X chromosome. Nature 2020;585(7823):79–84.

[4] Schwartz DC, Li X, Hernandez LI, et al. Ordered restriction maps of Saccharomyces cerevisiae chromosomes constructed by optical mapping. Science 1993; 262(5130):110–4.

[5] Bogas D, Nyberg L, Pacheco R, et al. Applications of optical DNA mapping in microbiology. Biotechniques 2017;62(6):255–67.

[6] Jo K, Schramm TM, Schwartz DC. A single-molecule barcoding system using nanoslits for DNA analysis : nanocoding. Methods Mol Biol 2009;544:29–42.

[7] Jing J, Reed J, Huang J, et al. Automated high resolution optical mapping using arrayed, fluid-fixed DNA molecules. Proc Natl Acad Sci U S A 1998;95(14):8046–51.

[8] Jain A, Sheats J, Reifenberger JG, et al. Modeling the relaxation of internal DNA segments during genome mapping in nanochannels. Biomicrofluidics 2016;10(5):054117.

[9] Lam ET, Hastie A, Lin C, et al. Genome mapping on nanochannel arrays for structural variation analysis and sequence assembly. Nat Biotechnol 2012;30(8):771–6.

[10] Ballouz S, Dobin A, Gillis JA. Is it time to change the reference genome? Genome Biol 2019;20(1):159.

[11] Barseghyan H, Tang W, Wang RT, et al. Next-generation mapping: a novel approach for detection of pathogenic structural variants with a potential utility in clinical diagnosis. Genome Med 2017;9:90.

[12] Neveling K, Mantere T, Vermeulen S, et al. Next-generation cytogenetics: Comprehensive assessment of 52 hematological malignancy genomes by optical genome mapping. Am J Hum Genet 2021;108(8):1423–35.

[13] Roses AD, Akkari PA, Chiba-Falek O, et al. Structural variants can be more informative for disease diagnostics, prognostics and translation than current SNP mapping and exon sequencing. Expert Opin Drug Metab Toxicol 2016;12(2):135–47.

[14] Chiang C, Scott AJ, Davis JR, et al. The impact of structural variation on human gene expression. Nat Genet 2017;49(5):692–9.

[15] Mostovoy Y, Yilmaz F, Chow SK, et al. Genomic regions associated with microdeletion/microduplication syndromes exhibit extreme diversity of structural variation. Genetics 2021;217(2):iyaa038.

[16] Vollger MR, Dishuck PC, Sorensen M, et al. Long-read sequence and assembly of segmental duplications. Nat Methods 2019;16(1):88–94.

[17] Levy-Sakin M, Pastor S, Mostovoy Y, et al. Genome maps across 26 human populations reveal population-specific patterns of structural variation. Nat Commun 2019; 10(1):1025.

[18] Wang H, Jia Z, Mao A, et al. Analysis of balanced reciprocal translocations in patients with subfertility using single-molecule optical mapping. J Assist Reprod Genet 2020;37(3):509–16.

[19] Aristidou C, Koufaris C, Theodosiou A, et al. Accurate breakpoint mapping in apparently balanced translocation families with discordant phenotypes using whole genome mate-pair sequencing. PLoS One 2017;12(1): e0169935.

[20] Warburton D. De novo balanced chromosome rearrangements and extra marker chromosomes identified at prenatal diagnosis: clinical significance and distribution of breakpoints. Am J Hum Genet 1991;49(5):995–1013.

[21] Sharim H, Grunwald A, Gabrieli T, et al. Long-read single-molecule maps of the functional methylome. Genome Res 2019;29(4):646–56.

[22] Zhang Y, Broach J. Abstract 5125: a novel method for isolating high-quality UHMW DNA from 10 mg of freshly frozen or liquid-preserved animal and human tissue including solid tumors. Cancer Res 2019;79(13 Supplement):5125.

[23] Goldrich DY, LaBarge B, Chartrand S, et al. Identification of somatic structural variants in solid tumors by optical genome mapping. J Pers Med 2021;11(2):142.

[24] Peng Y, Yuan C, Tao X, et al. Integrated analysis of optical mapping and whole-genome sequencing reveals intratumoral genetic heterogeneity in metastatic lung squamous cell carcinoma. Transl Lung Cancer Res 2020;9(3): 670–81.

[25] Dai Y, Li P, Wang Z, et al. Single-molecule optical mapping enables quantitative measurement of D4Z4 repeats in facioscapulohumeral muscular dystrophy (FSHD). J Med Genet 2020;57(2):109–20.

[26] Hewitt JE, Lyle R, Clark LN, et al. Analysis of the tandem repeat locus D4Z4 associated with facioscapulohumeral muscular dystrophy. Hum Mol Genet 1994;3(8): 1287–95.

[27] Sacconi S, Salviati L, Desnuelle C. Facioscapulohumeral muscular dystrophy. Biochim Biophys Acta 2015; 1852(4):607–14.

[28] Sharim H, Grunwald A, Gabrieli T, et al. Long-read single-molecule maps of the functional methylome. Genome Res 2019;29:646–56.

[29] Zheng Y, Kong L, Xu H, et al. Rapid prenatal diagnosis of facioscapulohumeral muscular dystrophy 1 by combined Bionano optical mapping and karyomapping. Prenat Diagn 2020;40(3):317–23.

[30] Sherman S, Pletcher BA, Driscoll DA. Fragile X syndrome: diagnostic and carrier testing. Genet Med 2005;7(8): 584–7.

[31] Villate O, Ibarluzea N, Maortua H, et al. Effect of AGG interruptions on FMR1 maternal transmissions. Front Mol Biosci 2020;7:135.

[32] Ardui S, Race V, de Ravel T, et al. Detecting AGG interruptions in females with a FMR1 premutation by long-

read single-molecule sequencing: a 1 year clinical experience. Front Genet 2018;9:150.

[33] Optical genome mapping as a next-generation cytogenomic tool for detection of structural and copy number variations for prenatal genomic analyses | medRxiv. Available at: https://www.medrxiv.org/content/10.1101/2021.02.19.21251714v1. Accessed March 16, 2021.

[34] Dols-Icardo O, García-Redondo A, Rojas-García R, et al. Characterization of the repeat expansion size in C9orf72 in amyotrophic lateral sclerosis and frontotemporal dementia. Hum Mol Genet 2014;23(3):749–54.

[35] Gijselinck I, Van Mossevelde S, van der Zee J, et al. The C9orf72 repeat size correlates with onset age of disease, DNA methylation and transcriptional downregulation of the promoter. Mol Psychiatry 2016;21(8):1112–24.

[36] Ebbert MTW, Farrugia SL, Sens JP, et al. Long-read sequencing across the C9orf72 "GGGGCC" repeat expansion: implications for clinical use and genetic discovery efforts in human disease. Mol Neurodegener 2018;13(1):46.

[37] Balachandran P, Beck CR. Structural variant identification and characterization. Chromosome Res 2020;28(1):31–47.

[38] Seo J-S, Rhie A, Kim J, et al. De novo assembly and phasing of a Korean human genome. Nature 2016;538(7624):243–7.

[39] Zook JM, Hansen NF, Olson ND, et al. A robust benchmark for detection of germline large deletions and insertions. Nat Biotechnol 2020;38(11):1347–55.

[40] Mantere T, Kersten S, Hoischen A. Long-read sequencing emerging in medical genetics. Front Genet 2019;10:426.

[41] Mukherjee K, Washimkar D, Muggli MD, et al. Error correcting optical mapping data. Gigascience 2018;7(6):giy061.

[42] Long walk to genomics: history and current approaches to genome sequencing and assembly - PubMed. Available at: https://pubmed.ncbi.nlm.nih.gov/31890139/. Accessed March 19, 2021.

[43] Howe K, Wood JMD. Using optical mapping data for the improvement of vertebrate genome assemblies. Gigascience 2015;4:10.

[44] Tang H, Lyons E, Town CD. Optical mapping in plant comparative genomics. Gigascience 2015;4:3.

[45] Amarasinghe SL, Su S, Dong X, et al. Opportunities and challenges in long-read sequencing data analysis. Genome Biol 2020;21(1):30.

[46] Gao G, Smith DI. Mate-pair sequencing as a powerful clinical tool for the characterization of cancers with a DNA viral etiology. Viruses 2015;7(8):4507–28.

Hematopathology

Advances in Molecular Pathology 4 (2021) 37–48
ADVANCES IN MOLECULAR PATHOLOGY

Diagnosis of Variant Translocations in Acute Promyelocytic Leukemia

Brittany B. Coffman, MD, Devon Chabot-Richards, MD*
University of New Mexico Department of Pathology, 1001 Woodward Place Northeast, Albuquerque, NM 87102, USA

KEYWORDS
• Acute promyelocytic leukemia • Acute myeloid leukemia • Variant • *PML* • *RARA*

KEY POINTS

- Acute promyelocytic leukemia (APL) is a distinct subtype of acute myeloid leukemia that is associated with the development of disseminated intravascular coagulopathy, which poses a medical emergency.
- APL is defined by the reciprocal translocation between PML nuclear body scaffold (PML) and retinoic acid receptor alpha (*RARA*), resulting in a t(15;17) translocation, which can be easily detected by cytogenetic or molecular methods.
- Case of variant and cryptic translocations exist, which may be negative for t(15;17) by traditional methods but present similarly. Such patients may require additional work-up in the molecular diagnostics laboratory.
- Prompt diagnosis and low suspicion for APL are necessary given its propensity to develop life-threatening coagulopathy. Given that APL is very sensitive to all-trans retinoic acid, patients should be started early to mitigated the underlying coagulopathy.

INTRODUCTION

Acute promyelocytic leukemia (APL) is a biologically, clinically, morphologically, and immunophenotypically distinct subtype of acute myeloid leukemia (AML). Rapid diagnosis of APL is important because of its association with disseminated intravascular coagulation (DIC), a medical emergency that can be mitigated with differentiating chemotherapeutic agents, all-trans retinoic acid (ATRA), and/or arsenic trioxide (ATO) [1]. Classic APL is defined by the presence of a balanced reciprocal translocation between the PML nuclear body scaffold (*PML*) gene and retinoic acid receptor alpha (*RARA*) gene, although variant translocations and cryptic cases exist. The prognosis of APL is very good, attributable to sensitivity to therapy with ATRA and/or ATO along with conventional chemotherapy. This article covers the clinical features of classic APL along with cryptic and variant cases, and reviews the molecular distinctions among them.

CLINICAL FEATURES

APL accounts for roughly 10% of AML cases [2]. Although APL can occur at any age, it is more common among middle-aged patients and is uncommon in children less than 10 years of age. Clinical symptoms are similar to those of other acute leukemias, including weakness, fatigue, infection, and weight loss. APL differs from other acute leukemias in its association with coagulopathy. Patients can present with bleeding, thrombosis, or occult DIC. Laboratory evaluation of hemostasis shows typical findings of DIC, including prolonged prothrombin time and activated partial thromboplastin time, low fibrinogen level, increased D-dimer level, and thrombocytopenia [3].

There are 2 common APL variants: hypergranular and hypogranular or microgranular [4]. On complete blood count, the hypergranular variant often presents with pancytopenia and rare circulating abnormal promyelocytes, whereas the microgranular variant typically

*Corresponding author, *E-mail address:* DChabot-Richards@salud.unm.edu

https://doi.org/10.1016/j.yamp.2021.06.002
2589-4080/21/

presents with a very high leukocyte count and numerous circulating abnormal promyelocytes [5].

MICROSCOPY

APL is morphologically distinct from other forms of AML in that it is defined by the presence of abnormal promyelocytes (Fig. 1), which are considered blast equivalents in APL [1]. Normal promyelocytes are larger than blasts but have slightly more cytoplasm, although the nuclear/cytoplasmic ratio is high [6]. The chromatin of the promyelocyte is immature and nucleoli may be present. The transition from myeloblast to promyelocyte is defined by the development of distinct primary granules. Although the neoplastic cell in both the hypergranular and microgranular variants is an abnormal promyelocyte, there are slightly different morphologic features [1,7]. Hypergranular APL typically shows promyelocytes with bilobed or kidney bean–shaped nuclei. The cytoplasm is densely packed with large granules, which may obscure the nucleus. Auer rods are typically present and are larger than those seen in other forms of AML. Cells filled with Auer rods may be seen. In the microgranular variant, the cytoplasm is not markedly granular; however, it is filled with submicroscopic granules that are easily identified on cytochemical stains [1]. Microgranular promyelocytes may be morphologically similar to monocytes. Helpful cytologic features include the presence of bilobed or sliding-plate nuclei and the presence of Auer rods, which may be numerous. Nuclear irregularity is typically more pronounced in the microgranular variant than the hypergranular variant. Occasional hypergranular promyelocytes may be present in cases of microgranular APL.

In addition to microgranular and hypergranular variants of APL, there are rare variants defined by variant translocations. Most APLs with variant translocations share morphologic features with the hypergranular and microgranular variants; however, some important distinctions are discussed in detail here.

IMMUNOPHENOTYPE AND SPECIAL STAINS

Cytochemical stains are a helpful tool in the diagnosis of all variants of APL [7]. In all forms of APL, myeloperoxidase (MPO) is strongly positive, often obscuring the nucleus in the abnormal promyelocyte (Fig. 2). MPO can be helpful in distinguishing abnormal promyelocytes from monocytes, which are typically MPO negative or have only occasional scattered MPO-positive granules. In some cases, the nonspecific esterase (NSE) cytochemical stain may be helpful. NSE identifies monocytes and is usually negative in promyelocytes. However, NSE can be positive in up to 25% of APL cases and should not be used alone as evidence against the diagnosis [1].

The characteristic immunophenotype of APL is often a clue to the diagnosis (Fig. 3). There are immunophenotype differences between hypergranular and microgranular variants [8]. By flow cytometry, the hypergranular variant is characterized by high side scatter, attributed to cytoplasmic complexity, moderate cluster of differentiation (CD) 45, and positivity for CD13, CD33, CD117, and MPO. Aberrant expression of CD2, CD4, and CD56 may be seen. CD34 and human leukocyte antigen, DR isotype (HLA-DR), are dim to negative. The microgranular variant has low side scatter; moderate CD45 expression; and expression of CD33, CD117, CD13, and MPO. CD34 may be dim, but HLA-DR is usually negative. Aberrant expression of CD2 has been reported in cases of the microgranular variant bearing *FLT3*-ITD [9]. CD2 expression is also associated with the microgranular bcr3 form of APL. These patients may also express CD34 [10]. CD56 is positive in a subset of APL, more commonly in the microgranular variant, and may be associated with worse prognosis [11].

GENETIC PROFILE

APL is defined by reciprocal translocation between the *PML* gene on chromosome 15q24 and *RARA* gene on chromosome 17q21 [1]. This disease-defining translocation event is found in greater than 90% of cases and is easily identified on fluorescence in situ hybridization (FISH) and conventional karyotype (Fig. 4) [2,12]. The resulting fusion gene product allows clonal proliferation of promyelocytes that lack differentiation capacity [13].

The classic form of APL includes 3 possible fusion transcripts, which vary based on heterogenous breakpoints in *PML* with constant breakpoints in intron 2 of *RARA* (Fig. 5). [14] Although standard FISH cannot differentiate, the different fusion products are distinguishable by molecular techniques. The long form, or bcr1, occurs in 50% to 60% of APL cases. This fusion protein results from breakpoints in intron 6 of *PML*, causing a fusion of *PML* exon 6 and *RARA* exon 3. The variable form, or bcr2, is identified in 5% of APL cases and results from the fusion of *RARA* exon 3 and exon 6 of *PML*. The breakpoint within exon 6 of *PML* is variable and results in variable-sized fusion products. The short form, or bcr3, is seen in up to 45% of APL cases. The fusion product in this form results from *PML* exon 3 fusion with *RARA* exon 3. Some variation may be seen in transcripts

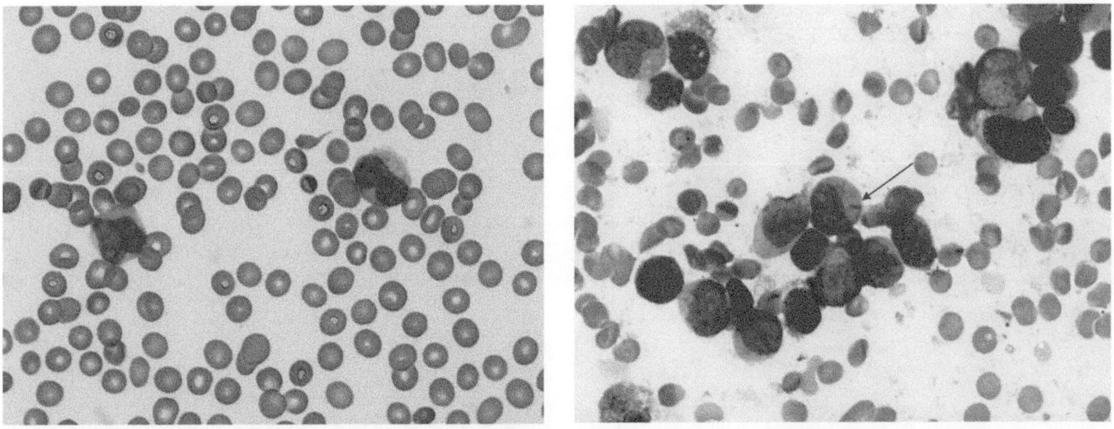

FIG. 1 Abnormal promyelocytes, peripheral blood (*left*), and bone marrow (*right*) with nuclear sliding plate morphology (*left*) and Auer rods (*right*, *arrow*) [Wright-Giemsa stained].

of the long form caused by alternative splicing. These translocation events are detected by conventional karyotype, FISH, and reverse transcriptase polymerase chain reaction (RT-PCR) (Fig. 6). FISH is widely available and can provide rapid results. Many laboratories can also perform rapid polymerase chain reaction (PCR). Advantages of PCR include identification of the specific fusion type (ie, bcr1, bcr2, or bcr3) by using fusion-specific primers and the ability to detect low transcript levels. This information is important for disease monitoring. PCR is the most readily available and sensitive method for determination of measurable residual disease or early relapse [15].

Another advantage of PCR compared with FISH is its ability to identify patients with so-called cryptic APL [16]. These patients carry the *PML-RARA* translocation but are negative by FISH. These specimens are often positive by PCR. These cases are of significant importance because they could be missed if PCR is not performed. It is recommended that any patient with clinical or morphologic suspicion of APL should undergo complete evaluation with both cytogenetics and molecular analysis. Patients with cryptic APL have clinical and morphologic presentation indistinguishable from classic APL and their biological behavior is analogous. These cases account for only 2% to 4% of all APL [2]. Most are caused by cryptic translocations resulting in the submicroscopic insertion of *RARA* into *PML* or vice versa [17]. Other possibilities include complex translocations not identified by traditional FISH probes.

In addition to cryptic APL, variant translocation cases resulting from translocations between *RARA* and

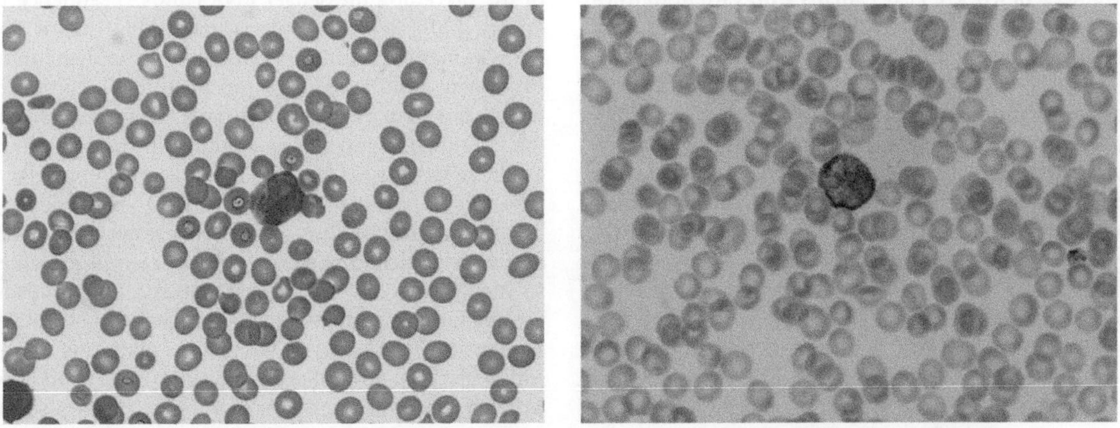

FIG. 2 Abnormal promyelocytes, peripheral blood (*left*), and positive MPO stain (*left*) [Wright-Giemsa stained].

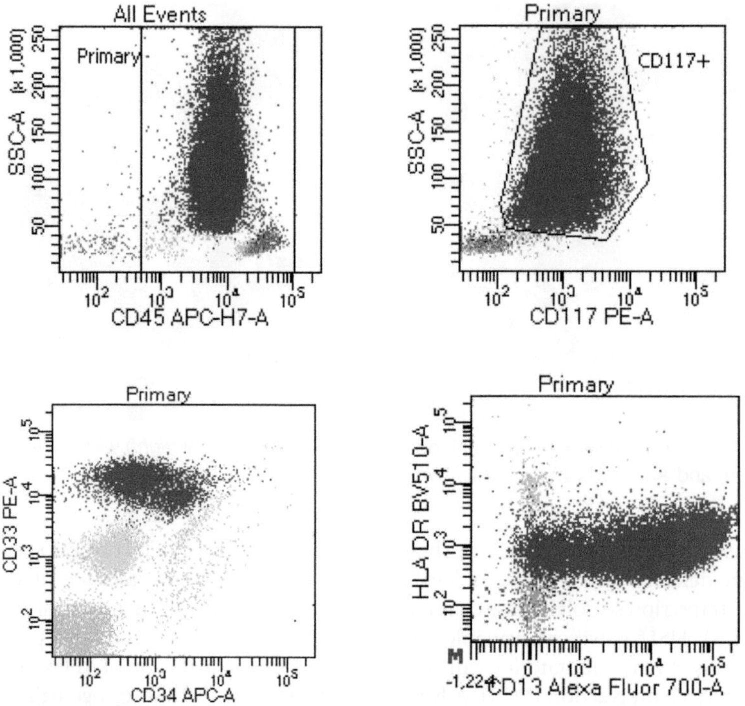

FIG. 3 Flow cytometry histograms, abnormal promyelocytes labeled red, which are positive for cluster of differentiation (CD) 117, CD33, CD13 (spectrum), dim CD45 and with high side scatter and negative for CD34 and human leukocyte antigen, DR isotype. APC, allophycocyanin.

genes other than *PML* occur. [13] Such variant translocations are rare, accounting for 1% to 2% of cases [18]. There are no reports of variant translocations involving *PML* resulting in the clinical entity of APL. However, very rare cases involving other members of the retinoic acid receptor superfamily *RARB* and *RARG* have been described. [13] Patients with variant translocations may present with clinical features of APL but are negative for t(15;17) by karyotype, FISH, and traditional PCR, because a *PML-RARA* fusion product does not exist. The discrepancy between clinical presentation/morphologic evaluation favoring APL with negative cytogenetic/molecular work-up indicates that additional testing may be required. Traditional dual-color dual-fusion FISH probes for t(15;17) may show atypical patterns such as additional *RARA* signals when *RARA* is fused with a variant partner [19]. If available, a breakapart probe for *RARA*, which detects a *RARA* translocation but does not identify the fusion partner, may be helpful. Conventional karyotype can also detect some variant translocations; however, some are cryptic by karyotype.

Variant APL cases are not detected by traditional RT-PCR studies for *PML-RARA* transcripts. However, other testing modalities may prove useful in this scenario. One option is the use of rapid amplification of complementary ends (RACE). RACE allows full-length complementary DNA (cDNA) sequencing when only a portion of the preceding messenger RNA (mRNA) sequence is known [20]. In the case of variant APL, use of the 5′RACE method with a reverse primer complementary to known exon 3 of RARA can yield a PCR product, which can then be sequenced [21]. Once sequenced, the unknown region can be identified by using various available databases, such as GenBank. However, given advances in next-generation sequencing (NGS), it may be more routine to perform massively parallel sequencing, including whole exome or whole genome, to identify fusions in atypical patients. In addition, variant fusion products can be detected through RNA sequencing (RNA-seq), via NGS platforms [22]. Although RNA-seq follows the same basic workflow as DNA, using RNA as a starting point requires some additional steps [23]. Following RNA isolation from

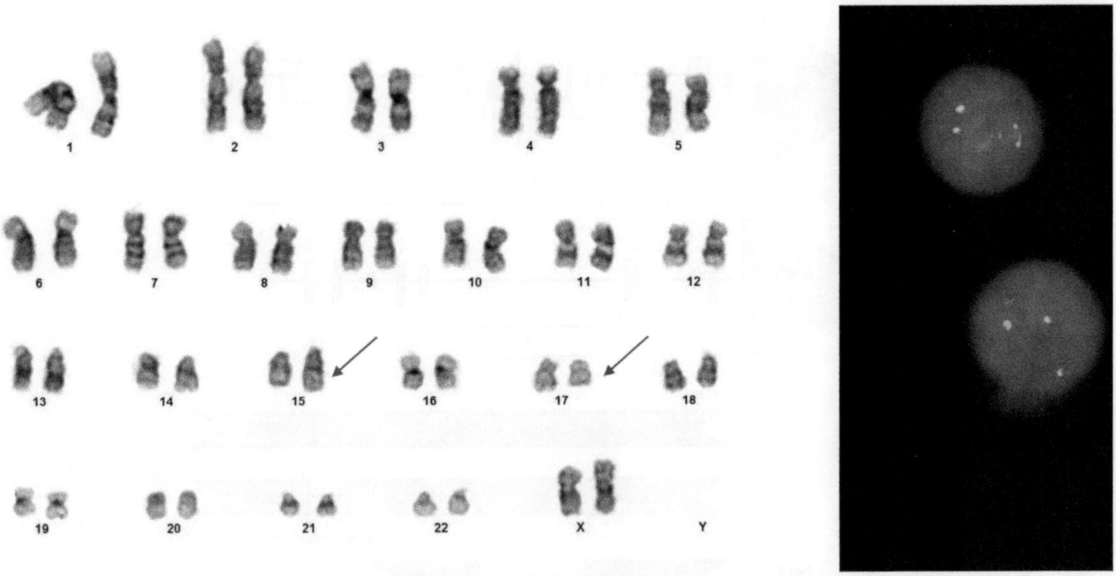

FIG. 4 Conventional karyotype (*left*) and FISH for t(15;17) (*right*). The t(15;17) is identified by karyotype (*arrows*) and by dual-color dual-fusion FISH. For FISH *PML* is labeled orange and *RARA* is labeled green; the presence of 2 fusion signals along with 1 orange and 1 green is consisted with the translocation.

the sample, the RNA should be enriched for mRNA because other types of RNA, transfer and ribosomal, may be present at higher levels in an individual cell [24]. This process can generally be done through depletion of ribosomal RNA and/or selection of mRNA. Following enrichment, the RNA sample is converted to cDNA for library preparation and later sequencing. At this point, the varying-length RNA strands should be fragmented to prevent 3′:5′ bias during the conversion of RNA to cDNA. Using strand-specific library preparation allows the sense and antisense strands to be accurately identified. Library preparation is laboratory and platform dependent, but an important consideration is the use of single-end versus paired-end sequencing. In NGS with DNA-based samples, duplicate reads can be filtered out as technical bias during PCR; however, in RNA-based samples, this may represent biological variation and should not be automatically excluded as noise. Use of single-end sequencing may be more prone to duplication of sequences compared with paired-end sequencing.

Once sequenced, FASTQ files can then be mapped to a known transcriptome for fusion detection. There are different approaches to analysis, including genome-based alignment or transcriptome assembly. Genome-based analysis uses read alignment and compares it with a reference genome. Numerous analysis programs are available for alignment and include TopHat, STAR, and HISAT [25]. Transcriptome analysis can by aided by assembly tools, including StringTie and SOAPdenovo-Trans.

VARIANT TRANSLOCATIONS

ZBTB16-RARA t(11;17)(q23;q21)

Although many variant translocations have been identified, the most common is *ZBTB16* and *RARA*, t(11;17)(q23;q21) [13,26]. *ZBTB16*, or zinc finger and BTB domain containing 16, encodes a transcription factor important many cellular processes, including proliferation, differentiation, stem cell development, and innate immunity [27]. *ZBTB16*, also known as *PLZF* (promyelocytic leukemia zinc finger), is located on chromosome 11, and the resultant translocation is t(11;17)(q23;21) [18]. This variant has been reported in young children and adults [28,29]. Patients may present with increased numbers of microgranular neutrophils with pelgeroid morphology in the peripheral blood [18]. The promyelocytes show regular nuclei with fine cytoplasmic granules, and usually lack Auer rods. These patients typically have usual APL immunophenotype, and may express CD56. This variant is negative for t(15;17) by FISH but shows variant transcripts by RARA breakapart probe. In addition, conventional

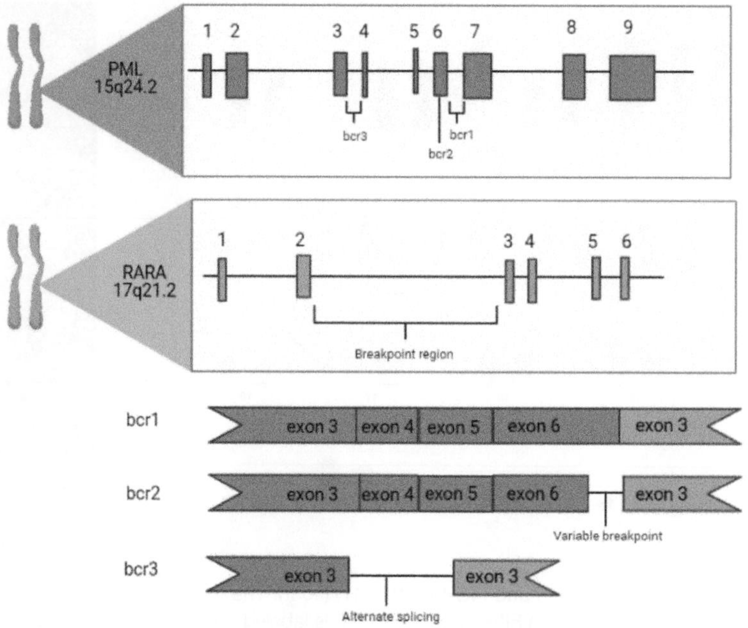

FIG. 5 The breakpoint in *RARA* is in intron 2, whereas the breakpoint of *PML* can occur at 3 different locations leading to different fusion products (bcr1, bcr2, and bcr3). Additional variability occurs in bcr2 and bcr3 because of alternate splicing (bcr3) and variable breakpoints within exon 6 of *PML* (bcr2).

karyotype reveals the translocation. RT-PCR for *PML-RARA* is negative, but primers designed for the *ZBTB16-RARA* transcripts could be used for detection if available [26]. This variant is important because patients show poor response to both ATRA and ATO [30]. However, other studies have shown some response when ATRA is used in combination with other therapeutic agents [31].

IRF2BP2-RARA t(1;17)(q42;q21)

A few case reports of variant APL with *IRF2BP2-RARA* have been described [32,33]. *IRF2BP2*, or interferon regulatory factor 2–binding protein 2, is a transcriptional corepressor that acts by repressing NFAT1-dependent promotors [34]. Adult patients with cytopenias and circulating promyelocytes with typical features of APL have been reported [18]. This translocation results in a t(1;17)(q42;q21) fusion, but without reciprocal transcripts [13]. The breakpoint in *IRF2BP2* tends to occur within the first or second exon or intron [35]. The breakpoint of *RARA* is the typical intron 2 location. In some of the reported cases, the karyotype is normal, whereas others show t(1;17) [32,36]. The cases with normal karyotype are attributed to a cryptic insertion forming the *IRF2BP2-RARA* fusion [36,37]. These cases usually show a typical APL immunophenotype, although expression of CD34 and HLA-DR have been described [33,38]. Of the few patients treated with this variant, most have been responsive to ATRA-containing chemotherapy and are reported to be sensitive to ATO treatment as well [30]. However, 3 of the 6 patients reported have died, but details are not known.

NPM1-RARA t(5;17)(q35;q21)

Translocations of *RARA* and *NPM1* (nucleophosmin) are the second most common cause of variant APL. [18] *NPM1* is located on chromosome 5 and is important in the regulation of tumor suppressor genes and protein synthesis. In addition to APL, genetic alterations involving *NPM1* have been described in lymphomas and other subtypes of AML [13]. The fusion gene joins exon 3 of *RARA* and the first 4 exons of *NPM1*, resulting in t(5;17)(q35;q21). Patients have a similar clinical presentation to classic APL, and remain at risk for DIC. Although data on this variant are limited, it may be more common in children [39]. The morphologic features of this variant are similar to classic APL, and the immunophenotype may show diminished CD13 expression [18]. Patients may show abnormal FISH signals, and the translocation is detected by conventional

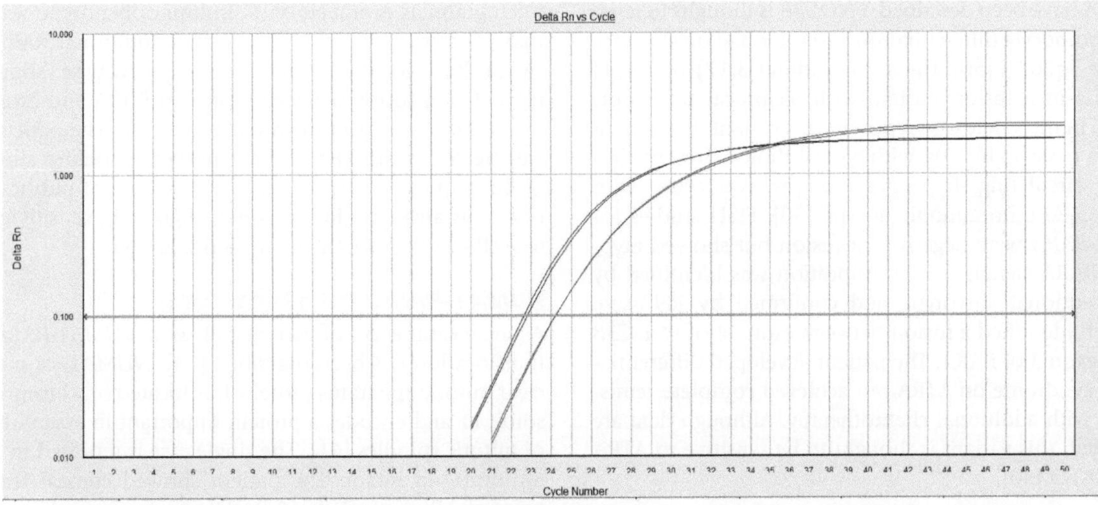

FIG. 6 Quantitative real-time polymerase chain reaction shows high copy number of *PML-RARA*, bcr3 form, fusion transcripts (*blue*) at time of diagnosis. Internal control, ABL1, is also present (*black*).

karyotype [40]. Patients with this variant are sensitive to ATRA but their response to ATO is not known [39].

STAT5B-RARA t(17;17)(q21;q21)

The *STAT5B* gene is located on chromosome 17 and encodes a signal transducer and activator of transcription important for signal transduction of cytokines and growth factors [41]. Fusions of *RARA* (exon 3) and *STAT5B* exon 15 result in typical APL clinical presentation and morphology and have been reported in more than 10 patients [18]. A significant proportion of patients present with DIC [42]. The immunophenotype is that of typical APL; however, rare expression of CD34 has been reported [43]. The translocation is typically cryptic, although, in rare cases, abnormalities of chromosome 17 or other chromosomes may be identified on karyotype. FISH for t(15;17) is negative. There are no reciprocal fusion transcripts present. This variant seems to be resistant to ATRA and ATO therapy.

BCOR-RARA t(X;17)(p11;q21)

BCOR-RARA is a rarely reported APL variant. The *BCOR*, or BCL6 corepressor gene, is located on the X chromosome and its gene product is a corepressor of BCL6 that functions in germinal center formation and immune cell regulation [44]. The resulting fusion in APL is between exon 3 of *RARA* and the first 12 exons of *BCOR*. [13] In the few case reports, patients present with typical APL clinical features, including DIC. One case report is notable for atypical cytoplasmic inclusions described as "round inclusions with rectangular cytoplasmic bodies." [45] However, Auer rods have also been reported [46]. The immunophenotype is similar to classic APL [18]. FISH studies for *PML-RARA* translocation may be negative or show an atypical *RARA* signal pattern. The translocation can be identified by routine karyotype. These cases are reportedly sensitive to ATRA but may be insensitive to ATO [30].

FIP1L1-RARA t(4;17)(q12;q21)

FIP1L1 has been implicated in translocations in other myeloid neoplasms, specifically chronic eosinophilic leukemia [18]. In APL, the fusion product between *FIP1L1* and *RARA* occurs at either exon 13 or 15 of *FIP1L1* and at exon 3 of *RARA*, and reciprocal transcripts have been identified. *FIP1L1*, or factor interacting with PAPOLA and CPSF1, is located on chromosome 4 and plays a role in mRNA processing [13]. Only 2 case reports of this variant exist [47–49]. Both patients were older and did not present with DIC, but otherwise had typical APL presentation. The promyelocytes in 1 patient were reportedly HLA-DR positive. In 1 patient, the translocation was identified by karyotype and abnormal *PML-RARA* FISH pattern. The other patient had a complex karyotype at diagnosis, including derivative chromosome 17 translocation [21]. This variant is thought to be sensitive to ATRA, but there are no data regarding ATO sensitivity [30].

FNDC3B-RARA t(3;17)(q26;q21)

Translocations between exon 24 of *FNDC3B* (fibronectin type III domain–containing 3B) and exon 3 of

RARA have been described. *FNDC3B* is thought to regulate adipocyte differentiation and is located on chromosome 3q26.31 [50]. The translocation t(3;17)(q26;q21) results in a fusion protein with reciprocal transcripts [13]. In the single case report of this variant, the patient was a male, in his 30s, with typical clinical presentation and circulating hypergranular promyelocytes with typical APL immunophenotype [50]. FISH studies for *PML-RARA* were negative for fusion but showed atypical RARA signals. The translocation was identified by conventional karyotype and confirmed by RNA-seq, which identified a fusion between exon 24 of *FNDC3B* and exon 3 of *RARA*. The patient developed differentiation syndrome on ATRA but achieved complete remission with additional chemotherapy. Although data are limited, this variant is thought to be sensitive to ATRA and ATO [30].

GTF2I-RARA t(7;17)(q11;q21)

A single case report of variant APL caused by translocation between exon 3 of *RARA* and exon 6 of *GTF2I* (general transcription factor IIi) has also been reported. This variant does not seem to have reciprocal transcripts [13]. The patient in this case report was a 35-year-old man who presented with fatigue and ecchymosis [51]. He was found to have an increased leukocyte count with a significant population of hypergranular promyelocytes. The promyelocytes showed cytochemical MPO positivity and typical APL immunophenotype. PCRs for *PML-RARA*, *ZBTB16-RARA*, and *NPM1-RARA* were negative. FISH revealed a split RARA signal without *PML* involvement. Karyotype showed deletion of 7q, which was confirmed by FISH. The *GTF2I* and *RARA* fusion was confirmed by 5′RACE and PCR. The patient was treated initially with ATRA, which stabilized his underlying coagulopathy but did not cause differentiation of the promyelocytes. He was then started on combination chemotherapy and ATO. He eventually succumbed to his disease without achieving remission. Therefore, in this single case, the variant show resistance to ATRA and ATO.

NABP1-RARA t(2;17)(q32;q21)

Again, a single case report of this variant exists. The translocation occurs between exon 3 of *RARA* and exon 5 of *NABP1*, or nucleic acid–binding protein 1 (also known as *OBFC2A* or oligonucleotide/oligosaccharide-binding fold–containing protein 2A), located on chromosome 2q32. The *NABP1* gene product plays a role in DNA damage response [13]. The adult patient presented with night sweats and petechiae [52]. Morphologic examination show a high percentage of microgranular promyelocytes. Immunophenotype was that of classic APL. FISH revealed an additional RARA signal but no *PML-RARA* fusion. Karyotype show t(2;17), and fusion between exon 3 of *RARA* and exon 5 of *NABP1* was confirmed by sequencing. The patient was treated with ATRA and chemotherapy before allogenic stem cell transplant and, at the time of publication, was alive and in remission, suggesting sensitivity to ATRA [30]. ATO sensitivity is not known.

NUMA1-RARA t(11;17)(q13;q21)

A single case report of variant APL with *NUMA1-RARA* translocation has been described [53]. *NUMA1*, or nuclear mitotic apparatus protein 1, is located on chromosome 11 and encodes a protein important in assembly of mitotic spindles [41]. The single case is reported in a 6-month-old infant. The patient showed clinical features of APL with *ZBTB16-RARA* translocation. Karyotype revealed t(11;17) but molecular did not support a fusion with *PML* or *ZBTB16* (PLZF). Sequencing of the fusion transcripts later detected the *NUMA1-RARA* without reciprocal transcripts. The patient was started on ATRA and achieved remission.

PRKAR1A-RARA t(17;17)(q21;q24)

The *PRKAR1A*, or protein kinase cyclic AMP–dependent type I regulatory subunit alpha, located on chromosome 17q24, has also been described as a translocation partner in variant APL. This gene product is important in cell signaling in cellular processes, including proliferation, differentiation, and cell death [13]. The single male patient described with this translocation presented without DIC but with leukoerythroblastic blood smear [54]. Hypergranular promyelocytes without Auer rods were identified. This variant showed a typical APL immunophenotype. Karyotype revealed an additional chromosome 22 in a subset of cells. FISH revealed a split RARA signal, and *RARA* breakapart showed a del17q. PCR confirmed the variant translocation and identified 2 PCR products, both involving exon 3 of *RARA* but different exons of *PRKAR1A*: a longer transcript with exon 3 and a shorter transcript with exon 2. The patient was treated with ATRA and achieved complete remission, suggesting ATRA sensitivity [30].

STAT3-RARA t(17;17)(q21;q21)

Two patients with *STAT3-RARA* variant translocation in a single case series have been reported. *STAT3* is part of the superfamily of STAT cytosolic transcription factors [55]. *STAT3*, in particular, is important in signal transduction to the nucleus. The *STAT3* gene is located on chromosome 17q21. The patients presented with a predominance of hypergranular promyelocytes with usual APL immunophenotype. FISH and PCR for *PML-RARA* were negative. One patient showed a normal karyotype, whereas the other had a loss of chromosome Y in a subset of analyzed cells. Whole-genome sequencing identified a breakpoint in intron 23 or intron 21 of *STAT3* along with 2 breakpoints, intron 2 and telomere of exon 9, of *RARA*, resulting in a *RARA* exon 3 to exon 9 fusion with exon 1 to exon 21 or 23 with *STAT3*. Both patients underwent therapy with ATRA and/or ATO along with combination chemotherapy. One patient achieved remission, but later relapsed and died. The other patient did not achieve remission and also expired. These findings suggest that this variant may be insensitive to traditional APL therapies.

TBL1XR1-RARA t(3;17)(q26;q21)

In this variant, APL *RARA* fuses with *TBL1XR1* (formerly *TBLR1*), or TBL1X receptor 1, located on chromosome 3q26. This gene and its larger family play a role in regulation of cellular processes. The fusion product results from *TBL1XR1* exon 5 and *RARA* exon 3 and exists without reciprocal transcripts [13]. The reported patients presented with hypergranular promyelocytes with usual immunophenotype [56,57]. This variant is reported in adults and 1 pediatric patient. The pediatric patient was found to have a cryptic insertion of *RARA* between exon 5 and exon 6 of *TBL1XR1* [56]. In published case reports, FISH and PCR for *PML-RARA* are negative, but karyotype revealed complex changes often involving chromosomes 3 and 17. Of note, FISH for *PML-RARA* has not shown atypical RARA signals. This variant seems to be insensitive to ATRA but responsive to ATO.

TFG-RARA t(3;14;17)(q12;q11;21)

The *TFG* (trafficking from endoplasmic reticulum to Golgi regulator) gene is located on chromosome 3q12 and is important in normal function of the endoplasmic reticulum [18]. A single variant APL case has been reported involving a *TFG-RARA* translocation [58]. The patient was an adolescent who presented with leukopenia and hypergranular promyelocytes in the bone marrow. Immunophenotype was typical of APL. FISH for *PML-RARA* translocation identified an abnormal RARA signal pattern. Karyotype identified a complex rearrangement: t(3;14;17)(q12;q11;q21). The fusion between *TFG* and *RARA* was confirmed by RNA-seq. The patient responded well to ATRA, but idarubicin was added for consolidation. The patient achieved remission and was reported to be on maintenance therapy with ATRA.

MOLECULAR PROGNOSTIC MARKERS

In addition to the *PML-RARA* translocation in typical cases of APL, other secondary mutations can occur. Studies have shown that greater than 50% of patients with APL have additional mutations, and nearly a third of those have more than 1 additional mutation [59]. *FLT3* mutations are among the most common, with *FLT3*-ITD being more common than *FLT3*-TKD [60]. *FLT3*-ITD is associated with increased occurrence of thrombotic events and higher leukocyte counts, and is more common with the short or bcr3 isoform [61]. These cases may show some degree of CD34 expression. It is thought that *FLT3*-ITD mutation in the setting of APL is associated with worse overall and disease-free survival, but it does not seem to affect rates of remission. However, note that the presence or absence of additional mutations has not been incorporated into existing guidelines and prognostic scales. Other studies have shown that patients with APL may also harbor mutations in *WT1*, *KRAS*, and less commonly *ASXL1*, *CBL*, *DNMT3A*, *NRAS*, *RUNX1*, *SF3B1*, and *TET2* [59,62,63]. The significance of these secondary mutations is not clear. Additional mutations may be detected by large panels, which are commonly performed for other types of AML. The utility of these panels in APL is less clear given the lack of information regarding the implications of such mutations.

TREATMENT

For treatment purposes, patients are risk stratified based on white blood cell count (WBC), with WBC equal to or less than 10,000/μL being low risk and greater than 10,000/μL being high risk. The cornerstone of APL treatment, regardless of risk status, is ATRA and ATO. Some patients may have addition or substitution of ATO with chemotherapy including idarubicin or gemtuzumab. Following induction, most low-risk patients can be followed for peripheral blood cell count recoveries without follow-up bone marrow biopsy. In contrast, high-risk patients should undergo bone marrow biopsy at day 28 to document remission before continuing to consolidation.

In both groups, following consolidation, molecular remission must be documented. This documentation is commonly done via PCR performed on peripheral blood. If patients are confirmed to be in molecular remission, they may proceed to maintenance therapy. The treating physician can decide what frequency and duration to monitor peripheral blood by PCR for possible relapse. A positive PCR result during this time should be repeated within 2 to 4 weeks, and a positive result on confirmatory testing should prompt treatment of relapsed disease. If confirmatory PCR is negative, the patient can remain on the current maintenance regimen and follow up with frequent PCR.

Testing for molecular remission is done via quantitative PCR at many laboratories. It is recommended that testing in individual patients be done at the same laboratory, which maintains consistency in PCR sensitivity. New studies show a higher level of sensitivity through the use of droplet digital PCR [15]. Such methods may allow earlier detection of relapse and faster initiation of therapy.

PROGNOSIS

With advances in diagnostics and therapeutics, APL has gone from a frequently fatal disease to a highly curable form of acute leukemia [23]. This favorable prognosis is caused by the sensitivity of APL to ATRA in combination with ATO and/or anthracycline chemotherapy. With these combined therapies, the remission rate is greater than 90% [64,65]. In 2000, Sanz and colleagues [66] proposed a risk stratification model for patients with APL. In this model, WBC and platelet count are used to assign patients to 3 categories: low risk, intermediate risk, and high risk. Simpler classifications incorporating just the WBC are now used by the National Comprehensive Cancer Network (NCCN). Other possible adverse prognostic markers, including *FLT3* mutations, expression of CD56 and CD2, and older age, are currently not incorporated into a formal risk stratification [9,11,60,67].

SUMMARY

Although almost all patients with APL present with classic clinical, morphologic, cytogenetic, and molecular features, there are a subset of patients who do not. This variation may be caused by cryptic translations of *PML-RARA* or *RARA* variant gene translocations causing similar disease. In these cases, it is imperative that negative cytogenetic and molecular diagnostic tests, which traditionally focus on *PML-RARA* translocation, not be used to exclude a diagnosis of APL. Instead, the discrepancy between the clinical/morphologic presentation and genomic findings should trigger additional testing. A high degree of suspicion is necessary to ensure that patients are promptly treated with appropriate therapies to reduce the risk of developing DIC and early death.

DISCLOSURE

The authors have nothing to disclose.

REFERENCES

[1] Arber D, Brunning R, Le Beau M, et al. WHO classification of tumours of haematopoietic and lymphoid tissues (Revised 4th Edition). Lyon: IRAC; 2017.
[2] Adams J, Nassiri M. Acute promyelocytic leukemia: a review and discussion of variant translocations. Arch Pathol Lab Med 2015;139(10):1308–13.
[3] Toh CH, Alhamdi Y, Abrams ST. Current pathologic and laboratory considerations in the diagnosis of disseminated intravascular coagulation. Ann Intern Med 2016; 36(6):505–12.
[4] Bennett J, Catovsky D, Daniel M, et al. Proposed revised criteria for the classification of acute myeloid leukemia. A report of the French-American-British Cooperative Group. Ann Intern Med 1985;103(4):620–5.
[5] Bennett J, Catovsky D, Daniel M, et al. Proposals for the classification of acute leukaemias. French-American-British (FAB) cooperative group. Br J Haematol 1976; 33(4):1365–2141.
[6] George T, Wilson CS. Promyelocytes. In: Color atlas of hematology: an illustrated field guide based on proficiency testing. 2nd edition. Northfield, Illinois: CAP; 2018. p. p170–1.
[7] Foucar K, Reichard K, Czuchlewski D. Acute myeloid leukemia. In: Bone marrow pathology, vol. 1, 4th edition. Chicago: ASCP; 2020. p. 397–443.
[8] Gorczyca W. Acute myeloid leukemia with recurrent genetic changes. In: Flow cytometry in neoplastic hematology. 3rd ed. Boca Raton, Florida: CRC Press; 2017. p. 392–8.
[9] Lin P, Hao S, Medeiros LJ, et al. Expression of CD2 in acute promyelocytic leukemia correlates with short form of PML-RARA transcripts and poorer prognosis. Am J Clin Pathol 2004;121(3):402–7.
[10] Foley R, Soamboonsrup P, Carter RF, et al. CD34-positive acute promyelocytic leukemia is associated with leukocytosis, microgranular/hypogranular morphology, expression of CD2 and bcr3 isoform. Am J Hematol 2001;67(1):34–41.
[11] Ono T, Takeshita A, Kishimoto Y, et al. Expression of CD56 is an unfavorable prognostic factor for acute promyelocytic leukemia with higher initial white blood cell counts. Cancer Sci 2014;105(1):97–104.
[12] Sainty D, Liso V, Cantù-Rajnoldi A, et al. A new morphologic classification system for acute promyelocytic leukemia distinguishes cases with underlying PLZF/RARA gene rearrangements. Blood 2000;96(4):1287–96.
[13] Geoffroy M-C, de Thé H. Classic and variants APLs, as viewed from a therapy response. Cancers 2020;12(4): 967.
[14] Choppa PC, Gomez J, Vall HG, et al. A novel method for the detection, quantitation, and breakpoint cluster

region determination of t(15;17) fusion transcripts using a one-step real-time multiplex RT-PCR. Am J Clin Pathol 2001;119(1):137–44.

[15] Jiang X, Chen S, Zhu X, et al. Development and validation of a droplet digital PCR assay for the evaluation of PML-RARα fusion transcripts in acute promyelocytic leukemia. Mol Cell Probes 2020;53:101617.

[16] Kim MJ, Cho SY, Kim MH, et al. FISH-negative cryptic PML-RARA rearrangement detected by long-distance polymerase chain reaction and sequencing analyses: a case study and review of the literature. Cancer Genet Cytogenet 2010;203(2):278–83.

[17] Koshy J, Qian YW, Bhagwath G, et al. Microarray, gene sequencing, and reverse transcriptase-polymerase chain reaction analyses of a cryptic *PML-RARA* translocation. Cancer Genet 2012;2015(10):537–40.

[18] Mannan A, Muhsen IB, Barragan E, et al. Genotypic and phenotypic characteristics of acute promyelocytic leukemia translocation variants. Hematol Oncol Stem Cell Ther 2020;13(4):189–201.

[19] Singh MK, Parihar M, Arora N, et al. Diagnosis of variant *RARA* translocation using standard dual-color dual-fusion PML/RARA FISH probes: An illustrative report. Hematol Oncol Stem Cell Ther 2019;12(1):50–3.

[20] Zhang Y, Frohman MA. Using rapid amplification of cDNA ends (RACE) to obtain full-length cDNAs. Methods Mol Biol 1997;69:61–87.

[21] Menezes J, Acquadro F, Perez-Pons de la Villa C, et al. *FIP1L1/RARA* with breakpoint at *FIP1L1* intron 13: a variant translocation in acute promyelocytic leukemia. Haematologica 2011;96(10):1565–6.

[22] Stark R, Grzelak M, Hadfield J. RNA sequencing: the teenage years. Nat Rev Genet 2019;20(11):631–56.

[23] Kukurba KR, Montgomery SB. RNA sequencing and analysis. Cold Spring Harb Protoc 2015;2015(11):951–69.

[24] Heyer EE, Deveson IW, Wooi D, et al. Diagnosis of fusion genes using targeted RNA sequencing. Nat Commun 2019;10(1):1388.

[25] Piskol R, Ramaswami G, Li JB. Reliable identification of genomic variants from RNA-Seq data. Am J Hum Genet 2013;93(4):641–51.

[26] Langabeer SE, Preston L, Kelly J, et al. Molecular profiling: a case of *ZBTB16-RARA* acute promyelocytic leukemia. Case Rep Hematol 2017;2017:7657393.

[27] Jin Y, Nenseth HZ, Saatcioglu F. Role of *PLZF* as a tumor suppressor in prostate cancer. Oncotarget 2017;8(41):71317–24.

[28] Lechevalier N, Dulucq S, Bidet A. A case of acute promyelocytic leukemia with unusual cytological features and a *ZBTB16-RARA* fusion gene. Br J Haematol 2016;174(4):502.

[29] Wells RA, Hummel JL, De Koven A, et al. A new variant translocation in acute promyelocytic leukemia: molecular characterization and clinical correlation. Leukemia 1996;10(4):735–40.

[30] Sanz MA, Fenaux P, Tallman MS, et al. Management of acute promyelocytic leukemia: updated recommendations from an expert panel of the European Leukemia Net. Blood 2019;133(15):1630–43.

[31] Rabade N, Raval G, Chaudhary S, et al. Molecular heterogeneity in acute promyelocytic leukemia-A single center experience form India. Mediterr J Hematol Infect Dis 2018;10(1):e2018002.

[32] Liu Y, Xu F, Hu H, et al. A rare case of acute promyelocytic leukemia with *IRF2BP2-RARA* fusion and literature review. Oncotargets Ther 2019;12:6157–63.

[33] Alotaibi AS, Abdulrazzaq M, Patel KP, et al. Acute promyelocytic leukemia (APL) with an IRF2BP2-RARA fusion transcript: an aggressive APL variant. Leuk Lymphoma 2020;61(12):3018–20.

[34] Carneiro FRG, Ramalho-Oliveira R, Mognol GP, et al. Interferon Regulatory Factor 2 Binding Protein 2 is a new NFAT1 partner and represses its transcriptional activity. Mol Cell Biol 2011;31(14):2889–901.

[35] Jovanovic JV, Chillon MC, Vincent-Fabert CV, et al. The cryptic *IRF2BP2-RARA* fusion transforms hematopoietic stem/progenitor cells and induces retinoid-sensitive acute promyelocytic leukemia. Leukemia 2017;31(3):747–51.

[36] Mazharuddin S, Chattopadhyay A, Levy MY, et al. IRF2BP2-RARA t(15;17)(q42.3;q21.2) APL blasts differentiate in response to all-trans retinoic acid. Leuk Lymphoma 2018;59(9):2246–9.

[37] Yan W, Zhang G. Molecular characteristics and clinical significance of 12 fusion genes in acute promyelocytic leukemia: a systematic review. Acta Haematol 2016;136(1):1–15.

[38] Shimomura Y, Mitsuii H, Yamashita Y, et al. New variant of acute promyelocytic leukemia with *IRF2BP2-RARA* fusion. Cancer Sci 2016;107(8):1165–8.

[39] Sobas M, Talarn-Forcadell MC, Martinez-Cuadron D, et al. PLZF-RARα, NPM1-RARα, and other acute promyelocytic leukemia variants: the PETHEMA registry experience and systematic literature review. Cancers 2020;21(12):1313.

[40] Nicci C, Ottaviani E, Luatti S, et al. Molecular and cytogenetic characterization of a new case of t(5;17)(q35;q21) variant acute promyelocytic leukemia. Leukemia 2005;19(3):470–2.

[41] Mannan A, Muhsen IN, Barragán E, et al. Genotypic and phenotypic characteristics of acute promyelocytic leukemia translocation variants. Hematol Oncol Stem Cell Ther 2020;13(4):189–201.

[42] Zhang C, Wang Y, Liu B, et al. Clinical characteristics of acute promyelocytic leukemia with the *STAT5B-RARA* fusion gene. Blood Cells Mol Dis 2018;69:71–3.

[43] Peterson JF, He RR, Nayer H, et al. Characterization of a rarely reported *STAT5B/RARA* gene fusion in a young adult with newly diagnosed acute promyelocytic leukemia with resistance to ATRA therapy. Cancer Genet 2019;237:51–4.

[44] Kang JH, Lee SH, Lee J, et al. The mutation of *BCOR* is highly recurrent and oncogenic in mature T-cell lymphoma. BMC Cancer 2021;21:1.

[45] Yamamoto Y, Tsuzuki S, Tsuzuki M, et al. *BCOR* as a novel fusion partner of retinoic acid receptor alpha in a t(X;17)(p11;q12) variant of acute promyelocytic leukemia. Blood 2010;116(20):4274–83.

[46] Ichikawa S, Takahashi T, Fujiwara T, et al. Successful treatment of acute promyelocytic leukemia with a t(X; 17)(p11.4;q21) and *BCOR-RARA* fusion gene. Cancer Genet 2015;208(4):162–3.

[47] Iwasaki J, Kondo T, Darmanin S, et al. *FIP1L1* presence in *FIP1L1-RARA* or *FIP1L1-PDGFRA* differentially contributes to the pathogenesis of distinct types of leukemia. Ann Hematol 2014;93(9):1473–81.

[48] Kondo T, Mori A, Darmanin S, et al. The seventh pathogenic fusion gene *FIP1L1-RARA* was isolated from a t(4; 17)-positive acute promyelocytic leukemia. Haematologica 2008;93(9):1414–6.

[49] Nakanishi T, Nakaya A, Nishio Y, et al. A variant acute promyelocytic leukemia with t(4;17)(q12;q21) showed two different clinical symptoms. Hematol Rep 2019; 11(3):49–51.

[50] Cheng CK, Wang AZ, Wong THY, et al. *FNDC3B* is another novel partner fused to RARA in the t(3; 17)(q26;q21) variant of acute promyelocytic leukemia. Blood 2017;129(19):2705–9.

[51] Li J, Zhong H-Y, Zhang Y, et al. GTF2I-RARA is a novel fusion transcript in a t(7;17) variant of acute promyelocytic leukaemia with clinical resistance to retinoic acid. Br J Haematol 2015;168(6):904–8.

[52] Won D, Shin SY, Park CJ, et al. *OBFC2A/RARA*: A novel fusion gene in variant acute promyelocytic leukemia. Blood 2013;121(8):1432–5.

[53] Wells RA, Catzavelos C, Kamel-Reid S. Fusion of retinoic acid receptor a to NuMA, the nuclear mitotic apparatus protein, by a variant translocation in acute promyelocytic leukaemia. Nat Genet 1997;17(1):109–13.

[54] Catalano A, Dawson MA, Somana K, et al. The *PRKAR1A* gene is fused to *RARA* in a new variant. Acute promyelocytic leukemia. Blood 2007;110(12):4073–6.

[55] Yao L, Wen L, Wang N, et al. Identification of novel recurrent *STAT3-RARA* fusion in acute promyelocytic leukemia lacking t(15;17)(q22;q12)/*PML-RARA*. Blood 2018;131(8):935–9.

[56] Osumi T, Watanabe A, Okamura K, et al. Acute promyelocytic leukemia with a cryptic insertion of RARA into Tbl1xr1. Genes Chromosomes Cancer 2019;58(11): 820–3.

[57] Chen Y, Shouyun L, Zhou C, et al. TBLR1 fuses to retinoid acid receptor α in a variant t(3;17)(q26;q21) translocation of acute promyelocytic leukemia. Blood 2014; 124(6):936–45.

[58] Chong M-L, Cheng H, Xu P, et al. TFG-RARA: a novel fusion gene in acute promyelocytic leukemia that is responsive to all-trans retinoic acid. Leuk Res 2018;74: 51–4.

[59] Fasan A, Haferlach C, Perglerovà K, et al. Molecular landscape of acute promyelocytic leukemia at diagnosis and relapse. Haematologica 2017;102(6):e222–4.

[60] Beitinjaneh A, Jang S, Roukoz H, et al. Prognostic significance of *FLT3* internal tandem duplication and tyrosine kinase domain mutations in acute promyelocytic leukemia: a systematic review. Leuk Res 2010;34(7):831–6.

[61] Testa U, Lo-Coco F. Prognostic factors in acute promyelocytic leukemia: strategies to define high-risk patients. Ann Hematol 2016;95(5):673–80.

[62] Iaccarino L, Ottone T, Alfonso V, et al. Mutational landscape of patients with acute promyelocytic leukemia at diagnosis and relapse. Am J Hematol 2019;94(10): 1091–7.

[63] Yedla RP, Bala SC, Pydi VR, et al. Outcomes in adult acute promyelocytic leukemia: a decade experience. Clin Lymphoma Myeloma Leuk 2020;20(4):e158–64.

[64] Sanz MA, Coco FL, Martin G, et al. Retinoic trioxide in the treatment of acute promyelocytic leukemia. A review of current evidence. Haematologica 2005;1231-5.

[65] Lo-Coco F, Avvisati G, Vignetti M, et al. Retinoic acid and arsenic trioxide for acute promyelocytic leukemia. N Engl J Med 2013;369(2):111–21.

[66] Sanz MA, Coco FL, Martin G, et al. Definition of relapse risk and role of non-anthracycline drugs for consolidation in patients with acute promyelocytic leukemia: a joint study of the PETHEMA and GIMEMA cooperative groups: Presented in part at the 41st meeting of the American Society of Hematology, New Orleans, LA, 1999. Blood 2000;96(4):1247–53.

[67] Jin B, Zhang Y, Hou W, et al. Comparative analysis of causes and predictors of early death in elderly and young patients with acute promyelocytic leukemia treated with arsenic trioxide. J Cancer Res Clin Oncol 2020;146(2): 485–92.

Advances in Molecular Pathology 4 (2021) 49–63
ADVANCES IN MOLECULAR PATHOLOGY

Next-Generation Sequencing for Measurable Residual Disease Assessment in Acute Leukemia

Alexandra E. Kovach, MD[a,*], Gordana Raca, MD, PhD[b], Deepa Bhojwani, MD[c], Brent L. Wood, MD, PhD[a]
[a]Division of Hematopathology, Department of Pathology and Laboratory Medicine, Children's Hospital Los Angeles, 4650 Sunset Boulevard, Mailstop #32, Los Angeles, CA 90027, USA; [b]Clinical Cytogenomics Laboratory, Center for Personalized Medicine, Children's Hospital Los Angeles, 4650 Sunset Boulevard, Mailstop #32, Los Angeles, CA 90027, USA; [c]Division of Hematology/Oncology, Children's Hospital Los Angeles, Keck School of Medicine, University of Southern California, 4650 Sunset Boulevard, Mailstop #54, Los Angeles, CA 90027, USA

KEYWORDS
• Minimal residual disease • Measurable residual disease • MRD • Next-generation sequencing • NGS
• Acute leukemia • ALL • AML

KEY POINTS

- Minimal residual disease, or measurable residual disease (MRD), is a strong independent adverse prognostic factor in acute leukemia and is now an essential component of standard-of-care post-therapeutic monitoring.
- Next-generation sequencing (NGS)-based MRD detection is emerging as an adjunct or replacement to immunophenotypic (flow cytometric) and quantitative polymerase chain reaction (qPCR) assays because of its high sensitivity and multiplexing potential, but complex laboratory and bioinformatics infrastructure are required.
- Clonal immunoglobulin heavy chain (IgH) and T-cell receptor (TCR) gene sequences are the basis for NGS-based MRD assessment in lymphoblastic leukemias.
- Acute myeloid leukemia is a genetically heterogeneous group of related neoplasms for which a universal molecular MRD marker is not available at present, but many genetic subtypes of AML may ultimately be amenable to NGS-based MRD monitoring as the analytical approaches evolve.

INTRODUCTION

Minimal residual disease, or measurable residual disease (MRD), has emerged as one of the most important independent prognostic factors in acute leukemia. Extrapolating from successes in molecular monitoring of diseases like chronic myeloid leukemia, *BCR-ABL1* [1], and acute promyelocytic leukemia [2–4], "molecular remission" has been recognized as crucial for cure in all acute leukemias even before highly sensitive methodologies such as next-generation sequencing (NGS) were available [5]. Indeed, re-emergence of clonal sequences over time detectable by standard polymerase chain reaction (PCR) [6] (such as *BCR-ABL1* transcripts in *BCR-ABL1*-associated acute lymphoblastic and myeloid leukemia [ALL and AML] [3], diagnostic sample-associated clonal sequences of the IgH hypervariable region in B-lymphoblastic leukemia [B-ALL] [7], and relevant core-binding factor [CBF] transcripts in CBF-associated AML [8,9]) is harbingers of impending morphologic and clinical relapse [5,10].

In the current era, MRD assessment is incorporated into the clinical standard of care of patients with ALL [11,12–17], including those undergoing hematopoietic stem cell transplantation (HSCT) [18–20], and is

*Corresponding author, *E-mail address:* akovach@chla.usc.edu

https://doi.org/10.1016/j.yamp.2021.07.011
2589-4080/21/

increasingly being used in AML [15]; thus, emerging as a primary endpoint in early-phase therapeutic clinical trials [21]. In B-ALL, the prognostic significance of MRD has been shown to hold true across studies, patient age, and MRD methodologies [22] as well as in the peri-HSCT period [23,24]. Data are similar but more recent in AML [25–27]; thus, genetic investigation of its heterogeneous biology has yielded cytogenetic and molecular-based reclassification [28,29], catalog of preleukemic subclones [30] and age-related subclinical myeloid mutations [31,32], and identification of appropriate NGS targets for MRD [26,33]. NGS MRD results have shown strong concordance with MRD results from established methodologies (immunophenotypic and PCR-based strategies) at early post-treatment time points in ALL. Owing to increased sensitivity and independence from phenotypic shifts, NGS-MRD is detected in a subset of post-therapy samples that are not detectable by the established methods and there is emerging evidence of its prognostic impact [34,35]. With the ongoing refinement of techniques, the significance of NGS MRD methods for monitoring AML will continue to develop.

This review summarizes and contextualizes the current state of NGS-based approaches to acute leukemia MRD assessment.

NEXT GENERATION SEQUENCING-BASED MEASURABLE RESIDUAL DISEASE ASSESSMENT: PERFORMANCE CHARACTERISTICS AND COMPARISON WITH OTHER ASSESSMENT METHODOLOGIES

Broadly used methodologies for MRD monitoring currently include flow cytometry, real-time quantitative PCR (RQ-PCR), and NGS. The advantages and limitations of NGS-based MRD assessment in comparison to more traditional approaches are discussed in the following and summarized in Table 1. Associated terms and concepts are defined in Table 2.

Flow cytometry-based MRD assays for acute leukemias rely on the understanding of the normal immunophenotypic maturational patterns of hematopoietic precursors (B, T, or myeloid precursors) for the recognition of "different from normal" or "leukemia-associated" immunophenotype in small populations [36,37]. The immunophenotypic analysis is amenable to all samples, does not require a diagnostic comparison sample (in the "difference from normal" interpretive approach), rapid (same day or next day data generation compared with a week or more for batched-run NGS testing), and relatively cost-effective. However, flow cytometry-based MRD assessment is less sensitive than NGS with the validated limits of quantitation of 0.01% for ALL and 0.1% for AML. Other limitations consist of interobserver variability and requiring practitioner experience, particularly for the interpretation of the immunophenotypic features of myeloid precursors. These analyses are difficult to standardize and require detailed knowledge of targeted immunotherapies that patients may have received, which alter the immunophenotype of normal and abnormal populations.

RQ-PCR is a powerful approach for monitoring specific individual markers, including some abnormal gene fusions and "hot-spot" mutations. It uses a PCR technology in which the inclusion of a fluorescent reporter molecule in the reaction functions to quantify the amplification product as the reaction progresses, allowing to extrapolate the initial number of copies of template DNA (the amplification target sequence). The RQ-PCR assays can be designed for RNA or DNA input and are sensitive, widely available, and relatively easy to perform. Standardized PCR protocols and primer-probe sets are available for B and T-ALL (BIOMED-2) [38–41], as well as for several AML-associated fusions including *RUNX1-RUNX1T1*, *CBFB-MYH11*, and *PML-RARA*, and also for *NPM1* mutations [42–50]. However, target quantification requires a standard, obtained by the amplification of serial dilutions of a calibrator (typically the target sequence cloned into a plasmid). The intersample difference in RNA quality and quantity is accounted for by parallel amplification of one or more housekeeping/endogenous reference genes. In addition to its targeted nature, the most important limitation of the RQ-PCR approach for MRD assessment is that the initial optimization and standardization of the assay for each molecular marker are very labor-intensive. Calibrators necessary to accurately quantify the target may not be readily available, and the choice of endogenous reference genes may affect the results [16,51].

NGS, also referred to as massively parallel sequencing, high-throughput sequencing, or deep sequencing, facilitates highly sensitive and specific detection of sequence(s) of interest [52,53]. Briefly, DNA is extracted from fresh, frozen, or formalin-fixed paraffin-embedded (FFPE) tissue and quantified. (The DNA may be fragmented if the target sequences are not known or a large panel is used, but this is generally not needed for amplicon-based sequencing as is more typical for MRD.) Flanking adaptor sequences are ligated to the fragments (library preparation). At this

TABLE 1
Overview of Common Markers and Techniques for MRD Detection

Disease	MRD Marker*	Assessment Technique	Applicability (Proportion of Cases)	Sensitivity	Advantages	Limitations	Reference
B-ALL	Abnormal immunophenotype	Flow cytometry	All patients	0.01%	Broadly available, fast, allows cellular level information and absolute quantitation	Requires expertise, difficult to standardize, medium sensitivity, changes in antigen expression can result in false negatives	[36,37]
	Clonal IGH/TCR sequence	NGS	High (>95%)	0.001%	High sensitivity, standardized assays commercially available	Costly, requires specialized equipment infrastructure and bioinformatics resources; not broadly clinically available	[69,76]
AML	Abnormal immunophenotype	Flow cytometry	All patients	0.1%	Fast, allows cellular level information and absolute quantitation	Interpretive complexity and interobserver variability greater than in ALL; not available at all institutions	[16]
	PML-RARA	RQ-PCR	5%–8% of AML cases	At least 0.1%	Both technical and clinical standards described; fast, affordable, and clinically available	Applicable to a small proportion of cases	[9,16]
	RUNX1-RUNX1T1	RQ-PCR	1%–5% of AML cases	0.001%	Both technical and clinical standards described; fast, affordable, and clinically available	Applicable to a small proportion of cases	[9,16]

(*continued on next page*)

TABLE 1
(*continued*)

Disease	MRD Marker*	Assessment Technique	Applicability (Proportion of Cases)	Sensitivity	Advantages	Limitations	Reference
	CBFB-MYXH11	RQ-PCR	5%–8% of younger AML patients	0.001%	Both technical and clinical standards described; fast, affordable, and clinically available	Applicable to a small proportion of cases	[9,16]
	NPM1 mutations	RQ-PCR and NGS	27%–35% adult patients	0.010%	Both technical and clinical standards described; fast, affordable, and clinically available	Applicable to a small proportion of cases	[16,45–50]
	Multiple DNA (sequence) variants	NGS	High	0.001%	High sensitivity if error-corrected methods applied; could be applicable for a high proportion of cases	Not standardized and not broadly clinically available; CHIP mutations not predictive; secondary mutations may be unstable; costly, requires specialized equipment, infrastructure, and bioinformatics resources	[123]

Desired characteristics of molecular MRD markers are as follows: (1) applicable for most of the patients; (2) stable throughout the disease course; (3) able to differentiate between the malignant clone and nonmalignant disorders or normal cells; and (4) detectable and quantifiable with high sensitivity using broadly available, simple, and robust assays.

point, the DNA may be enriched by PCR or probe hybridization for targets of interests. Next, the library is applied to a solid-phase platform that immobilizes the DNA-adaptor fragments. Individual DNA bases, with either a fluorescence- or ion-based emission signal associated with each base type, are added and many immobilized DNA-adaptor fragments are sequenced simultaneously (multiplex) to a prescribed depth of coverage based on the application and capabilities of the instrument [54]. Using a bioinformatics pipeline, the fragments are reassembled, compared with reference sequences, classified as normal or abnormal, and quantified [55,56].

An advantage of NGS compared with other methodologies for MRD assessment includes multiplex design, allowing laboratories to develop one NGS-based MRD assay applicable for a larger number of patients.

The sensitivity of conventional NGS for the detection of variants with low allele frequencies is roughly 1% to 0.1% under optimal conditions due to inherent errors in PCR amplification and NGS sequencing [57]. This initial limitation has been addressed more recently by the development of a variety of "error-corrected" NGS techniques [57–61]. One increasingly common approach that has been successfully applied to MRD in acute leukemia uses molecular barcoding

TABLE 2
Important Concepts in NGS-Based MRD Detection

Depth of coverage	Number of sequencing reads that span (or cover) a particular reference sequence
Unique coverage	Reads that come from distinct DNA molecules in the sample; only unique reads should be used for calculating sensitivity for variant detection. The number of unique reads can be increased by the following: (1) increasing the amount of input DNA; (2) increasing the amount of produced sequence and coverage depths (to ensure all DNA molecules are sequenced); and (3) using efficient enrichment methods for target regions to recover high % of target molecules from input DNA.
Duplicate reads	Library/PCR duplicates are copies of the original target molecule created during PCR steps in library preparation; they do not add new information and are generally discarded by routine NGS analysis pipelines. PCR-only enrichment methods may not allow to distinguish between unique vs duplicate reads and may not be appropriate for MRD analysis unless additional steps are implemented (eg, unique molecular identifiers) to distinguish duplicate reads.
VAF	Fraction of reads containing a mutation, divided by the total number of reads at a given locus; a measure of mutational abundance.
Sensitivity	Calculated for NGS based on VAF; sensitivity of 0.1% means detection of 1 variant molecule out of 1000 molecules, corresponding to 1/500 cells with a heterozygous mutation.
Required DNA input	MRD detection requires high DNA input to ensure the representation of a large number of cells; 1 ng and 1 μg of DNA correspond to approximately 10^{-2} to 10^{-5} human cells, respectively; sensitivity can be increased by increasing the amount of input DNA.
UMIs or barcodes	Short oligonucleotides that are added to the fragments of genomic DNA before enrichment to allow for the tracking of individual DNA molecules throughout the sequencing process; allow distinguishing real low-level mutations from sequencing error and increase sensitivity for MRD detection beyond intrinsic sequencing error rate of NGS platforms.

Abbreviations: UMI, unique molecular identifier; VAF, variant allele fraction.

or "unique molecular identifiers" (UMIs) [62–64]. UMIs are highly diverse mixtures of oligonucleotides, each having a unique sequence, that are ligated to sample DNA molecules in the first steps of library preparation before PCR amplification. This allows for each sequenced read to be tracked back to a single individual input DNA molecule. During analysis, reads with shared UMI that track back to the same original molecule are consolidated, so that only sequence variants present in all members of the family are considered true positives. This greatly reduces the frequency of false-positive mutations due to PCR and sequencing errors, allowing the detection of single base-pair mutations at frequencies of 10^{-4} to 10^{-7} or lower depending on the implementation. A single-molecule molecular inversion probe approach has also been described, which combines amplicon targeting and UMI incorporation steps [65]. The basic concept of tag-based error correction has been extended with a variety of other error-correction approaches to allow increasingly sensitive detection of single-base pair mutations [57]. An approach that greatly increases accuracy and specificity is duplex sequencing, where both strands of the DNA molecule are labeled with a UMI and an asymmetric strand-defining element followed by the sequencing of each of the duplex strands. This increases the capability for identifying both early and late PCR and sequencing errors, allowing the detection of mutations theoretically at $\sim 10^{-9}$ and approaching the biologically observed mutation rate of 10^{-7} to 10^{-8} for the fidelity of DNA replication in newborns.

Limitations of NGS-based MRD testing are that it is costly and the turn-around time may be longer than is optimal for clinical decision making; however, both the sequencing cost and bioinformatics challenges are decreasing over time [56]. Other limitations include availability and testing is concentrated at specialized centers with the infrastructure and bioinformatics resources and expertise, which can increase the turnaround time and cost of testing for ordering clinicians. Finally, NGS-based quantitative [66].

DISEASE-SPECIFIC APPLICATIONS OF NEXT GENERATION SEQUENCING-BASED MEASURABLE RESIDUAL DISEASE ASSESSMENT

Acute lymphoblastic leukemia (B-ALL and T-ALL)

Most cases of ALL (95% of B-ALL and 70% of T-ALL [67]), pediatric and adult, are amenable to NGS-based MRD assessment using clonal leukemia-associated Ig or TCR sequences. The immunoglobulin heavy chain (IgH) and T-cell receptor (TCR) genes in normal lymphoid progenitors show intrinsic biological diversity at these loci because of genetic rearrangement during maturation that is unique to each B or T lymphocyte. Clonal expansion of individual lymphoid cells as a consequence of neoplastic transformation results in clonally rearranged IgH and/or TCR genes. These leukemia-associated clonal rearrangements are generally stable over time, although clonal evolution may occur after therapy or as a result of other selection pressures [68]. Consensus PCR primers for IgH and TCR sequences have long been used for clonality assessment in mature lymphoid neoplasms at diagnosis. Their application for MRD quantitation in acute leukemia of B and T lineage requires sequencing of the PCR products at diagnosis to identify leukemia-specific sequence(s) followed by the construction and validation of patient-specific PCR primers before the assessment of post-therapy samples. The process is laborious and costly, taking 3 to 4 weeks, but has been standardized and is the principal method used in European clinical trials [41]. False-positive results because of nonspecific primer binding, particularly when normal B cell precursors are increased, and false-negative results because of ongoing mutation or clonal evolution are known to occur.

NGS-based MRD detection in lymphoid leukemia is based on the same principle, using either consensus primers or a large, multiplexed family of allele-specific primers for the initial PCR-based amplification of the VDJ loci, but relies on the direct sequence analysis of the products for detection. The approach improves the specificity of detection and abrogates the need for the creation and validation of patient-specific primers. High-level primer multiplexing also allows for improved amplification of a broader range of rearranged targets, as well as biostatistical correction for differential amplification of specific primer pairs [69]. In addition, reference sequences may be included with the sample at a known frequency to allow improved quantitation of leukemic sequences. In B-ALL, this method has been shown to be technically robust [34,70], comparable to other molecular and immunophenotypic methods [71], and the results are predictive of clinical behavior similar to, and in certain situations, superior to flow cytometry-based methodology [72,73]. Similarly, NGS-based MRD assessment of the TCR beta and gamma chain variable regions in a cohort of T-ALL samples showed concordance and increased sensitivity compared with concurrent flow cytometry-based MRD assessment [74]. However, a clonal TCRB sequence was detected in only ~70% of T-ALL, those lacking a clonal TCRB sequence being immunophenotypically immature (ETP, early thymic precursor, or Near-ETP), and less than half of those contained a clonal TCRG sequence. Thus, ~15% of T-ALL cannot be monitored for MRD using this method, and other complementary approaches are needed. Standardized assays based on multi-institutional validation in ALL (EuroClonality-NGS working group) are now published [75], and proprietary assays (clonoSEQ, Adaptive Biotechnologies) based on this approach have received FDA clearance in the United States for MRD monitoring in B-ALL [69,76]. At a lower limit of detection of 0.001% or perhaps 0.0001%, these NGS methods are at least 10-fold more sensitive than standard flow cytometry-based MRD for B-ALL [73,75,77], although flow cytometry methods acquiring larger numbers of events and incorporating additional antibodies have been developed that can routinely reach a sensitivity of 0.001%, albeit with increased effort [78]. A whole-genome amplification step may be helpful for cases with limited amounts of material to identify clonal IgH and TCR sequences at diagnosis [79]. Studies are emerging that show NGS can identify additional clonal markers not seen with standard PCR-based screening approaches and may be suitable for future disease tracking [80], including in patients whose leukemia does not show applicable sequences by routine methods [58].

With NGS-based monitoring of clonal IgH and TCR sequences becoming an increasingly accepted method for molecular MRD assessment in B-ALL, one remaining question revolves around the significance of very low levels of detectable disease (<0.01%) in modifying the clinical management [76,81]. Data showing concordance between NGS- and flow cytometry-based MRD methods in B-ALL are based in part on pediatric cohorts, which have an overall low relapse rate [34,35,82]. However, there is growing evidence that MRD of less than 0.01% detected by NGS is predictive of future flow cytometry-based positivity [73] and useful as a clinical trigger for treatment refinement [24]. In particular, an absence of detectable MRD by NGS at a level of roughly 0.0001% (1 cell in a million) at end of induction has been associated with an excellent outcome and very low relapse rate in standard risk pediatric B-ALL patients, allowing the identification of a subset of patients early after treatment that are destined to be cured by standard therapy [79]. These patients may be candidates for exclusion from further therapy intensification, as is being studied in a frontline Children's Oncology Group (COG) trial (NCT03914625) [24,83]. However, in high-risk pediatric B-ALL, a subset of patients continue to relapse despite an absence of detectable MRD even at a sensitivity of 0.0001%, suggesting that small numbers of residual leukemic cells below the limit of detection of the assay are still capable of producing relapse, a reflection of the inherent biology of the disease [79]. The implication is that the clinical significance of MRD thresholds depends on the underlying biological and clinical risk groups. FDA approval of blinatumomab for adult patients with MRD-positive B-ALL marks significant progress toward the development of MRD-targeted intervention [84–86]. Based on the data of excellent outcomes for patients without detectable NGS-MRD pre-HSCT [24], another ongoing trial is also studying the elimination of TBI conditioning to reduce toxicities for selected subsets of pediatric patients undergoing HSCT [87].

Discordance between flow cytometric and molecular B-ALL MRD has been noted in a subset of patients having MRD greater than 0.01%. These discordances are predominantly an absence of MRD detected by flow cytometry in the presence of MRD identified by either PCR or NGS MRD assays and have a clinical outcome intermediate between concordantly MRD positive and concordantly MRD-negative patients [34,88]. The reasons for these discrepancies appear heterogeneous, although monocytic differentiation following therapy for patients with *DUX4*, *ZNF384*, and *PAX5*-P80R genetic abnormalities has emerged as a major contributor [89], leading to the leukemic population not identified by standard B-ALL MRD flow cytometric assays but with the persistence of the clonal molecular marker. Whether leukemic cells undergoing such immunophenotypic shifts retain relapse potential is unclear, but this highlights an intrinsic limitation of flow cytometry-based MRD, in that leukemic progenitors may undergo immunophenotypic change after therapy that may complicate MRD detection unless a suitably comprehensive assay is used. Cases that are flow-MRD-positive and NGS-MRD-negative are even rarer and may be attributable to loss or mutation of the clonal molecular marker, sampling differences, or technical and bioinformatic factors related to the NGS platform. Consequently, flow cytometric and NGS MRD are complementary in that they assess different characteristics of the leukemic population and are hence able to compensate for each other's limitations. Now, a step-wise testing approach, that is, the reflex to NGS-MRD if flow-based MRD is negative at defined clinical time points, appears to make optimal use of the relative speed and sensitivity of these techniques.

In addition to IgH and TCR, some other disease-associated gene mutations have been exploited for NGS-based MRD assessment. The *PTEN* gene is recurrently mutated in T-ALL, leading to the loss of PTEN expression [90], and has been shown to be associated with an increased risk of relapse [91]. High-throughput sequencing of the *PTEN* gene samples from patients with known *PTEN* mutations has been reported as a feasible NGS-MRD strategy in this subset of patients [92]. Separately, a heterogeneous and growing group of genetic drivers (mutations, deletions, fusion transcripts) with relatively poor prognosis is recognized in B-ALL, together termed *BCR-ABL1*-like, or Philadelphia-like (Ph-like) B-ALL, given that their gene expression profiles mimic that of Ph + B-ALL [93,94]. Studies are emerging that harness NGS to characterize unique mutations in these leukemias at diagnosis for personalized MRD detection [95].

Acute myeloid leukemia

Although the field of MRD detection in AML is earlier in its development than in ALL, MRD in AML and other myeloid neoplasms is also now recognized as a strong prognostic factor across patient age and disease subtype, largely based on flow cytometric MRD data [14,15,41], and is being integrated into standard-of-care therapeutic monitoring algorithms [14,15,96–99]. The allogeneic HSCT community has been one of the earliest adopters and advocates of AML MRD, including by NGS-based methods [100–103]. NGS-MRD positivity before HSCT has been reported as an independent predictor of relapse [104] and may guide post-HSCT disease monitoring or interventions. In addition, for patients in first clinical remission who remain NGS-MRD positive, treatment intensification with HSCT was found to decrease relapse rates compared with patients who received chemotherapy alone, demonstrating the utility of NGS-MRD to guide treatment decisions [103]. Preanalytic sample protocols [105] and the first consensus document from the European LeukemiaNet MRD Working Party [16], on AML MRD technical and interpretive standardization across methods, highlight the growing maturity of this testing.

Some disease-defining recurrent genetic abnormalities in AML [29] are excellent targets for MRD assessment, as they are often driver mutations or obligatory for the maintenance of the neoplastic state [98]. CBF fusions, t(8;21) (q22;q22.1);*RUNX1-RUNX1T1* and inv(16) (p13.1q22) or t(16;16) (p13.1;q22);*CBFB-MYH11*, and *PML-RARA* fusions, t(15;17) (q22;q11–12) are well-established prognostically significant RQ-PCR-based MRD targets [42–44]. More recently recognized recurrent single base-pair mutations or short insertions or deletions are particularly amenable to NGS-based MRD assessment. A prominent example is the family of nucleophosmin 1 (*NPM1*) mutations, which are considered driver mutations in roughly one-third of AML cases and have served as a target for precise, sensitive MRD quantitation by both RQ-PCR and NGS, in part due to the ease in detecting the typical 4 base-pair insertion with high sensitivity [45–50,59,106,107]. NGS-based NPM1 MRD assessment has been shown to improve post-HSCT relapse risk assessment [108] and to serve as an independent prognostic factor across monitoring time points [109,110]. The optimal clinical time points for NPM1 and CBF MRD evaluation have been debated [111], but consensus guidelines have recently begun to address this [16]. *FLT3* internal tandem duplications (ITD) or tyrosine kinase domain (TKD) mutations often co-occur with *NPM1* mutations or independently, but their presence tends to be transient and subclonal [112], such that FLT3 may not be a reliable MRD target outside of an NGS panel design strategy [106,113,114], although some strategies using *FLT3* for MRD assessment are emerging [115].

The remaining subsets of AML are genetically diverse and contain a wide variety of disease-associated mutations [116] whose biological importance is not well understood [117] and whose suitability for MRD assessment is unclear. The heterogeneity in these remaining molecular targets necessitates the use of a panel design for efficient MRD testing, something well suited to the high-level multiplexing capabilities of NGS. However, many of these residual mutations in AML are single base-pair mutations, so error-correction approaches are required for sensitive and specific mutation detection [57–61]. Of particular importance is the recognition that AML in older patients often evolves from pre-existing age-related clonal hematopoiesis or clonal hematopoiesis of indeterminate potential (CHIP), which is associated with mutations in *DNMT3A*, *TET2*, and *ASXL1*(so-called DTA variants). Such clonal hematopoiesis is not eradicated by current AML therapies, so these mutations often persist in remission. Although this may represent some increased risk for the development of future myeloid neoplasia, their presence does not appear to be associated with prognostic significance post-therapy in AML and may confound MRD analysis of NGS data [31,32,118–121]. AML cases with DTA-type mutations frequently carry secondary oncogenic mutations in signaling or cell cycle genes like *NRAS*, *KRAS*, *PTPN11*, and *FLT3*, which being subclonal may also be suboptimal for MRD assessment, as they are unstable through the course of the disease and changeable between the diagnosis and relapse [121,122]. MRD assessment by NGS in AML evolving from clonal hematopoiesis might be performed by following the concurrence of multiple variants (eg, mutation patterns) rather than individual mutations, but, in general, relies primarily on the persistence of non-DTA mutations [123]. A related issue is that the optimal level of sensitivity required for MRD assays in AML and the clinically relevant levels of MRD have yet to be established for many mutations, the latter likely being dependent on the particular genetic subtype of AML, the time point where testing is performed, and the therapies used. Consequently, NGS-based MRD assays for AML must be carefully designed for an appropriate level of sensitivity using error-corrected approaches, and the clinical significance of the data is cautiously interpreted with an understanding of CHIP-type mutations and knowledge of patient mutational history.

Another significant category of AML with limited options for molecular MRD monitoring is leukemias driven by rare abnormal gene fusions for which standardized, clinically validated quantitative assays are not broadly available. Such fusions are particularly common in pediatric AML [124–126], and general strategies for sensitive MRD detection in this patient population remain to be developed [127]. The achievable sensitivity level for MRD assessment for less prevalent fusions is not known, but will likely vary depending on their expression levels in leukemia cells if RNA-based strategies are used.

In comparison, flow cytometry-based MRD for AML and myeloid neoplasms, while applicable to the large majority of patients, has greater interpretive complexity and interobserver variability than in ALL and its adoption outside of specialized centers may, therefore, be hampered. Nevertheless, flow cytometry provides a broader, independent, and integrated assessment of the impact of underlying molecular abnormalities on cellular function, and hence is complementary to molecular approaches for MRD assessment [34,35,67,73,77,88,89,128]. A multifaceted approach, for example, flow cytometry-based MRD assessment performed at the centers of excellence with reflex to NGS-based testing for flow cytometry-negative samples or where highly sensitive MRD detection is clinically relevant for a specific disease subtype or time point in therapy is likely to emerge as a best practice [16].

ADDITIONAL METHODOLOGIES AND CONSIDERATIONS

Transcriptome analysis through RNA sequencing (RNA-Seq) has been exploited for the identification of leukemia-associated IgH clonal sequences, which can then be used in NGS-based MRD analysis [129]. Furthermore, gene expression profiling of MRD-positive and MRD-negative pediatric ALL samples show distinct differences [130]; while these could be exploited for MRD detection, they are labor-intensive, more highly dependent on sample quality, and likely lack the sensitivity of conventional MRD methods, making RNA-Seq and gene expression profiling unlikely to become clinical assays for MRD assessment. Separately, digital droplet PCR (ddPCR) may be appropriate for ultrasensitive point mutation detection [131,132], but mutation-specific assay design is required [133] that may be cost- and labor-prohibitive in clinical practice [134]. Other approaches, including circulating microRNA profiling and microfluidic chip platforms [135] are under investigation but of unproven utility at present.

The feasibility of using peripheral blood instead of more invasive and traumatic BM samples for molecular MRD assessment in acute leukemia is being explored. Although the MRD level in blood is generally found to be significantly lower than in BM for B-ALL and AML [99], and hence less optimal for the quantitation of disease burden, false-negative MRD results in the blood are infrequent when MRD is detected in marrow [42,136–139]. Consequently, it may be possible to use NGS of blood to detect the presence or absence of MRD with a reflex to obtaining and testing marrow only when more accurate quantitation is desired. Now, the use of PB for MRD assessment is not recommended to maximize assay sensitivity [16].

On a final note, although MRD assessment in acute leukemia has emerged as the standard of care at referral centers in developed countries, barriers to accessibility of these techniques in global and community settings deserve attention [140]. Additional international standardization of technologies and automation pipelines [16,38,141], feasible for resource-limited environments as the costs of these technologies continue to decrease, is needed for these clinically predictive assays to be accessible to more patients.

SUMMARY

MRD is an important independent adverse prognostic factor in acute leukemias across subtypes. NGS-based MRD detection is emerging as an adjunct or replacement to immunophenotypic (flow cytometric) and RQ-PCR assays because of its high sensitivity, but a complex laboratory and bioinformatics infrastructure are required. Clonal IgH and TCR gene sequences are the basis for NGS-based MRD assessment in ALL. AML is a more heterogeneous group of related neoplasms, many of which may ultimately be amenable to NGS-based MRD approaches as the analytical approaches evolve. Advantages and challenges in the feasibility and interpretation of NGS-based MRD dictate the need for an improved understanding of the specific disease characteristics and optimal clinical time points to which it is best suited. As data are gathered using the first edition consensus guidelines for ALL and AML MRD assessment incorporated NGS [16,75], further refinement of the current recommendations will emerge.

CLINICS CARE POINTS

- Next-generation sequencing using "error correction" and "unique molecular identifiers" (UMIs) has markedly improved its sensitivity for minimal residual disease detected, allowing the detection of mutations theoretically at 10^{-9}.
- The optimal approach to minimal residual disease testing in acute leukemia depends on the leukemia biology (immunophenotypic, recurrent genetic fusions, and mutational features amenable to testing) and the

clinical question at hand (eg, end of induction chemotherapy, prehematopoietic stem cell transplant evaluation, post-therapy evaluation for deep remission).

- In certain biological and clinical scenarios, peripheral blood is emerging as an alternative to bone marrow aspirate material for minimal residual disease assessment.

DISCLOSURE

The authors have nothing to disclose.

REFERENCES

[1] Alikian M, Gale RP, Apperley JF, et al. Molecular techniques for the personalised management of patients with chronic myeloid leukaemia. Biomol Detect Quantif 2017;11:4–20.

[2] Laczika K, Mitterbauer G, Korninger L, et al. Rapid achievement of PML-RAR alpha polymerase chain reaction (PCR)-negativity by combined treatment with all-trans-retinoic acid and chemotherapy in acute promyelocytic leukemia: a pilot study. Leukemia 1994;8:1–5.

[3] Takatsuki H, Umemura T, Sadamura S, et al. Detection of minimal residual disease by reverse transcriptase polymerase chain reaction for the PML/RAR alpha fusion mRNA: a study in patients with acute promyelocytic leukemia following peripheral stem cell transplantation. Leukemia 1995;9:889–92.

[4] Grimwade D. The significance of minimal residual disease in patients with t(15;17). Best Pract Res Clin Haematol 2002;15:137–58.

[5] Ito Y, Miyamura K. Clinical significance of minimal residual disease in leukemia detected by polymerase chain reaction: is molecular remission a milestone for achieving a cure? Leuk Lymphoma 1994;16:57–64.

[6] van Dongen JJ, Breit TM, Adriaansen HJ, et al. Detection of minimal residual disease in acute leukemia by immunological marker analysis and polymerase chain reaction. Leukemia 1992;6(Suppl 1):47–59.

[7] Jacquy C, Delepaut B, Van Daele S, et al. A prospective study of minimal residual disease in childhood B-lineage acute lymphoblastic leukaemia: MRD level at the end of induction is a strong predictive factor of relapse. Br J Haematol 1997;98:140–6.

[8] Krauter J, Gorlich K, Ottmann O, et al. Prognostic value of minimal residual disease quantification by real-time reverse transcriptase polymerase chain reaction in patients with core binding factor leukemias. J Clin Oncol 2003;21:4413–22.

[9] van Dongen JJ, Macintyre EA, Gabert JA, et al. Standardized RT-PCR analysis of fusion gene transcripts from chromosome aberrations in acute leukemia for detection of minimal residual disease. Report of the BIOMED-1 Concerted Action: investigation of minimal residual disease in acute leukemia. Leukemia 1999;13:1901–28.

[10] Miyamura K, Tanimoto M, Morishima Y, et al. Detection of Philadelphia chromosome-positive acute lymphoblastic leukemia by polymerase chain reaction: possible eradication of minimal residual disease by marrow transplantation. Blood 1992;79:1366–70.

[11] National comprehensive cancer network clinical practice guidelines in Oncology (NCCN guidelines): acute lymphoblastic leukemia. NCCN; 2020.

[12] Brown PA, Wieduwilt M, Logan A, et al. Guidelines Insights: Acute Lymphoblastic Leukemia, Version 1.2019. J Natl Compr Canc Netw 2019;17(5):414–23.

[13] Brown P, Inaba H, Annesley C, et al. Pediatric Acute Lymphoblastic Leukemia, Version 2.2020, NCCN Clinical Practice Guidelines in Oncology. J Natl Compr Canc Netw 2020;18(1):81–112.

[14] Ossenkoppele G, Schuurhuis GJ. MRD in AML: does it already guide therapy decision-making? Hematol Am Soc Hematol Educ Program 2016;2016:356–65.

[15] Ossenkoppele G, Schuurhuis GJ, van de Loosdrecht A, et al. Can we incorporate MRD assessment into clinical practice in AML? Best Pract Res Clin Haematol 2019;32:186–91.

[16] Schuurhuis GJ, Heuser M, Freeman S, et al. Minimal/measurable residual disease in AML: a consensus document from the European LeukemiaNet MRD Working Party. Blood 2018;131:1275–91.

[17] Pollyea DA, Bixby D, Perl A, et al. NCCN Guidelines Insights: Acute Myeloid Leukemia, Version 2.2021. J Natl Compr Canc Netw 2021;19(1):16–27.

[18] Campana D, Leung W. Clinical significance of minimal residual disease in patients with acute leukaemia undergoing haematopoietic stem cell transplantation. Br J Haematol 2013;162:147–61.

[19] Cloos J, Ossenkoppele GJ, Dillon R. Minimal residual disease and stem cell transplantation outcomes. Hematol Am Soc Hematol Educ Program 2019;2019:617–25.

[20] Nagler A, Baron F, Labopin M, et al. Measurable residual disease (MRD) testing for acute leukemia in EBMT transplant centers: a survey on behalf of the ALWP of the EBMT. Bone Marrow Transpl 2021;96(1):218–24.

[21] BLAST MRD AML-2: BLockade of PD-1 added to standard therapy to target measurable residual disease in acute myeloid leukemia 2- a randomized phase 2 study of anti-PD-1 pembrolizumab in combination with azacitidine and venetoclax as frontline therapy in unfit patients with acute myeloid leukemia. 2021 Availble at: https://clinicaltrials.gov/ct2/show/NCT04284787?term=ETC-+Zeidan&recrs=a&cond=acute+myeloid+leukemia&cntry=US&draw=2&rank=1. Accessed March 12, 2021.

[22] Berry DA, Zhou S, Higley H, et al. Association of minimal residual disease with clinical outcome in pediatric and adult acute lymphoblastic leukemia: a meta-analysis. JAMA Oncol 2017;3:e170580.

[23] Pulsipher MA, Bader P, Klingebiel T, et al. Allogeneic transplantation for pediatric acute lymphoblastic leukemia: the emerging role of peritransplantation minimal residual disease/chimerism monitoring and novel chemotherapeutic, molecular, and immune approaches aimed at preventing relapse. Biol Blood Marrow Transpl 2009;15:62–71.

[24] Pulsipher MA, Carlson C, Langholz B, et al. IgH-V(D)J NGS-MRD measurement pre- and early post-allotransplant defines very low- and very high-risk ALL patients. Blood 2015;125:3501–8.

[25] Hantel A, Stock W, Kosuri S. Molecular minimal residual disease testing in acute myeloid leukemia: a review for the practicing clinician. Clin Lymphoma Myeloma Leuk 2018;18:636–47.

[26] Othus M, Wood BL, Stirewalt DL, et al. Effect of measurable ('minimal') residual disease (MRD) information on prediction of relapse and survival in adult acute myeloid leukemia. Leukemia 2016;30:2080–3.

[27] Coustan-Smith E, Campana D. Should evaluation for minimal residual disease be routine in acute myeloid leukemia? Curr Opin Hematol 2013;20:86–92.

[28] Papaemmanuil E, Dohner H, Campbell PJ. Genomic classification in acute myeloid leukemia. N Engl J Med 2016;375:900–1.

[29] Arber DA, Brunning RD, Le Beau MM, et al. Acute myeloid leukaemia with recurrent genetic abnormalities. In: Swerdlow SH, Harris NL, Jaffe ES, et al, editors. World health organization (WHO) classification of tumuors of haematopoietic and lymphoid tissues. 4th edition. Lyon: International Agency for Research on Cancer; 2017.

[30] Theunissen PMJ, de Bie M, van Zessen D, et al. Next-generation antigen receptor sequencing of paired diagnosis and relapse samples of B-cell acute lymphoblastic leukemia: clonal evolution and implications for minimal residual disease target selection. Leuk Res 2019; 76:98–104.

[31] Hasserjian RP, Steensma DP, Graubert TA, et al. Clonal hematopoiesis and measurable residual disease assessment in acute myeloid leukemia. Blood 2020;135:1729–38.

[32] Jaiswal S, Fontanillas P, Flannick J, et al. Age-related clonal hematopoiesis associated with adverse outcomes. N Engl J Med 2014;371:2488–98.

[33] Kayser S, Walter RB, Stock W, et al. Minimal residual disease in acute myeloid leukemia–current status and future perspectives. Curr Hematol Malig Rep 2015;10: 132–44.

[34] Wu D, Emerson RO, Sherwood A, et al. Detection of minimal residual disease in B lymphoblastic leukemia by high-throughput sequencing of IGH. Clin Cancer Res 2014;20:4540–8.

[35] Kotrova M, Trka J, Kneba M, et al. Is next-generation sequencing the way to go for residual disease monitoring in acute lymphoblastic leukemia? Mol Diagn Ther 2017;21:481–92.

[36] Borowitz MJ, Wood BL, Devidas M, et al. Prognostic significance of minimal residual disease in high risk B-ALL: a report from Children's Oncology Group study AALL0232. Blood 2015;126:964–71.

[37] Borowitz MJ, Pullen DJ, Shuster JJ, et al. Minimal residual disease detection in childhood precursor-B-cell acute lymphoblastic leukemia: relation to other risk factors. A Children's Oncology Group study. Leukemia 2003;17:1566–72.

[38] Brüggemann M, Kotrová M, Knecht H, et al. Standardized next-generation sequencing of immunoglobulin and T-cell receptor gene recombinations for MRD marker identification in acute lymphoblastic leukaemia; a EuroClonality-NGS validation study. Leukemia 2019;33:2241–53.

[39] Langerak AW, Groenen PJ, Bruggemann M, et al. EuroClonality/BIOMED-2 guidelines for interpretation and reporting of Ig/TCR clonality testing in suspected lymphoproliferations. Leukemia 2012;26:2159–71.

[40] Scheijen B, Meijers RWJ, Rijntjes J, et al. Next-generation sequencing of immunoglobulin gene rearrangements for clonality assessment: a technical feasibility study by EuroClonality-NGS. Leukemia 2019;33:2227–40.

[41] van Dongen JJ, Langerak AW, Bruggemann M, et al. Design and standardization of PCR primers and protocols for detection of clonal immunoglobulin and T-cell receptor gene recombinations in suspect lymphoproliferations: report of the BIOMED-2 Concerted Action BMH4-CT98-3936. Leukemia 2003;17:2257–317.

[42] Rucker FG, Agrawal M, Corbacioglu A, et al. Measurable residual disease monitoring in acute myeloid leukemia with t(8;21)(q22;q22.1): results from the AML Study Group. Blood 2019;134:1608–18.

[43] Yin JA, Frost L. Monitoring AML1-ETO and CBFbeta-MYH11 transcripts in acute myeloid leukemia. Curr Oncol Rep 2003;5:399–404.

[44] Stentoft J, Hokland P, Ostergaard M, et al. Minimal residual core binding factor AMLs by real time quantitative PCR–initial response to chemotherapy predicts event free survival and close monitoring of peripheral blood unravels the kinetics of relapse. Leuk Res 2006; 30:389–95.

[45] Barragan E, Pajuelo JC, Ballester S, et al. Minimal residual disease detection in acute myeloid leukemia by mutant nucleophosmin (NPM1): comparison with WT1 gene expression. Clin Chim Acta 2008;395:120–3.

[46] Bacher U, Badbaran A, Fehse B, et al. Quantitative monitoring of NPM1 mutations provides a valid minimal residual disease parameter following allogeneic stem cell transplantation. Exp Hematol 2009;37: 135–42.

[47] Papadaki C, Dufour A, Seibl M, et al. Monitoring minimal residual disease in acute myeloid leukaemia with NPM1 mutations by quantitative PCR: clonal evolution is a limiting factor. Br J Haematol 2009;144:517–23.

[48] Dvorakova D, Racil Z, Jeziskova I, et al. Monitoring of minimal residual disease in acute myeloid leukemia

with frequent and rare patient-specific NPM1 mutations. Am J Hematol 2010;85:926–9.

[49] Pettersson L, Leveen P, Axler O, et al. Improved minimal residual disease detection by targeted quantitative polymerase chain reaction in Nucleophosmin 1 type a mutated acute myeloid leukemia. Genes Chromosomes Cancer 2016;55:750–66.

[50] Salipante SJ, Fromm JR, Shendure J, et al. Detection of minimal residual disease in NPM1-mutated acute myeloid leukemia by next-generation sequencing. Mod Pathol 2014;27:1438–46.

[51] Gabert J, Beillard E, van der Velden VH, et al. Standardization and quality control studies of 'real-time' quantitative reverse transcriptase polymerase chain reaction of fusion gene transcripts for residual disease detection in leukemia - a Europe Against Cancer program. Leukemia 2003;17:2318–57.

[52] Goodwin S, McPherson JD, McCombie WR. Coming of age: ten years of next-generation sequencing technologies. Nat Rev Genet 2016;17:333–51.

[53] Reuter JA, Spacek DV, Snyder MP. High-throughput sequencing technologies. Mol Cell 2015;58:586–97.

[54] Sims D, Sudbery I, Ilott NE, et al. Sequencing depth and coverage: key considerations in genomic analyses. Nat Rev Genet 2014;15:121–32.

[55] Yohe S, Thyagarajan B. Review of clinical next-generation sequencing. Arch Pathol Lab Med 2017;141:1544–57.

[56] Behjati S, Tarpey PS. What is next generation sequencing? Arch Dis Child Educ Pract Ed 2013;98:236–8.

[57] Salk JJ, Schmitt MW, Loeb LA. Enhancing the accuracy of next-generation sequencing for detecting rare and subclonal mutations. Nat Rev Genet 2018;19:269–85.

[58] Cavagna R, Guinea Montalvo ML, Tosi M, et al. Capture-based next-generation sequencing improves the identification of immunoglobulin/T-cell receptor clonal markers and gene mutations in adult acute lymphoblastic leukemia patients lacking molecular probes. Cancers (Basel) 2020;12:1505.

[59] Ritterhouse LL, Parilla M, Zhen CJ, et al. Clinical validation and implementation of a measurable residual disease assay for NPM1 in acute myeloid leukemia by error-corrected next-generation sequencing. Mol Diagn Ther 2019;23:791–802.

[60] Balagopal V, Hantel A, Kadri S, et al. Measurable residual disease monitoring for patients with acute myeloid leukemia following hematopoietic cell transplantation using error corrected hybrid capture next generation sequencing. PLoS One 2019;14:e0224097.

[61] Kennedy SR, Schmitt MW, Fox EJ, et al. Detecting ultralow-frequency mutations by Duplex Sequencing. Nat Protoc 2014;9:2586–606.

[62] Hiatt JB, Pritchard CC, Salipante SJ, et al. Single molecule molecular inversion probes for targeted, high-accuracy detection of low-frequency variation. Genome Res 2013;23:843–54.

[63] Gregory MT, Bertout JA, Ericson NG, et al. Targeted single molecule mutation detection with massively parallel sequencing. Nucleic Acids Res 2016;44:e22.

[64] Kinde I, Wu J, Papadopoulos N, et al. Detection and quantification of rare mutations with massively parallel sequencing. Proc Natl Acad Sci U S A 2011;108:9530–5.

[65] Waalkes A, Penewit K, Wood BL, et al. Ultrasensitive detection of acute myeloid leukemia minimal residual disease using single molecule molecular inversion probes. Haematologica 2017;102:1549–57.

[66] Dillon LW, Hayati S, Roloff GW, et al. Targeted RNA-sequencing for the quantification of measurable residual disease in acute myeloid leukemia. Haematologica 2019;104:297–304.

[67] Xu C, Studer A, Chen X, et al. Comprehensive evaluation and validation of a next-generation sequencing assay for minimal residual disease detection in T-Lymphoblastic Leukemia/Lymphoma. Blood 2019; 134(Supplement_1):1475.

[68] Shahkarami S, Mehrasa R, Younesian S, et al. Minimal residual disease (MRD) detection using rearrangement of immunoglobulin/T cell receptor genes in adult patients with acute lymphoblastic leukemia (ALL). Ann Hematol 2018;97:585–95.

[69] Ching T, Duncan ME, Newman-Eerkes T, et al. Analytical evaluation of the clonoSEQ Assay for establishing measurable (minimal) residual disease in acute lymphoblastic leukemia, chronic lymphocytic leukemia, and multiple myeloma. BMC Cancer 2020;20:612.

[70] Monter A, Nomdedéu JF. ClonoSEQ assay for the detection of lymphoid malignancies. Expert Rev Mol Diagn 2019;19:571–8.

[71] Ladetto M, Brüggemann M, Monitillo L, et al. Next-generation sequencing and real-time quantitative PCR for minimal residual disease detection in B-cell disorders. Leukemia 2014;28:1299–307.

[72] Sekiya Y, Xu Y, Muramatsu H, et al. Clinical utility of next-generation sequencing-based minimal residual disease in paediatric B-cell acute lymphoblastic leukaemia. Br J Haematol 2017;176:248–57.

[73] Cheng S, Inghirami G, Cheng S, et al. Simple deep sequencing-based post-remission MRD surveillance predicts clinical relapse in B-ALL. J Hematol Oncol 2018;11:105.

[74] Wu D, Sherwood A, Fromm JR, et al. High-throughput sequencing detects minimal residual disease in acute T lymphoblastic leukemia. Sci Transl Med 2012;4: 134ra63.

[75] Bruggemann M, Kotrova M, Knecht H, et al. Standardized next-generation sequencing of immunoglobulin and T-cell receptor gene recombinations for MRD marker identification in acute lymphoblastic leukaemia; a EuroClonality-NGS validation study. Leukemia 2019;33:2241–53.

[76] Monter A, Nomdedeu JF. ClonoSEQ assay for the detection of lymphoid malignancies. Expert Rev Mol Diagn 2019;19:571–8.

[77] Faham M, Zheng J, Moorhead M, et al. Deep-sequencing approach for minimal residual disease detection in acute lymphoblastic leukemia. Blood 2012;120:5173–80.
[78] Theunissen P, Mejstrikova E, Sedek L, et al. Standardized flow cytometry for highly sensitive MRD measurements in B-cell acute lymphoblastic leukemia. Blood 2017;129:347–57.
[79] Della Starza I, De Novi LA, Nunes V, et al. Whole-genome amplification for the detection of molecular targets and minimal residual disease monitoring in acute lymphoblastic leukaemia. Br J Haematol 2014;165:341–8.
[80] Wright G, Watt E, Inglott S, et al. Clinical benefit of a high-throughput sequencing approach for minimal residual disease in acute lymphoblastic leukemia. Pediatr Blood Cancer 2019;66:e27787.
[81] Reyes-Barron C, Burack WR, Rothberg PG, et al. Next-Generation Sequencing for Minimal Residual Disease Surveillance in Acute Lymphoblastic Leukemia: An Update. Crit Rev Oncog 2017;22:559–67.
[82] Chen X, Wood BL. How do we measure MRD in ALL and how should measurements affect decisions. Re: Treatment and prognosis? Best Pract Res Clin Haematol 2017;30:237–48.
[83] McNeer JL, Rau RE, Gupta S, et al. Cutting to the Front of the Line: Immunotherapy for Childhood Acute Lymphoblastic Leukemia. Am Soc Clin Oncol Educ Book 2020;40:1–12.
[84] Gokbuget N, Dombret H, Bonifacio M, et al. Blinatumomab for minimal residual disease in adults with B-cell precursor acute lymphoblastic leukemia. Blood 2018;131:1522–31.
[85] Kantarjian H, Stein A, Gokbuget N, et al. Blinatumomab versus chemotherapy for advanced acute lymphoblastic leukemia. N Engl J Med 2017;376:836–47.
[86] Jen EY, Xu Q, Schetter A, et al. FDA approval: blinatumomab for patients with B-cell precursor acute lymphoblastic leukemia in morphologic remission with minimal residual disease. Clin Cancer Res 2019; 25:473–7.
[87] The EndRAD trial: eliminating total body irradiation (TBI) for NGS-MRD negative children, adolescents, and young adults with B-ALL Availble at: https://clinicaltrials.gov/ct2/show/NCT03509961?term=ENDrad&cond=Leukemia&draw=2&rank=1. Accessed March 14, 2021.
[88] Group M-A-BS, Langebrake C, Creutzig U, Dworzak M, et al. Residual disease monitoring in childhood acute myeloid leukemia by multiparameter flow cytometry: the MRD-AML-BFM Study Group. J Clin Oncol 2006; 24:3686–92.
[89] Novakova M, Zaliova M, Fiser K, et al. DUX4r, ZNF384r and PAX5-P80R mutated B-cell precursor acute lymphoblastic leukemia frequently undergo monocytic switch. Haematologica 2021;106(8):2066–75.
[90] Palomero T, Sulis ML, Cortina M, et al. Mutational loss of PTEN induces resistance to NOTCH1 inhibition in T-cell leukemia. Nat Med 2007;13:1203–10.
[91] Paganin M, Grillo MF, Silvestri D, et al. The presence of mutated and deleted PTEN is associated with an increased risk of relapse in childhood T cell acute lymphoblastic leukaemia treated with AIEOP-BFM ALL protocols. Br J Haematol 2018;182:705–11.
[92] Germano G, Valsecchi MG, Buldini B, et al. Next-generation sequencing of PTEN mutations for monitoring minimal residual disease in T-cell acute lymphoblastic leukemia. Pediatr Blood Cancer 2020;67:e28025.
[93] Roberts KG, Pei D, Campana D, et al. Outcomes of children with BCR-ABL1-like acute lymphoblastic leukemia treated with risk-directed therapy based on the levels of minimal residual disease. J Clin Oncol 2014;32:3012–20.
[94] Roberts KG, Reshmi SC, Harvey RC, et al. Genomic and outcome analyses of Ph-like ALL in NCI standard-risk patients: a report from the Children's Oncology Group. Blood 2018;132:815–24.
[95] Sherali N, Hamadneh T, Aftab S, et al. Integration of next-generation sequencing in diagnosing and minimal residual disease detection in patients with philadelphia chromosome-like acute lymphoblastic leukemia. Cureus 2020;12:e10696.
[96] Getta BM, Devlin SM, Levine RL, et al. Multicolor flow cytometry and multigene next-generation sequencing are complementary and highly predictive for relapse in acute myeloid leukemia after allogeneic transplantation. Biol Blood Marrow Transpl 2017;23:1064–71.
[97] Chen X, Wood BL. Monitoring minimal residual disease in acute leukemia: technical challenges and interpretive complexities. Blood Rev 2017;31:63–75.
[98] Zhou Y, Wood BL. Methods of detection of measurable residual disease in AML. Curr Hematol Malig Rep 2017; 12:557–67.
[99] Grimwade D, Freeman SD. Defining minimal residual disease in acute myeloid leukemia: which platforms are ready for "prime time"? Hematol Am Soc Hematol Educ Program 2014;2014:222–33.
[100] Araki D, Wood BL, Othus M, et al. Allogeneic hematopoietic cell transplantation for acute myeloid leukemia: time to move toward a minimal residual disease-based definition of complete remission? J Clin Oncol 2016; 34:329–36.
[101] Shapiro RM, Kim DDH. Next-generation sequencing-based minimal residual disease monitoring in patients receiving allogeneic hematopoietic stem cell transplantation for acute myeloid leukemia or myelodysplastic syndrome. Curr Opin Hematol 2018;25:425–32.
[102] Thol F, Gabdoulline R, Liebich A, et al. Measurable residual disease monitoring by NGS before allogeneic hematopoietic cell transplantation in AML. Blood 2018; 132:1703–13.
[103] Ahn JS, Kim T, Jung SH, et al. Allogeneic transplant can abrogate the risk of relapse in the patients of first remission acute myeloid leukemia with detectable measurable residual disease by next-generation sequencing. Bone Marrow Transpl 2021;56(5):1159–70.

[104] Press RD, Eickelberg G, Froman A, et al. Next-generation sequencing-defined minimal residual disease before stem cell transplantation predicts acute myeloid leukemia relapse. Am J Hematol 2019;94:902–12.
[105] Cloos J, Harris JR, Janssen J, et al. Comprehensive protocol to sample and process bone marrow for measuring measurable residual disease and leukemic stem cells in acute myeloid leukemia. J Vis Exp 2018; 133:56386.
[106] Thol F, Kolking B, Damm F, et al. Next-generation sequencing for minimal residual disease monitoring in acute myeloid leukemia patients with FLT3-ITD or NPM1 mutations. Genes Chromosomes Cancer 2012; 51:689–95.
[107] Radich JP, Zelenetz AD, Chan WC, et al. NCCN task force report: molecular markers in leukemias and lymphomas. J Natl Compr Canc Netw 2009;7(Suppl 4): S1–34 [quiz S5–6].
[108] Zhou Y, Othus M, Walter RB, et al. Deep NPM1 sequencing following allogeneic hematopoietic cell transplantation improves risk assessment in adults with NPM1-mutated AML. Biol Blood Marrow Transpl 2018;24:1615–20.
[109] Patkar N, Kodgule R, Kakirde C, et al. Clinical impact of measurable residual disease monitoring by ultradeep next generation sequencing in NPM1 mutated acute myeloid leukemia. Oncotarget 2018;9: 36613–24.
[110] Guolo F, Minetto P, Clavio M, et al. Longitudinal minimal residual disease (MRD) evaluation in acute myeloid leukaemia with NPM1 mutation: from definition of molecular relapse to MRD-driven salvage approach. Br J Haematol 2019;186:e223–5.
[111] Forghieri F, Comoli P, Marasca R, et al. Minimal/measurable residual disease monitoring in NPM1-mutated acute myeloid leukemia: a clinical viewpoint and perspectives. Int J Mol Sci 2018;19:3492.
[112] Bibault JE, Figeac M, Helevaut N, et al. Next-generation sequencing of FLT3 internal tandem duplications for minimal residual disease monitoring in acute myeloid leukemia. Oncotarget 2015;6:22812–21.
[113] Dillon R, Potter N, Freeman S, et al. How we use molecular minimal residual disease (MRD) testing in acute myeloid leukaemia (AML). Br J Haematol 2021; 193(2):231–44.
[114] Fasan O. Using minimal (measurable) residual disease assessments to guide decision-making for timing of allogeneic transplantation in acute myeloid leukemia. Curr Opin Hematol 2019;26:413–20.
[115] Levis MJ, Perl AE, Altman JK, et al. A next-generation sequencing-based assay for minimal residual disease assessment in AML patients with FLT3-ITD mutations. Blood Adv 2018;2:825–31.
[116] Mardis ER, Ding L, Dooling DJ, et al. Recurring mutations found by sequencing an acute myeloid leukemia genome. N Engl J Med 2009;361:1058–66.
[117] Welch JS, Ley TJ, Link DC, et al. The origin and evolution of mutations in acute myeloid leukemia. Cell 2012;150:264–78.
[118] Xie M, Lu C, Wang J, et al. Age-related mutations associated with clonal hematopoietic expansion and malignancies. Nat Med 2014;20:1472–8.
[119] Genovese G, Kahler AK, Handsaker RE, et al. Clonal hematopoiesis and blood-cancer risk inferred from blood DNA sequence. N Engl J Med 2014;371:2477–87.
[120] Steensma DP, Bejar R, Jaiswal S, et al. Clonal hematopoiesis of indeterminate potential and its distinction from myelodysplastic syndromes. Blood 2015;126:9–16.
[121] Buccisano F, Dillon R, Freeman SD, et al. Role of minimal (measurable) residual disease assessment in older patients with acute myeloid leukemia. Cancers (Basel) 2018;10:215.
[122] Buccisano F, Maurillo L, Del Principe MI, et al. Minimal residual disease as a biomarker for outcome prediction and therapy optimization in acute myeloid leukemia. Expert Rev Hematol 2018;11:307–13.
[123] Jongen-Lavrencic M, Grob T, Hanekamp D, et al. Molecular minimal residual disease in acute myeloid leukemia. N Engl J Med 2018;378:1189–99.
[124] Farrar JE, Schuback HL, Ries RE, et al. Genomic profiling of pediatric acute myeloid leukemia reveals a changing mutational landscape from disease diagnosis to relapse. Cancer Res 2016;76:2197–205.
[125] Maxson JE, Ries RE, Wang YC, et al. CSF3R mutations have a high degree of overlap with CEBPA mutations in pediatric AML. Blood 2016;127:3094–8.
[126] Bolouri H, Farrar JE, Triche T Jr, et al. The molecular landscape of pediatric acute myeloid leukemia reveals recurrent structural alterations and age-specific mutational interactions. Nat Med 2018;24:103–12.
[127] Brunner AM, Graubert TA. Genomics in childhood acute myeloid leukemia comes of age. Nat Med 2018; 24:7–9.
[128] Bruggemann M, Kotrova M. Minimal residual disease in adult ALL: technical aspects and implications for correct clinical interpretation. Blood Adv 2017;1:2456–66.
[129] Li Z, Jiang N, Lim EH, et al. Identifying IGH disease clones for MRD monitoring in childhood B-cell acute lymphoblastic leukemia using RNA-Seq. Leukemia 2020;34:2418–29.
[130] Sitthi-Amorn J, Herrington B, Megason G, et al. Transcriptome analysis of minimal residual disease in subtypes of pediatric B cell acute lymphoblastic leukemia. Clin Med Insights Oncol 2015;9:51–60.
[131] Brambati C, Galbiati S, Xue E, et al. Droplet digital polymerase chain reaction for DNMT3A and IDH1/2 mutations to improve early detection of acute myeloid leukemia relapse after allogeneic hematopoietic stem cell transplantation. Haematologica 2016;101: e157–61.
[132] Waterhouse M, Pfeifer D, Duque-Afonso J, et al. Droplet digital PCR for the simultaneous analysis of minimal residual disease and hematopoietic chimerism after

allogeneic cell transplantation. Clin Chem Lab Med 2019;57:641–7.

[133] Coccaro N, Anelli L, Zagaria A, et al. Droplet digital PCR is a robust tool for monitoring minimal residual disease in adult philadelphia-positive acute lymphoblastic leukemia. J Mol Diagn 2018;20:474–82.

[134] Cilloni D, Petiti J, Rosso V, et al. Digital PCR in myeloid malignancies: ready to replace quantitative PCR? Int J Mol Sci 2019;20:2249.

[135] Liu Y, Zhang H, Du Y, et al. Highly sensitive minimal residual disease detection by biomimetic multivalent aptamer nanoclimber functionalized microfluidic chip. Small 2020;16:e2000949.

[136] Maurillo L, Bassan R, Cascavilla N, et al. Quality of Response in acute myeloid leukemia: the Role of minimal residual disease. Cancers (Basel) 2019;11:1417.

[137] Coustan-Smith E, Sancho J, Hancock ML, et al. Use of peripheral blood instead of bone marrow to monitor residual disease in children with acute lymphoblastic leukemia. Blood 2002;100:2399–402.

[138] Schumich A, Maurer-Granofszky M, Attarbaschi A, et al. Flow-cytometric minimal residual disease monitoring in blood predicts relapse risk in pediatric B-cell precursor acute lymphoblastic leukemia in trial AIEOP-BFM-ALL 2000. Pediatr Blood Cancer 2019;66:e27590.

[139] Skou AS, Juul-Dam KL, Ommen HB, et al. Peripheral blood molecular measurable residual disease is sufficient to identify patients with acute myeloid leukaemia with imminent clinical relapse. Br J Haematol 2021.

[140] Kim C, Delaney K, McNamara M, et al. Cross-sectional physician survey on the use of minimal residual disease testing in the management of pediatric and adult patients with acute lymphoblastic leukemia. Hematology 2019;24:70–8.

[141] Ni W, Hu B, Zheng C, et al. Automated analysis of acute myeloid leukemia minimal residual disease using a support vector machine. Oncotarget 2016;7:71915–21.

Advances in Molecular Pathology 4 (2021) 65–79
ADVANCES IN MOLECULAR PATHOLOGY

Molecular Profile of *BCR-ABL1* Negative Myeloproliferative Neoplasms and Its Impact on Prognosis and Management

Ayman Qasrawi, MD[a,b], Ranjana Arora, MD[c,*]
[a]Assistant Professor, Division of Hematology, Blood and Marrow Transplantation & Cellular Therapy, University of Kentucky, Lexington, Kentucky 40536, USA; [b]University of Kentucky Markey Cancer Center, 800 Rose Street, Markey Cancer Center CC412, Lexington, KY 40536, USA; [c]Associate Professor, Department of Pathology and Laboratory Medicine, University of Kentucky, 800 Rose Street, Lexington, KY 40536, USA

KEYWORDS
• Calreticulin • Janus kinase • *JAK2* • Molecular • Mutations • MPN • *MPL*

KEY POINTS

- Myeloproliferative neoplasms are mainly driven by the driver mutations *JAK2*, *CALR*, and *MPL*, which activate the JAK-STAT pathway.
- More than 50% of myeloproliferative neoplasm patients harbor additional nondriver mutations, which could be associated with increased risk of leukemic transformation and worse survival.
- Nondriver mutations generally effect the genes responsible for epigenetic modulation, spliceosome function, signaling pathways, and transcription regulations.
- Modern prognostic models in myeloproliferative neoplasm incorporate molecular mutations with clinical information to predict survival and the need for allogenic transplantation in primary myelofibrosis.
- The use of high-throughput next-generation sequencing in myeloproliferative neoplasm allows the discovery of new mutations in MPN and the investigation of new therapeutics.

INTRODUCTION

Myeloproliferative neoplasms (MPNs) or disorders are a group of clonal disorders of multipotent hematopoietic progenitors characterized by expansion of the myeloid cell line in the bone marrow and peripheral blood with or without liver and spleen. These disorders have many overlapping clinical, genetic, and molecular features. Under the 2016 World Health Organization classification for tumors of the hematopoietic and lymphoid tissues, MPNs include chronic myeloid leukemia, chronic neutrophilic leukemia, polycythemia vera (PV), primary myelofibrosis (PMF), essential thrombocythemia (ET), chronic eosinophilic leukemia–not otherwise specified, and MPN, unclassifiable [1].

MPNs have multiple overlapping molecular and clinical features. The hallmark of PV is the excessive production of functionally normal red cells blood cells that leads to erythrocytosis. However, given the fact that PV arises from multipotent hematopoietic progenitors, it

*Corresponding author. 800 Rose Street, MS 117 Wm R Willard Med Ed Bldg, Lexington, KY 40536. *E-mail address:* ranjana.arora@uky.edu

https://doi.org/10.1016/j.yamp.2021.06.001
2589-4080/21/

can also lead to leukocytosis, thrombocytosis, and/or splenomegaly [2]. The distinctive clinical feature of ET is thrombocytosis, but can also be accompanied by leukocytosis [3]. PMF causes bone marrow reticulin fibrosis and dysregulated cytokine expression, which leads to constitutional symptoms, extramedullary hematopoiesis, cytopenias, and/or leukocytosis. Despite common presentations, erythrocytosis is only seen in PV [2]. MPNs generally have increased risk of venous and arterial thromboembolism and variably increased risk of transformation to acute myeloid leukemia (AML) [4]. Chronic myeloid leukemia is characterized by the *BCR-ABL1* fusion, and although it is classified as an MPN, the management of chronic myeloid leukemia is completely different from other subtypes of MPNs. For the purposes of this review, we focus on the common MPNs, which include PV, ET, and PMF.

At the molecular level, Philadelphia chromosome-negative MPNs are driven by various molecular mutations that lead to constitutive activation of the JAK-signal transducer and activator of transcription (STAT) signaling pathway. These driver mutations are found in the Janus kinase 2 domain (*JAK2*), calreticulin (*CALR*), and myeloproliferative leukemia virus oncogene (*MPL*) genes [5]. These mutations, which can impact clinical presentation, prognosis and treatment decisions, are generally mutually exclusive; however, rare cases with co-occurrence of more than one of these mutations have been reported [6].

Two types of *JAK2* mutations are seen in MPNs. The most common is *JAK2* p.V617F seen in exon 14 and reported in 95% of PV and 50% to 60% cases of ET and PMF [7,8]. The other type are *JAK2* exon 12 mutations, which have been reported in 2% to 3% patients with PV who lack the *JAK2* p.V617F [9,10]. Mutations of the *CALR* gene in exon 9 have been reported in approximately 20% to 35% of patients with ET and myelofibrosis (MF) [11,12]. Gain-of-function activating mutations in *MPL*, which encodes the cell surface receptor thrombopoietin, are seen in 3% to 8% of patients with ET and PMF [13,14]. Patients with PMF who lack all 3 driver mutations comprise approximately 10% of cases and are referred to as triple negative. These patients often have a worse prognosis than those who have driver gene mutations [15,16].

Advances in the application of high-throughput next-generation sequencing (NGS) has expanded our knowledge of genomic profile of MPNs. More than 50% of these patients harbor additional mutations often associated with disease progression and advanced age [5]. These mutations affect multiple pathways that play a role in regulating DNA methylation, histone modification, messenger RNA (mRNA) splicing, signaling pathways, and transcription factors. Fig. 1 summarizes the suggested algorithm for molecular testing in suspected MPNs [1,17]. In this article, we evaluate the importance of comprehensive molecular profiling, not only for the driver mutations (*JAK2*, *CALR*, and *MPL*) associated with MPNs, but also for other myeloid clones. Regular follow-up for acquired new mutant clones using comprehensive NGS panels in patients showing clinical features of disease progression would better help clinicians in risk assessment and consideration of newer therapeutic agents.

DRIVER MUTATIONS IN MYELOPROLIFERATIVE NEOPLASMS

Janus Kinase 2 Structure and Function

The *JAK2* gene is located on the short arm of chromosome 9 at the band 9p24.1 and was first cloned from a murine hematopoietic cell line by Wilks and colleagues in 1989 [18]. *JAK2* is a member of the Janus kinase family of nonreceptor protein tyrosine kinases, which includes the 4 kinases *JAK1*, *JAK2*, *JAK3*, and TYK2 [19]. Multiple studies demonstrated that *JAK2* is the principal JAK activated in response to type I cytokines including erythropoietin, granulocyte macrophage-colony stimulating factor, and thrombopoietin [19,20].

JAKs have 7 defined regions of homology that have been termed JAK homology (JH) domains (JH1-7). Both the JH1 and JH2 domains are almost identical in amino acid sequence, but have different functions. The JH1 domain is located near the carboxyl terminus of the kinase and incorporates the catalytic activity. The JH2, or the pseudokinase domain, lacks any catalytic activity and acts as a negative kinase regulatory motif [7,19]. In addition, the JH2 domain mediates interaction with STAT family members and the deletion of JH2 domain results in constitutive activation of the kinase [19]. The JH6 and JH7 domains, or the FERM domain, mediate the association of JAK kinases with cytokine receptors.

The JAKs are integral parts of the JAK-STAT signaling pathway. When a type I cytokine binds to its corresponding receptor, a conformational change is induced in the receptor, which leads to receptor dimerization. The JAK2 protein from each individual receptor subsequently phosphorylates the other, activating the kinase pair. The activated kinases phosphorylate tyrosine residues on intracellular domains of the cytokine receptors. STAT transcription factors subsequently bind to the

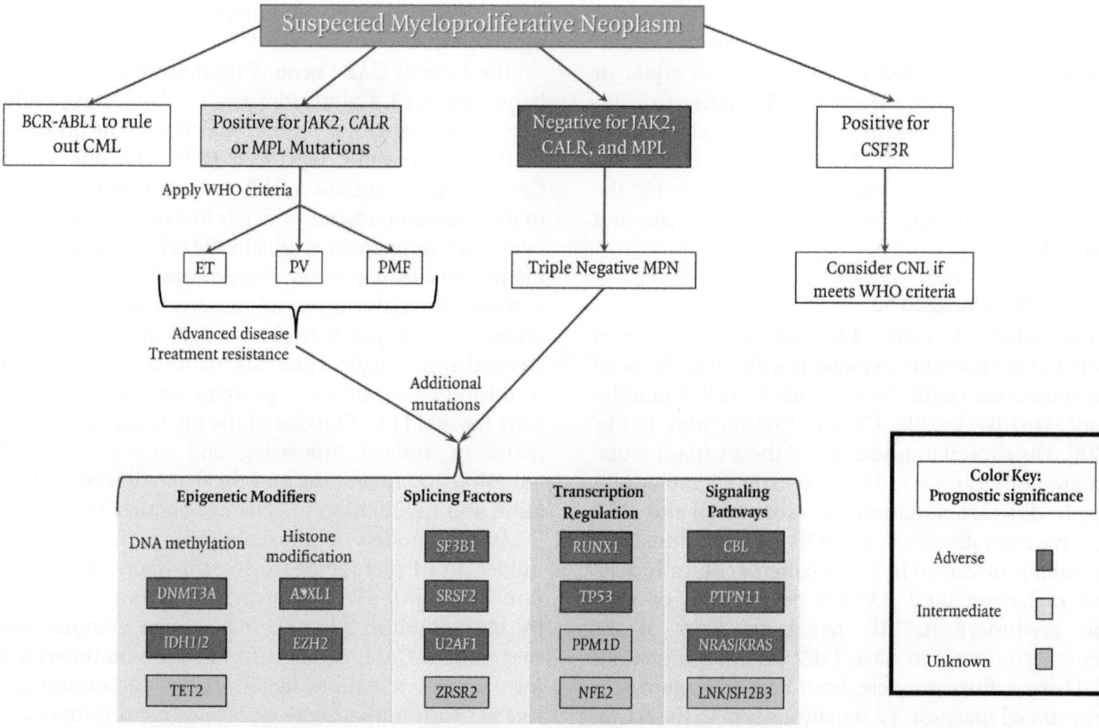

FIG. 1 Suggested molecular testing algorithm for suspected MPNs for diagnosis, prognostic stratification, and in advanced disease or treatment resistance.

cytokine receptor–JAK2 complex, and they are also phosphorylated by activated JAK2. This process activates the STAT factors, which dimerize and enter the nucleus, where they alter the transcription of target genes [7,8].

Chromosomal translocations involving the *JAK2* gene have been implicated in various hematologic malignancies. These rearrangements lead to the formation of a new fusion protein where the JH1 domain is fused to an *N*-terminal domain derived from the partner gene that contains a dimerization or oligomerization domain. These fusion proteins are constitutively activated in the absence of cytokine signaling [21]. Examples of such fusions include *ETV6-JAK2* t(9;12) (p24;p13); *PCM1-JAK2* t(8;9) (p22;p24); and *BCR-JAK* t(9;22) (p24;q11.2) [1].

More important, *JAK2* mutations are implicated in the pathogenesis of *BCR-ABL1* negative MPNs.

JAK2 V617F Mutation

The prototype mutation in the *JAK2* gene is p.V617F, which is caused by a c.1849 G > T missense alteration in exon 14 (JH2 domain) of *JAK2* and was first described in 2005 [22,23]. Earlier work by Kralovics and colleagues [24] demonstrated that approximately one-third of patients with PV had loss of heterozygosity (LOH) on chromosome 9p. In a subsequent study by the same group, microsatellite mapping of the 9p LOH region and DNA sequencing identified the presence of a *JAK2* p.V617F mutation in all patients with MPN with 9p LOH. Patients without the 9p LOH also had the mutation identified, but in smaller frequencies [23]. Several studies strongly implicated the *JAK2* p.V617F in the pathophysiology of MPNs. In these studies, the mutation was found to be heterozygous in most patients, but could be homozygous in a subset because of mitotic recombination of the telomeric region of 9p. Homozygosity was most prevalent in patients with PV relative to those with ET and PMF [25]. At least in PV, homozygosity for the *JAK2* mutation leads to a higher mutation burden favoring erythroid differentiation [8]. Differences in the mutation burden could partly explain the phenotype manifestations of the MPN subtypes [21]. This outcome has been demonstrated in a murine model where mice with expression of *JAK2* p.V617F that was lower than the endogenous wild-type *JAK2* developed an ET phenotype without erythrocytosis. PV phenotypes with and without thrombocytosis were developed in mice that had equal or increased expression of *JAK2* p.V617F relative to wild-type *JAK2*, respectively [26]. A similar correlation was also found in patients with MPN [26]. Other than a correlation of allelic burden with erythrocytosis in PV, the reasons for phenotype variations in MPD are not defined clearly.

Other *JAK2* Mutations

There are other *JAK2* exon 14 mutations that have been reported in the literature in patients with MPN. Some of these mutations could coexist with V617F. Examples include D620E, E627E, C616Y, C618R, and L611V [27,28]. The clinical implications of these variant mutations are not clear. In addition to exon 14 mutations, multiple different mutations in exon 12 of the *JAK2* gene have been described. In 2007, exon 12 mutations were initially described in 3% of patients clinically diagnosed as having *JAK2* p.V617F-negative PV or idiopathic erythrocytosis. The remaining 97% of the patients were found to have *JAK2* p.V617F mutations [10]. Using cellular models, Scott and colleagues [10] demonstrated that exon 12 mutations lead to the activation of erythropoietin signaling pathways, which results in the MPN phenotype. In comparison with *JAK2* p.V617F+ patients with PV, those with exon 12 mutations were younger and had higher hemoglobin levels and lower platelet and leukocyte counts at diagnosis, but had similar incidences of thrombosis, MF, leukemia, and death [10,29]. These results suggest that virtually all patients with PV will have a *JAK2* mutation [8,10]. At least 17 different mutations have been described in the literature with N542_E543del, K539L, and E543_D544del being the most common [29].

CALR

CALR mutations were first identified in 2013 and have been detected in about 70% to 80% of MPN cases with wild-type *JAK2* [11,12]. Since then, at least 50 mutations have been identified in *CALR* gene in patients with MPN. The mechanism of these mutations is the same and involves a frameshift deletion or insertion of nucleotides within exon 9, shifting to the same novel reading frame to generate an abnormal mutant C-terminal amino acid sequence [12]. In about 50% of the cases, the mutation involves a 52-base deletion, which has been termed type I mutation. In another 30% of the cases, the mutation involves a 5-base insertion, which has been termed a type II mutation [11,12]. The remaining mutations can be generally classified based on similarity to either type I like, type II like, or others [30].

The human *CALR* gene is located on chromosome band 19p13.13. Calreticulin is a Ca^{2+}–binding multifunctional chaperone protein that is present primarily in the endoplasmic reticulum (ER). The nonmutant CALR protein contains an ER retention signal (KDEL) in the C-domain region, which is lost in the mutant variants. This differences results in the cells retaining varying amount of negatively charged amino acids. Type I variants eliminate almost all negatively charged amino acids, whereas type II retain one-half of the negatively charged amino acids. These fluctuations in the ER result in misfolded or unfolded proteins with selective cytosolic transfer [11]. Outside of the ER, CALR also participates in antigen processing and presentation, cell adhesion and migration, and the regulation of proliferation and modulation of gene expression [31].

Animal models demonstrated that *CALR* mutations induce an ET phenotype by an *MPL*-dependent activation of the JAK-STAT pathway, which can be blocked by JAK inhibitors [32,33]. It has been demonstrated that mutant CALR proteins form homomultimers and lose the ER retention signal. These homomultimers interact with immature *N*-glycans of the thrombopoietin receptor (TPOR, encoded by *MPL*) in the ER. The mutant CALR–TPOR complex is subsequently transported through the Golgi apparatus to the cell surface, where the mutant CALR leads to constitutive activation of TPOR and downstream signaling through the JAK-STAT pathway [34,35].

MPL

The human *MPL* gene is located on the band 1p34.2, and it encodes TPOR. Similar to the erythropoietin receptor, TPOR is a type I cytokine receptor that signals through the JAK-STAT pathway [36]. Through its interaction with its receptor, thrombopoietin induces megakaryocyte progenitor cell proliferation, megakaryocyte differentiation, and plays a role in hematopoietic stem cell maintenance, as well as platelet aggregation [37]. *MPL* mutations can be detected in approximately 3% of the cases of ET and approximately 10% of PMF [38]. There are multiple *MPL* mutations, but the most common are p.S505N and p.W515L/K in exon 10 of the gene, which result in thrombopoietin-independent signaling [39].

ADDITIONAL MUTATIONS IN MYELOPROLIFERATIVE NEOPLASMS

In addition to driver mutations in *JAK2*, *CALR*, and *MPL*, more than 50% of patients with MPN have other gene mutations. These mutations could provide prognostic and predictive information in MPN [5]. Notable affected genes are involved in epigenetic regulation of DNA methylation (*TET2*, *DNMT3A*, and *IDH1/2*), chromatin structure (*ASXL1* and *EZH2*), mRNA splicing (*SF3B1*, *SRSF2*, and *U2AF1*), signaling pathways (*LNK*, *CBL*, *NRAS/KRAS*, and *PTPN11*), and transcription regulation (*RUNX1*, *TP53*, and *PPM1D*) [12,17].

Genes Involved in Epigenetic Regulation by DNA Methylation

Genes that function in epigenetic regulation through cytosine methylation and histone methylation and acetylation are frequently mutated in hematologic malignancies. One of the most important epigenetic regulators is DNA methyltransferase 3A (*DNMT3A*). The *DNMT3A* gene encodes a DNA methyltransferase that functions as a catalyst in de novo DNA methylation. Somatic mutations in the *DNMT3A* gene generally result in impaired enzymatic methylation activity and can be frameshift, nonsense, or missense mutations, with codon R882 being the most commonly altered residue [17]. *DNMT3A* is commonly altered in clonal hematopoiesis, myelodysplastic syndromes (MDS), and AML [40–42]. Additionally, *DNMT3A* mutations have been detected in approximately 10% of patients with unselected MPN [43]. Interestingly, *DNMT3A* mutations can either precede or follow *JAK2* p.V617F or *MPL* mutation in MPN, and the order of mutation acquisition can influence the MPN phenotype. If *JAK2* p.V617F is acquired before *DNMT3A*, patients are found to more likely present with PV. In contrast, an ET phenotype is more likely if a *DNMT3A* mutation is acquired first [44]. The impact of *DNMT3A* mutations on the prognosis of MPN has been studied, but the data are not very clear. One study in patients with ET and PV found an increased risk of cytopenias after hydroxyurea use as well as decreased survival [45]. Additionally, *DNMT3A* mutations have been found to confer worse outcomes after allogeneic hematopoietic stem cell transplantation in patients with MF [46]. However, a more recent study demonstrated no increased risk of leukemic transformation in patients with MPN [47].

Human *Ten-eleven-translocation* 2 (*TET2*) encodes TET2, 1 of 3 human enzymes (TET1, TET2, and TET3) involved in epigenetic regulation by oxidation of 5-methylcytosine to 5-hydroxymethylcytosine promoting DNA demethylation [48,49]. Similar to *DNMT3A*, *TET2* mutations have been detected in clonal hematopoiesis and hematologic malignancies, and their overall frequency in unselected patients with MPN is approximately 12% to 14% [40,48,49]. The frequency seems to be higher in the *JAK2* p.V617F mutated patients compared with those with wild-type *JAK2* (approximately 17% vs 7%) [49]. *TET2* mutations have not been found to impact thrombotic risk, leukemic transformation risk, or survival of patients with MPN [48]. However, similar to *DNMT3A*, the order of *TET2* and *JAK2* p.V617F mutation acquisition can influence disease phenotype and response to *JAK2* inhibition in vitro. If *JAK2* p.V617F is acquired first, patients are more likely to present with PV and have an increased thrombotic risk. The acquisition of *TET2* before *JAK2* alters the gene transcription affected by *JAK2*. Hematopoietic stem cells obtain a self-renewal advantage and *JAK2*+/*TET2*+ mutant cells expand at the stem cell level [50].

In addition to inactivating *TET2* mutations, functional inhibition of *TET2* in the setting of isocitrate dehydrogenase (*IDH*) mutations has been described [51]. *IDH1/2* are important metabolic enzymes of the Krebs cycle and convert isocitrate to α-ketoglutarate, which in turn acts as a cofactor for TET2. Mutations at the R140 and R172 arginine residues of the *IDH* enzymes results in a neomorphic enzyme activity and production of the abnormal oncometabolite 2-hydroxyglutarate. The latter inhibits α-ketoglutarate–dependent enzymes, including TET dioxygenases, which blocks myeloid cell differentiation leading to leukemic transformation [51,52]. *IDH* mutations are rare in PV, ET, and PMF (approximately 1%–5%), but have increased frequency in blast phase MPN (approximately 20%) and have been associated with increased risk of leukemic transformation, increased risk of relapse after transplantation, and decreased survival [53–56].

Genes Involved in Histone Modification

Additional sex combs-like 1 (*ASXL1*) and enhancer of zeste homolog 2 (*EZH2*) are 2 important genes involved in epigenetic regulation through histone modifications. *ASXL1* regulates transcription through interaction with polycomb repressive complex proteins (PRC1 and 2) and various transcription activators and repressors [57]. PRC2, composed of 4 subunits including EZH2, catalyzes the dimethylation and trimethylation of lysine residue 27 on histone H3 (H3K27me2/3) and represses chromatin. Loss of function of *ASXL1* has been demonstrated to lead to loss of PRC2-mediated trimethylation of histone H3 (H3K27me3) and upregulation of target genes in hematopoietic cells, such as *HOXA*, a well-known leukemogenic focus [58]. Upregulation of *HOXA* has been shown to result from the exclusion of EZH2 from the

PRC2 complex [58]. These results suggest that *ASXL1* is necessary for the ability of EZH2 to occupy the PRC2 complex, which mediates the silencing of *HOXA*. *ASXL1* and *EZH2* mutations are common in hematologic malignancies. In one study, *ASXL1* mutations were mutually exclusive of *JAK2* p.V617F and detected in approximately 3% of ET cases and 30% of PMF cases [59]. Another study detected *ASXL1* mutations in 13% and 18% of PMF and blast phase MPN, respectively [60]. *EZH2* mutations can be detected in about approximately 3% of PV cases and approximately 7% to 13% of those with PMF [60,61]. In PMF, data suggest that both *ASXL1* and *EZH2* mutations precede and synergize to sustain the expansion of driver mutations in the chronic phase and could promote expansion of preleukemic clones [56]. In addition, loss of function of *EZH2* correlates with aberrant erythropoiesis in PMF [56]. *ASXL1* mutations have a significant adverse impact on the prognosis of PMF and could predict an increased leukemic transformation risk and shorter survival, including after transplantation [56,62]. Similarly, *EZH2* mutations have been found to be an independent risk factor for shorter survival in patients with PMF [54].

Genes Involved in Messenger RNA Splicing

The spliceosome is a large RNA–protein complex that is composed of 5 nuclear ribonucleoproteins and numerous other proteins and functions in removing noncoding introns from pre-mRNA [63]. *SF3B1*, *SRSF2*, and *U2AF1* are the most commonly mutated spliceosome genes in hematologic malignancies. These mutations are usually heterozygous and mutually exclusive [64]. The human *SF3B1* gene encodes subunit 1 of the splicing factor 3b protein complex, which is involved in encoding a core component of U2 small nuclear ribonucleoprotein [65]. Animal models and myeloid cell line studies demonstrated that *SF3B1* mutant erythroid progenitors display a G0/G1 cell cycle arrest, resulting in dysfunctional erythroid maturation and proliferation [65,66]. *SF3B1* is the most commonly mutated gene in MDS (>20%) and in a high percentage (approximately 70%) of cases of MDS with ringed sideroblasts [65]. *SF3B1* mutations are uncommon in MPN and can be detected in approximately 3% to 5% of patients with PV or ET and approximately 10% in those with PMF [67]. Patients with ET with *SF3B1* mutations were found to have older age, higher platelets counts, and decreased MF-free survival [68]. Interestingly, a recent study demonstrated that *SF3B1* mutations increase the risk of progression of MPN to fibrotic phase only if the mutation occurred in the driver clones, and not in subclones [67]. In the same study, *SF3B1* mutational status had no impact on overall survival (OS), leukemic transformation, or thrombotic/hemorrhagic event-free survival [67].

Another important splicing factor is serine and arginine rich splicing factor 2 (SRSF2) that belongs to the serine and arginine rich (SR) family of proteins. SRSF2 is involved in transcription elongation and spliceosome assembly at alternate splice sites to allow appropriate exon inclusion [69]. The most common hotspot for *SRSF2* gene mutations is in codon P95, and *SRSF2* mutations occur in approximately 4% to 18% of patients with MDS and approximately 25% to 45% of patients with chronic myelomonocytic leukemia [70]. They are generally rare in PV or ET (<1%), but have been found to be predictive of leukemia-free and MF-free survival in patients with PV [68,71]. The frequency increases to around 18% in patients with PMF and blast phase MPN [71,72]. The mutational status of *SRSF2* has been found to be predictive of leukemic transformation and worse leukemia-free and OS in PMF [54,73]. Additionally, it has been demonstrated that the presence of *SRSF2* mutations at first presentation of MPN is an independent risk factor for rapid blast phase transformation [47]. *SRSF2* mutations are also predictive of worse survival for patients with leukemic transformation of MPN [74].

U2 auxiliary factor (U2AF) complex is a non–small nuclear ribonucleoprotein protein required for binding U2 small nuclear ribonucleoprotein to the pre-mRNA branch site and is involved in the recognition of the 3′ splice site [75]. Somatic mutations in *U2AF1* can be identified in about 12% of patients with MDS [64]. *U2AF1* mutations generally affect either the S34 or the Q157 codons within the first and second CCCH-type zinc fingers of the protein [64]. Similar to *SRSF2*, mutations in *U2AF1* are rare in ET and PV and occur in about 9% to 16% of patients with PMF [68,71,72]. The presence of *U2AF1* mutations is predictive of anemia and thrombocytopenia in patients with PMF and inferior MF-free survival in patients with ET [64,68,72,76,77]. Additionally, the mutational status of *U2AF1* is also an important predictor of OS in patients with PMF. Those with the *U2AF1* p.Q157 variants have inferior survival compared with patients with *U2AF1* p.S34 variants or wild-type *U2AF1* [64]. Additionally, *U2AF1* mutations are predictive of inferior survival after transplantation [46]. Similar to *SRSF2*, *U2AF1* mutation at first presentation of MPN is an independent risk factor for rapid blast phase transformation [47].

Genes Involved in Signaling Pathways

Multiple genes control signaling pathways that are mutated in MPNs; the most notable are *CBL*, *NRAS/KRAS*, and *PTPN11*. The Casitas B-lineage lymphoma (*CBL*) gene encodes an E3 ubiquitin–protein ligase that is involved in numerous processes including down-regulation of activated tyrosine kinases by ubiquitination, including JAK/STAT and TPOR. Hematopoietic cells with a *CBL* mutation have decreased ubiquitination activity, leading to prolonged activation of tyrosine kinases after cytokine stimulation [78]. CBL mutations are not frequent in MPN and have been detected in approximately 5% of patients with PMF or blast phase MPN [72,79,80]. Research demonstrated that *CBL* mutations independently predict a decreased response to *JAK* inhibitors, increased risk of leukemic transformation, and decreased survival [80].

The RAS/mitogen-activated protein (MAP) kinase pathway is a serine/threonine-specific protein kinase that regulates numerous cellular processes including proliferation, differentiation and tissue development. Ras G-proteins, which regulate the MAP kinase pathways, are mutated in approximately 30% of all human cancers [81]. *KRAS/NRAS* mutations can be detected in close to 5% of patients with PMF or after ET or after PV MF and about 15% of those with blast phase MPN [79,82]. In patients with PMF, mutations involving the RAS pathway have been found to be associated with monocytosis, leukocytosis, thrombocytopenia, higher bone marrow blasts, a very high risk karyotype, and inferior OS [82–84]. Another important regulator of the MAP kinase pathway is protein–tyrosine phosphatase nonreceptor type 11 (*PTPN11*), also known as Src homology region 2 domain-containing phosphatase-2 (*SHP-2*). *PTPN11* is required for the activation of the RAS/MAP kinase cascade induced by various growth factors and is also a negative regulator of JAK/STAT signaling. *PTPN11* mutations are rare in MPN, and can be detected in about approximately 1% of PMF cases [82]. The rate of these mutations seems to be higher in blast phase MPN (approximately 8%) and are associated with inferior survival [79].

Genes Involved in Transcription Regulation

Notable genes regulating transcription that are involved in MPN and associated with inferior outcomes include RUNT-related transcription factor 1 (*RUNX1*) and *TP53*. *RUNX1*, also known as AML 1 protein (*AML1*) or core-binding factor subunit alpha-2 (*CBFA2*), is a member of the core-binding factor family of transcription factors that regulates numerous genes involved in hematopoietic differentiation [85]. Germline *RUNX1* mutations cause familial platelet disorder with a predisposition to AML (FPD/AML), whereas somatic mutations and rearrangements are commonly found in MDS and AML [1]. *RUNX1* mutations can be detected in less than 5% of PMF cases and about 15% in blast phase MPN and have been implicated in leukemic transformation and worse outcomes in patients with blast phase MPN [72,79,84,86]. Tumor protein p53 is a tumor-suppressor protein encoded by the *TP53* gene located on the short arm of chromosome 17 (17p13.1). *TP53* maintains genomic stability and activates DNA repair mechanisms in response to DNA damage. Mutations in *TP53* are common in all types of cancers and could mediate resistance to DNA-damaging chemotherapeutic agents [87]. Similar to *RUNX1*, *TP53* mutations can be detected in less than 5% of cases of chronic MPN and around 15% in blast phase MPN, and have been demonstrated to increase risk of leukemic transformation and worsen survival [68,72,79,88].

CLINICAL APPLICATIONS OF NEXT-GENERATION SEQUENCING IN MYELOPROLIFERATIVE NEOPLASMS

Mutational Allele Burden in Myeloproliferative Neoplasms

High-throughput NGS has allowed the incorporation of molecular mutations in the prognostication of patients with MPNs. NGS allows the simultaneous screening for mutations in all the myeloid genes commonly mutated in MPN. The identification of these mutations could help in risk stratification, monitoring response to therapy, predicting risk of leukemic or fibrotic transformation, and consideration of newer therapeutic agents. NGS does not merely identify mutations; it also provides a rough estimate of the allele burden of those mutations. As explained elsewhere in this article, the mutational burden of *JAK2* influences the phenotype of MPN. In addition, NGS may also predict the course of the disease. In patients with PV, *JAK2* p.V617F higher mutational allele burden (MAB) of greater than 50% has been correlated with increasing hematocrit, hemoglobin, white cell counts, bone marrow cellularity, and spleen size; and could be predictive of post-PV MF development [45,89,90]. Additionally, a very high MAB (>75%) at time of diagnosis is strongly correlated with major cardiovascular events [91]. Similarly, higher MAB of *JAK2* p.V617F in patients with ET could predict a higher red blood cell count, neutrophil count, organomegaly, and an increased risk of thrombotic complications and fibrotic transformation [45,89,92,93]. Additionally, in both PV and ET, *JAK2* p.V617F MAB between 26% and 50% and greater than 50% were the strongest independent predictors of subsequent vascular events, regardless of other factors or subtype of MPN [94]. A variant allele frequency of *JAK2* p.V617F of more than 50% in patients diagnosed clinically with ET has been strongly correlated with a diagnosis of prefibrotic PMF rather than ET [92]. In contrast, a low *JAK2* MAB in patients with PMF (<25%) is predictive of a myelodepletive rather than myeloproliferative phenotype and has been found to be an independent factor associated with inferior survival [95]. Finally, serial NGS monitoring of variant allele frequency in patients with MPD can identify clonal expansion of somatic mutations associated with leukemic transformation, such as *TP53* [96]. The serial monitoring of mutations is also important after transplantation in MF, because patients who fail to clear their mutations at day +100 or at day +180 after allogenic transplant are at higher risk of relapse [97].

TABLE 1
MIPSS for OS in patients with ET (MIPSS-ET) and PV (MIPSS-PV)

MIPS-ET		MIPSS-PV	
Risk Factor	**Points**	**Risk Factor**	**Points**
Adverse mutations (*SRSF2*, *SF3B1*, *U2AF1* and *TP53*)	2	*SRSF2* mutation	2
Age >60	3	Abnormal karyotype	1
Male sex	1	Age >67	3
		Leukocytosis ≥15,000/μL	2
Risk Groups (Median OS)	**Points**	**Risk Groups (Median OS)**	**Points**
Low (34.4 y)	0–1	Low (not reached)	0–1
Intermediate (14.1 y)	2–3	Intermediate (10.3 y)	2–4
High (8.3 y)	≥4	High (4.6 y)	≥5

Incorporation of Next-generation Sequencing in Prognostic Scores

The use of NGS has been applied to incorporate molecular information with clinical and cytogenetic data in prognostication of MPNs. Historically, survival prediction in patients with PV or ET has been based only on clinical factors. In a large recent multi-institutional study, Tefferi and colleagues [98] identified molecular prognostic information in PV and ET. The most common nondriver mutations in ET were *ASXL1* (20%), *TET2* (11%), *DNMT3A* (7%), and *SF3B1* (5%). In PV, the most frequent were *TET2* (18%), *ASXL1* (15%), and *SH2B3* (3%). Multivariate analyses identified adverse mutations in each MPN subcategory. In PV, *SRSF2* mutations were found in 2% of cases and was predictive of inferior OS. In ET, *SF3B1* and *SRSF2*, *U2AF1* and *SF3B1*, and *TP53* mutations were predictive of worse OS, MF-free survival, and leukemic transformation, respectively. The frequency of these 4 adverse mutations (*SF3B1*, *SRSF2*, *U2AF1*, and *TP53)* in ET was 10%. The incorporation of these adverse molecular mutations with clinical risk factors allowed the development of validated 3-tiered mutation-enhanced international prognostic systems (MIPSS) in both subtypes of MPN (Table 1) [98].

For patients with PMF, multiple prognostic systems can help to predict outcomes and the need for allogenic transplantation. The most widely used scores are (1) the genetically inspired prognostic scoring system (GIPSS), which is exclusively based on genetic markers, and (2) the MIPSS70+ Version 2 (revised mutation- and karyotype-enhanced international prognostic scoring system for transplant-age patients), which combines genetic and clinical information [99,100]. In the GIPSS score, adverse outcomes predictive of inferior OS are unfavorable or high-risk karyotype, absence of type I-like *CALR* mutations, and the presence of high-risk somatic mutations (*ASXL1*, *SRSF2*, and *U2AF1* Q157). The incorporation of this information allowed the development of a 4-tiered prognostic score (low, intermediate-1, intermediate-2, and high risk) with a 5-year OS ranging from 94% with zero points to 14% in patients with 3 or more points [99]. In the MIPSS-70+ v2.0, the score incorporates the severity of anemia, the presence of constitutional symptoms, and the presence of circulating blasts with the karyotype and molecular information. The score divides patients into 5 tiers from very low to very high risk for mortality, with the 10-year OS rates ranging from 86% to less than 3% [100]. In general, patients with a high-risk GIPSS score (>2) and/or MIPSS70+ v.2.0 (>4) should be evaluated for allogenic transplantation [101]. The 2 prognostic models are summarized in Table 2.

TABLE 2
GIPSS and MIPSS70+ v2.0 Scores for Predicting OS in MF

GIPSS		MIPSS70+ v.2.0	
Risk Factor	**Points**	**Risk Factor**	**Points**
VHR karyotype[a]	2	Constitutional symptoms	2
Unfavorable karyotype[a]	1	Hemoglobin <9 g/dL in men or <8 g/dL in women	2
Absent type I-like CALR	1	Hemoglobin 9.0–10.9 g/dL in men or 8.0–9.9 g dL in women	1
ASXL1	1	Circulating blasts ≥2%	1
SRSF2	1	VHR karyotype[a]	4
U2AF1 Q157	1	Unfavorable karyotype[a]	3
		>1 High-risk mutation[b]	3
		1 High-risk mutation[b]	2
		Absent type I-like CALR	2
Risk Groups (5-y OS)	**Points**	**Risk Groups (10-y OS)**	**Points**
Low (94%)	0	Very low (86%)	0
Intermediate-1 (73%)	1	Low (50%)	1–2
Intermediate-2 (40%)	2	Intermediate (30%)	3–4
High (14%)	≥3	High (10%)	5–8
		Very high (<3%)	≥9

[a] Cytogenetic classification: very high risk (VHR), single or multiple abnormalities of−7, i(17q), inv(3)/3q21, 12p−/12p11.2, 11q−/11q23,+21, or other autosomal trisomies, not including +8/+9 (eg, +21 or +19). Favorable, a normal karyotype or sole abnormalities of 13q−, +9, 20q− chromosome 1 translocation or duplication or sex chromosome abnormality including Y. Unfavorable, all other abnormalities.
[b] High-risk mutations in MIPSS70+ v.2.0 include *ASXL1*, *EZH2*, *IDH1/2*, *SRSF2*, and *U2AF1* Q157.

Therapeutic Targets

Given that the common driver mutations in MPN activate the JAK-STAT pathway, JAK1/2 inhibition has been thoroughly investigated in MPN with 2 JAK inhibitors currently approved by the US Food and Drug Administration. The first one is ruxolitinib, which targets both JAK1 and JAK2. The approval was based on the COMFORT studies. In COMFORT-I, patients with intermediate-2 or high-risk MF were randomly assigned to ruxolitinib or placebo. The primary end point was the proportion of patients with a decreased in spleen volume at 24 weeks and was reached in approximately 42% of patients in the ruxolitinib group. The response was maintained for 48 weeks or more in two-thirds of patients. In addition, 46% of patients who received ruxolitinib had a decrease in symptom burden [102]. Significant and prolonged decreases in spleen volume and symptom burden were confirmed in the COMFORT-II study [103]. Additionally, long-term follow-up demonstrated a one-third decrease in the risk of death with ruxolitinib [104]. The RESPONSE study investigated ruxolitinib in patients with PV resistant to hydroxyurea. Patients were randomized to receive either ruxolitinib or a standard therapy. When compared with standard therapy, ruxolitinib improved phlebotomy independence and spleen size reduction; achieved better control of PV symptoms such as fatigue, pruritus, and night sweats; and resulted in fewer thromboembolic events. However, ruxolitinib also increased rates of herpes zoster infection and nonmelanoma skin cancer [105,106]. Given that ruxolitinib targets both JAK1 and JAK2, its activity is independent of *JAK2* mutation [17]. Fedratinib is a selective JAK2 inhibitor and is the second drug approved by the US Food and Drug Administration for the treatment of MF. This finding was based on a placebo-controlled randomized phase II trial in patients with intermediate-2 or high-risk primary PMF, post-PV MF, or post-ET MF. Fedratinib therapy significantly decreased splenomegaly and symptom burden [107]. Other JAK1/2 inhibitors currently under clinical investigation include momelotinib and pacritinib [108,109]. Although JAK2 inhibition can decrease MAB in patients with MPN, the clinical significance of this decrease is unclear [110]. Given the frequent abnormalities in epigenetic modulation in patients with MPN, combining JAK inhibitors with DNA methyltransferase and histone deacetylase inhibitors has been investigated. The addition of azacitidine to ruxolitinib in patients with MF showed promising responses. The overall response rate was 72%, with one-fourth of the responses occurring after the addition of azacitidine. A 50% decrease in spleen size was achieved in 71% of the patients and was maintained in 95% of patients at 48 weeks. Treatment also led to improvements in bone marrow reticulin fibrosis grade in more than one-half of the patients [111]. The combination of ruxolitinib and the histone deacetylase inhibitor is being investigated and can lead to a decrease in spleen size and an improvement in bone marrow fibrosis [112].

Other therapeutic strategies targeting molecular mutations are also under investigation. Mouse models demonstrated that *JAK2* p.V617F and *IDH2* p.R140Q mutant MPNs were sensitive to small molecule inhibition of *IDH*. Combined *JAK2* and *IDH2* inhibitor treatment normalized the stem and progenitor cell compartments in a murine model and decreased disease burden to a greater extent than was seen with *JAK* inhibition alone [55]. Treatment of *IDH2*-mutant accelerated/blast phase MPN with enasidenib was studied retrospectively in 8 patients [113]. The overall response rate was 37.5% with the 2017 European LeukemiaNet criteria and 75% with 2012 MPN in blast phase criteria. The median OS for all 8 patients was not reached with a median follow-up time of approximately 9 months.

There are numerous other therapeutic strategies currently under investigation including combination therapy with ruxolitinib and poly-ADP-ribose polymerase inhibition and bromodomain and extraterminal inhibition, protein arginine methyltransferase 5 inhibition, and human double minute 2 inhibition. These strategies are reviewed elsewhere, including by Li and colleagues [114].

SUMMARY

Although MPNs are commonly driven by *JAK2*, *CALR*, or *MPL*, deep targeted sequencing has allowed us better to understand the pathophysiology and prognosis of MPN. Approximately one-half of the patients with MPN will display mutations in genes that control epigenetic modulation, spliceosome function and assembly, signal transduction, and/or transcription regulation. Some of these mutations increase the risk of leukemic or fibrotic transformation and/or death, including after transplantation. Recent research has validated enhanced international prognostic scoring systems that incorporate molecular mutations in each subtype of MPN [98–100]. These prognostic models can predict the survival outcomes and help to identify patients who could benefit from allogeneic transplantation. Therefore, NGS should be used routinely in the management of patients with MPN. Although JAK inhibitors improve the symptom burden in patients with MF, they might not change the disease course. Future research will allow us to identify appropriate molecular markers for targeted therapies.

DISCLOSURE

No conflicts. The authors have nothing to disclose.

ACKNOWLEDGMENTS

The authors thank Heather N. Russell-Simmons, MA, MBA, for her efforts in editing this article.

REFERENCES

[1] Arber DA, Orazi A, Hasserjian R, et al. The 2016 revision to the World Health Organization classification of myeloid neoplasms and acute leukemia. Blood 2016;127(20):2391–405. https://doi.org/10.1182/blood-2016-03-643544.

[2] Spivak JL. How I treat polycythemia vera. Blood 2019;134(4):341–52. https://doi.org/10.1182/blood.2018834044.

[3] Tefferi A, Pardanani A. Essential thrombocythemia. N Engl J Med 2019;381(22):2135–44. https://doi.org/10.1056/NEJMcp1816082.

[4] Arachchillage DR, Laffan M. Pathogenesis and management of thrombotic disease in myeloproliferative neoplasms. Semin Thromb Hemost 2019;45(6):604–11. https://doi.org/10.1055/s-0039-1693477.

[5] Grinfeld J, Nangalia J, Baxter EJ, et al. Classification and personalized prognosis in myeloproliferative neoplasms. N Engl J Med 2018;379(15):1416–30. https://doi.org/10.1056/NEJMoa1716614.

[6] Zamora L, Xicoy B, Cabezon M, et al. Co-existence of JAK2 V617F and CALR mutations in primary myelofibrosis. Leuk Lymphoma 2015;56(10):2973–4. https://doi.org/10.3109/10428194.2015.1015124.

[7] Smith CA, Fan G. The saga of JAK2 mutations and translocations in hematologic disorders: pathogenesis, diagnostic and therapeutic prospects, and revised World Health Organization diagnostic criteria for myeloproliferative neoplasms. Hum Pathol 2008;39(6):795–810. https://doi.org/10.1016/j.humpath.2008.02.004.

[8] Tefferi A. JAK and MPL mutations in myeloid malignancies. Leuk Lymphoma 2008;49(3):388–97. https://doi.org/10.1080/10428190801895360.

[9] Pietra D, Li S, Brisci A, et al. Somatic mutations of JAK2 exon 12 in patients with JAK2 (V617F)-negative myeloproliferative disorders. *Blood*. 2008;111(3):1686–9. https://doi.org/10.1182/blood-2007-07-101576.

[10] Scott LM, Tong W, Levine RL, et al. JAK2 exon 12 mutations in polycythemia vera and idiopathic

erythrocytosis. N Engl J Med 2007;356(5):459–68. https://doi.org/10.1056/NEJMoa065202.

[11] Klampfl T, Gisslinger H, Harutyunyan AS, et al. Somatic mutations of calreticulin in myeloproliferative neoplasms. N Engl J Med 2013;369(25):2379–90. https://doi.org/10.1056/NEJMoa1311347.

[12] Nangalia J, Massie CE, Baxter EJ, et al. Somatic CALR mutations in myeloproliferative neoplasms with nonmutated JAK2. N Engl J Med 2013;369(25):2391–405. https://doi.org/10.1056/NEJMoa1312542.

[13] Beer PA, Campbell PJ, Scott LM, et al. MPL mutations in myeloproliferative disorders: analysis of the PT-1 cohort. Blood 2008;112(1):141–9. https://doi.org/10.1182/blood-2008-01-131664.

[14] Pardanani AD, Levine RL, Lasho T, et al. MPL515 mutations in myeloproliferative and other myeloid disorders: a study of 1182 patients. *Blood.* 2006;108(10):3472–6. https://doi.org/10.1182/blood-2006-04-018879.

[15] Milosevic Feenstra JD, Nivarthi H, Gisslinger H, et al. Whole-exome sequencing identifies novel MPL and JAK2 mutations in triple-negative myeloproliferative neoplasms. Blood 2016;127(3):325–32. https://doi.org/10.1182/blood-2015-07-661835.

[16] Tefferi A, Lasho TL, Finke CM, et al. CALR vs JAK2 vs MPL-mutated or triple-negative myelofibrosis: clinical, cytogenetic and molecular comparisons. Leukemia 2014;28(7):1472–7. https://doi.org/10.1038/leu.2014.3.

[17] Loscocco GG, Guglielmelli P, Vannucchi AM. Impact of mutational profile on the management of myeloproliferative neoplasms: a short review of the emerging data. Onco Targets Ther 2020;13:12367–82. https://doi.org/10.2147/OTT.S287944.

[18] Wilks AF, Harpur AG, Kurban RR, et al. Two novel protein-tyrosine kinases, each with a second phosphotransferase-related catalytic domain, define a new class of protein kinase. Mol Cell Biol 1991;11(4):2057–65. https://doi.org/10.1128/mcb.11.4.2057.

[19] Vainchenker W, Dusa A, Constantinescu SN. JAKs in pathology: role of Janus kinases in hematopoietic malignancies and immunodeficiencies. Semin Cell Dev Biol 2008;19(4):385–93. https://doi.org/10.1016/j.semcdb.2008.07.002.

[20] Silvennoinen O, Witthuhn BA, Quelle FW, et al. Structure of the murine Jak2 protein-tyrosine kinase and its role in interleukin 3 signal transduction. Proc Natl Acad Sci U S A 1993;90(18):8429–33. https://doi.org/10.1073/pnas.90.18.8429.

[21] Ihle JN, Gilliland DG. Jak2: normal function and role in hematopoietic disorders. Curr Opin Genet Dev 2007;17(1):8–14. https://doi.org/10.1016/j.gde.2006.12.009.

[22] Baxter EJ, Scott LM, Campbell PJ, et al. Acquired mutation of the tyrosine kinase JAK2 in human myeloproliferative disorders. Lancet 2005;365(9464):1054–61. https://doi.org/10.1016/S0140-6736(05)71142-9.

[23] Kralovics R, Passamonti F, Buser AS, et al. A gain-of-function mutation of JAK2 in myeloproliferative disorders. N Engl J Med 2005;352(17):1779–90. https://doi.org/10.1056/NEJMoa051113.

[24] Kralovics R, Guan Y, Prchal JT. Acquired uniparental disomy of chromosome 9p is a frequent stem cell defect in polycythemia vera. Exp Hematol 2002;30(3):229–36. https://doi.org/10.1016/s0301-472x(01)00789-5.

[25] Kralovics R, Buser AS, Teo SS, et al. Comparison of molecular markers in a cohort of patients with chronic myeloproliferative disorders. *Blood.* 2003;102(5):1869–71. https://doi.org/10.1182/blood-2003-03-0744.

[26] Tiedt R, Hao-Shen H, Sobas MA, et al. Ratio of mutant JAK2-V617F to wild-type Jak2 determines the MPD phenotypes in transgenic mice. *Blood.* 2008;111(8):3931–40. https://doi.org/10.1182/blood-2007-08-107748.

[27] Schnittger S, Bacher U, Kern W, et al. Report on two novel nucleotide exchanges in the JAK2 pseudokinase domain: D620E and E627E. Leukemia 2006;20(12):2195–7. https://doi.org/10.1038/sj.leu.2404325.

[28] Cleyrat C, Jelinek J, Girodon F, et al. JAK2 mutation and disease phenotype: a double L611V/V617F in cis mutation of JAK2 is associated with isolated erythrocytosis and increased activation of AKT and ERK1/2 rather than STAT5. Leukemia 2010;24(5):1069–73. https://doi.org/10.1038/leu.2010.23.

[29] Passamonti F, Elena C, Schnittger S, et al. Molecular and clinical features of the myeloproliferative neoplasm associated with JAK2 exon 12 mutations. *Blood.* 2011;117(10):2813–6. https://doi.org/10.1182/blood-2010-11-316810.

[30] Pietra D, Rumi E, Ferretti VV, et al. Differential clinical effects of different mutation subtypes in CALR-mutant myeloproliferative neoplasms. Leukemia 2016;30(2):431–8. https://doi.org/10.1038/leu.2015.277.

[31] Merlinsky TR, Levine RL, Pronier E. Unfolding the role of calreticulin in myeloproliferative neoplasm pathogenesis. Clin Cancer Res 2019;25(10):2956–62. https://doi.org/10.1158/1078-0432.CCR-18-3777.

[32] Lim KH, Chang YC, Chiang YH, et al. Expression of CALR mutants causes mpl-dependent thrombocytosis in zebrafish. Blood Cancer J 2016;6(10):e481. https://doi.org/10.1038/bcj.2016.83.

[33] Shide K, Kameda T, Yamaji T, et al. Calreticulin mutant mice develop essential thrombocythemia that is ameliorated by the JAK inhibitor ruxolitinib. Leukemia 2017;31(5):1136–44. https://doi.org/10.1038/leu.2016.308.

[34] Araki M, Komatsu N. The role of calreticulin mutations in myeloproliferative neoplasms. Int J Hematol 2020;111(2):200–5. https://doi.org/10.1007/s12185-019-02800-0.

[35] Araki M, Yang Y, Imai M, et al. Homomultimerization of mutant calreticulin is a prerequisite for MPL binding and activation. Leukemia 2019;33(1):122–31. https://doi.org/10.1038/s41375-018-0181-2.

[36] Drachman JG, Griffin JD, Kaushansky K. The c-Mpl ligand (thrombopoietin) stimulates tyrosine phosphorylation of Jak2, Shc, and c-Mpl. J Biol Chem 1995;

270(10):4979–82. https://doi.org/10.1074/jbc.270.10.4979.

[37] Hitchcock IS, Kaushansky K. Thrombopoietin from beginning to end. Br J Haematol 2014;165(2):259–68. https://doi.org/10.1111/bjh.12772.

[38] Tefferi A. Primary myelofibrosis: 2019 update on diagnosis, risk-stratification and management. Am J Hematol 2018;93(12):1551–60. https://doi.org/10.1002/ajh.25230.

[39] Vainchenker W, Plo I, Marty C, et al. The role of the thrombopoietin receptor MPL in myeloproliferative neoplasms: recent findings and potential therapeutic applications. Expert Rev Hematol 2019;12(6):437–48. https://doi.org/10.1080/17474086.2019.1617129.

[40] Jaiswal S, Fontanillas P, Flannick J, et al. Age-related clonal hematopoiesis associated with adverse outcomes. N Engl J Med 2014;371(26):2488–98. https://doi.org/10.1056/NEJMoa1408617.

[41] Ley TJ, Ding L, Walter MJ, et al. DNMT3A mutations in acute myeloid leukemia. N Engl J Med 2010;363(25):2424–33. https://doi.org/10.1056/NEJMoa1005143.

[42] Walter MJ, Ding L, Shen D, et al. Recurrent DNMT3A mutations in patients with myelodysplastic syndromes. Leukemia 2011;25(7):1153–8. https://doi.org/10.1038/leu.2011.44.

[43] Stegelmann F, Bullinger L, Schlenk RF, et al. DNMT3A mutations in myeloproliferative neoplasms. Leukemia 2011;25(7):1217–9. https://doi.org/10.1038/leu.2011.77.

[44] Nangalia J, Nice FL, Wedge DC, et al. DNMT3A mutations occur early or late in patients with myeloproliferative neoplasms and mutation order influences phenotype. Haematologica 2015;100(11):e438–42. https://doi.org/10.3324/haematol.2015.129510.

[45] Senín A, Fernández-Rodríguez C, Bellosillo B, et al. Non-driver mutations in patients with JAK2V617F-mutated polycythemia vera or essential thrombocythemia with long-term molecular follow-up. Ann Hematol 2018;97(3):443–51. https://doi.org/10.1007/s00277-017-3193-5.

[46] Tamari R, Rapaport F, Zhang N, et al. Impact of high-molecular-risk mutations on transplantation outcomes in patients with myelofibrosis. Biol Blood Marrow Transplant 2019;25(6):1142–51. https://doi.org/10.1016/j.bbmt.2019.01.002.

[47] Bartels S, Vogtmann J, Schipper E, et al. Combination of myeloproliferative neoplasm driver gene activation with mutations of splice factor or epigenetic modifier genes increases risk of rapid blastic progression. Eur J Haematol 2021. https://doi.org/10.1111/ejh.13579.

[48] Tefferi A. Novel mutations and their functional and clinical relevance in myeloproliferative neoplasms: JAK2, MPL, TET2, ASXL1, CBL, IDH and IKZF1. Leukemia 2010;24(6):1128–38. https://doi.org/10.1038/leu.2010.69.

[49] Tefferi A, Pardanani A, Lim KH, et al. TET2 mutations and their clinical correlates in polycythemia vera, essential thrombocythemia and myelofibrosis. Leukemia 2009;23(5):905–11. https://doi.org/10.1038/leu.2009.47.

[50] Ortmann CA, Kent DG, Nangalia J, et al. Effect of mutation order on myeloproliferative neoplasms. N Engl J Med 2015;372(7):601–12. https://doi.org/10.1056/NEJMoa1412098.

[51] Haladyna JN, Yamauchi T, Neff T, et al. Epigenetic modifiers in normal and malignant hematopoiesis. Epigenomics 2015;7(2):301–20. https://doi.org/10.2217/epi.14.88.

[52] Losman JA, Looper RE, Koivunen P, et al. (R)-2-hydroxyglutarate is sufficient to promote leukemogenesis and its effects are reversible. Science 2013;339(6127):1621–5. https://doi.org/10.1126/science.1231677.

[53] Tefferi A, Lasho TL, Abdel-Wahab O, et al. IDH1 and IDH2 mutation studies in 1473 patients with chronic-, fibrotic- or blast-phase essential thrombocythemia, polycythemia vera or myelofibrosis. Leukemia 2010;24(7):1302–9. https://doi.org/10.1038/leu.2010.113.

[54] Vannucchi AM, Lasho TL, Guglielmelli P, et al. Mutations and prognosis in primary myelofibrosis. Leukemia 2013;27(9):1861–9. https://doi.org/10.1038/leu.2013.119.

[55] McKenney AS, Lau AN, Somasundara AVH, et al. JAK2/IDH-mutant-driven myeloproliferative neoplasm is sensitive to combined targeted inhibition. J Clin Invest 2018;128(2):789–804. https://doi.org/10.1172/JCI94516.

[56] Kröger N, Panagiota V, Badbaran A, et al. Impact of molecular genetics on outcome in myelofibrosis patients after allogeneic stem cell transplantation. Biol Blood Marrow Transplant 2017;23(7):1095–101. https://doi.org/10.1016/j.bbmt.2017.03.034.

[57] Gelsi-Boyer V, Brecqueville M, Devillier R, et al. Mutations in ASXL1 are associated with poor prognosis across the spectrum of malignant myeloid diseases. J Hematol Oncol 2012;5:12. https://doi.org/10.1186/1756-8722-5-12.

[58] Abdel-Wahab O, Adli M, LaFave LM, et al. ASXL1 mutations promote myeloid transformation through loss of PRC2-mediated gene repression. Cancer Cell 2012;22(2):180–93. https://doi.org/10.1016/j.ccr.2012.06.032.

[59] Carbuccia N, Murati A, Trouplin V, et al. Mutations of ASXL1 gene in myeloproliferative neoplasms. Leukemia 2009;23(11):2183–6. https://doi.org/10.1038/leu.2009.141.

[60] Abdel-Wahab O, Pardanani A, Patel J, et al. Concomitant analysis of EZH2 and ASXL1 mutations in myelofibrosis, chronic myelomonocytic leukemia and blast-phase myeloproliferative neoplasms. Leukemia 2011;25(7):1200–2. https://doi.org/10.1038/leu.2011.58.

[61] Ernst T, Chase AJ, Score J, et al. Inactivating mutations of the histone methyltransferase gene EZH2 in myeloid disorders. Nat Genet 2010;42(8):722–6. https://doi.org/10.1038/ng.621.

[62] Wang Z, Liu W, Wang M, et al. Prognostic value of ASXL1 mutations in patients with primary myelofibrosis and its relationship with clinical features: a

meta-analysis. Ann Hematol 2021;100(2):465–79. https://doi.org/10.1007/s00277-020-04387-7.

[63] Will CL, Lührmann R. Spliceosome structure and function. Cold Spring Harb Perspect Biol 2011;3(7). https://doi.org/10.1101/cshperspect.a003707.

[64] Tefferi A, Finke CM, Lasho TL, et al. U2AF1 mutation types in primary myelofibrosis: phenotypic and prognostic distinctions. Leukemia 2018;32(10):2274–8. https://doi.org/10.1038/s41375-018-0078-0.

[65] Dolatshad H, Pellagatti A, Fernandez-Mercado M, et al. Disruption of SF3B1 results in deregulated expression and splicing of key genes and pathways in myelodysplastic syndrome hematopoietic stem and progenitor cells. Leukemia 2015;29(5):1092–103. https://doi.org/10.1038/leu.2014.331.

[66] De La Garza A, Cameron RC, Gupta V, et al. The splicing factor Sf3b1 regulates erythroid maturation and proliferation via TGFβ signaling in zebrafish. Blood Adv 2019;3(14):2093–104. https://doi.org/10.1182/bloodadvances.2018027714.

[67] Zhao L-P, De Oliveira RD, Marcault C, et al. SF3B1 mutations in the driver clone increase the risk of evolution to myelofibrosis in patients with myeloproliferative neoplasms (MPN). Blood 2020;136(Supplement 1). https://doi.org/10.1182/blood-2020-141296.

[68] Tefferi A, Lasho TL, Guglielmelli P, et al. Targeted deep sequencing in polycythemia vera and essential thrombocythemia. Blood Adv 2016;1(1):21–30. https://doi.org/10.1182/bloodadvances.2016000216.

[69] Aujla A, Linder K, Iragavarapu C, et al. SRSF2 mutations in myelodysplasia/myeloproliferative neoplasms. Biomark Res 2018;6:29. https://doi.org/10.1186/s40364-018-0142-y.

[70] Arbab Jafari P, Ayatollahi H, Sadeghi R, et al. Prognostic significance of SRSF2 mutations in myelodysplastic syndromes and chronic myelomonocytic leukemia: a meta-analysis. Hematology 2018;23(10):778–84. https://doi.org/10.1080/10245332.2018.1471794.

[71] Song J, Hussaini M, Zhang H, et al. Comparison of the mutational profiles of primary myelofibrosis, polycythemia vera, and essential thrombocytosis. Am J Clin Pathol 2017;147(5):444–52. https://doi.org/10.1093/ajcp/aqw222.

[72] Tefferi A, Lasho TL, Finke CM, et al. Targeted deep sequencing in primary myelofibrosis. Blood Adv 2016;1(2):105–11. https://doi.org/10.1182/bloodadvances.2016000208.

[73] Lasho TL, Jimma T, Finke CM, et al. SRSF2 mutations in primary myelofibrosis: significant clustering with IDH mutations and independent association with inferior overall and leukemia-free survival. *Blood*. 2012;120(20):4168–71. https://doi.org/10.1182/blood-2012-05-429696.

[74] Zhang SJ, Rampal R, Manshouri T, et al. Genetic analysis of patients with leukemic transformation of myeloproliferative neoplasms shows recurrent SRSF2 mutations that are associated with adverse outcome. Blood 2012;119(19):4480–5. https://doi.org/10.1182/blood-2011-11-390252.

[75] Dutta A, Yang Y, Le BT, et al. U2af1 is required for survival and function of hematopoietic stem/progenitor cells. Leukemia 2021. https://doi.org/10.1038/s41375-020-01116-x.

[76] Barraco D, Elala YC, Lasho TL, et al. Molecular correlates of anemia in primary myelofibrosis: a significant and independent association with U2AF1 mutations. Blood Cancer J 2016;6:e416. https://doi.org/10.1038/bcj.2016.24.

[77] Tefferi A, Finke CM, Lasho TL, et al. U2AF1 mutations in primary myelofibrosis are strongly associated with anemia and thrombocytopenia despite clustering with JAK2V617F and normal karyotype. Leukemia 2014;28(2):431–3. https://doi.org/10.1038/leu.2013.286.

[78] Sanada M, Suzuki T, Shih LY, et al. Gain-of-function of mutated C-CBL tumour suppressor in myeloid neoplasms. Nature 2009;460(7257):904–8. https://doi.org/10.1038/nature08240.

[79] Lasho TL, Mudireddy M, Finke CM, et al. Targeted next-generation sequencing in blast phase myeloproliferative neoplasms. Blood Adv 2018;2(4):370–80. https://doi.org/10.1182/bloodadvances.2018015875.

[80] Coltro G, Rotunno G, Mannelli L, et al. RAS/CBL mutations predict resistance to JAK inhibitors in myelofibrosis and are associated with poor prognostic features. Blood Adv 2020;4(15):3677–87. https://doi.org/10.1182/bloodadvances.2020002175.

[81] Shapiro P. Ras-MAP kinase signaling pathways and control of cell proliferation: relevance to cancer therapy. Crit Rev Clin Lab Sci 2002;39(4–5):285–330. https://doi.org/10.1080/10408360290795538.

[82] Santos FPS, Getta B, Masarova L, et al. Prognostic impact of RAS-pathway mutations in patients with myelofibrosis. Leukemia 2020;34(3):799–810. https://doi.org/10.1038/s41375-019-0603-9.

[83] Tenedini E, Bernardis I, Artusi V, et al. Targeted cancer exome sequencing reveals recurrent mutations in myeloproliferative neoplasms. Leukemia 2014;28(5):1052–9. https://doi.org/10.1038/leu.2013.302.

[84] Patel KP, Newberry KJ, Luthra R, et al. Correlation of mutation profile and response in patients with myelofibrosis treated with ruxolitinib. *Blood*. 2015;126(6):790–7. https://doi.org/10.1182/blood-2015-03-633404.

[85] Sood R, Kamikubo Y, Liu P. Role of RUNX1 in hematological malignancies. Blood 2017;129(15):2070–82. https://doi.org/10.1182/blood-2016-10-687830.

[86] Ding Y, Harada Y, Imagawa J, et al. AML1/RUNX1 point mutation possibly promotes leukemic transformation in myeloproliferative neoplasms. Blood 2009;114(25):5201–5. https://doi.org/10.1182/blood-2009-06-223982.

[87] Kadia TM, Jain P, Ravandi F, et al. TP53 mutations in newly diagnosed acute myeloid leukemia: Clinicomolecular characteristics, response to therapy, and outcomes. *Cancer*. 2016;122(22):3484–91. https://doi.org/10.1002/cncr.30203.

[88] Rampal R, Ahn J, Abdel-Wahab O, et al. Genomic and functional analysis of leukemic transformation of myeloproliferative neoplasms. Proc Natl Acad Sci U S A 2014;111(50):E5401–10. https://doi.org/10.1073/pnas.1407792111.

[89] Kim DY, Tariq H, Brown AF, et al. JAK2 V617F mutation allele burden (MAB) and its correlation with hematologic characteristics in myeloproliferative neoplasms. Blood 2017;130(Supplement 1):5267. https://doi.org/10.1182/blood.V130.Suppl_1.5267.5267.

[90] Passamonti F, Rumi E, Pietra D, et al. A prospective study of 338 patients with polycythemia vera: the impact of JAK2 (V617F) allele burden and leukocytosis on fibrotic or leukemic disease transformation and vascular complications. Leukemia 2010;24(9):1574–9. https://doi.org/10.1038/leu.2010.148.

[91] Vannucchi AM, Antonioli E, Guglielmelli P, et al. Prospective identification of high-risk polycythemia vera patients based on JAK2(V617F) allele burden. Leukemia 2007;21(9):1952–9. https://doi.org/10.1038/sj.leu.2404854.

[92] Hussein K, Bock O, Theophile K, et al. JAK2(V617F) allele burden discriminates essential thrombocythemia from a subset of prefibrotic-stage primary myelofibrosis. Exp Hematol 2009;37(10):1186–93.e7. https://doi.org/10.1016/j.exphem.2009.07.005.

[93] Ha JS, Kim YK, Jung SI, et al. Correlations between Janus kinase 2 V617F allele burdens and clinicohematologic parameters in myeloproliferative neoplasms. Ann Lab Med 2012;32(6):385–91. https://doi.org/10.3343/alm.2012.32.6.385.

[94] Carobbio A, Finazzi G, Antonioli E, et al. JAK2V617F allele burden and thrombosis: a direct comparison in essential thrombocythemia and polycythemia vera. Exp Hematol 2009;37(9):1016–21. https://doi.org/10.1016/j.exphem.2009.06.006.

[95] Guglielmelli P, Barosi G, Specchia G, et al. Identification of patients with poorer survival in primary myelofibrosis based on the burden of JAK2V617F mutated allele. Blood 2009;114(8):1477–83. https://doi.org/10.1182/blood-2009-04-216044.

[96] Lundberg P, Karow A, Nienhold R, et al. Clonal evolution and clinical correlates of somatic mutations in myeloproliferative neoplasms. *Blood*. 2014;123(14):2220–8. https://doi.org/10.1182/blood-2013-11-537167.

[97] Wolschke C, Badbaran A, Zabelina T, et al. Impact of molecular residual disease post allografting in myelofibrosis patients. Bone Marrow Transplant 2017;52(11):1526–9. https://doi.org/10.1038/bmt.2017.157.

[98] Tefferi A, Guglielmelli P, Lasho TL, et al. Mutation-enhanced international prognostic systems for essential thrombocythaemia and polycythaemia vera. Br J Haematol 2020;189(2):291–302. https://doi.org/10.1111/bjh.16380.

[99] Tefferi A, Guglielmelli P, Nicolosi M, et al. GIPSS: genetically inspired prognostic scoring system for primary myelofibrosis. Leukemia 2018;32(7):1631–42. https://doi.org/10.1038/s41375-018-0107-z.

[100] Tefferi A, Guglielmelli P, Lasho TL, et al. MIPSS70+ version 2.0: mutation and karyotype-enhanced international prognostic scoring system for primary myelofibrosis. J Clin Oncol 2018;36(17):1769–70. https://doi.org/10.1200/JCO.2018.78.9867.

[101] Tefferi A, Guglielmelli P, Pardanani A, et al. Myelofibrosis treatment algorithm 2018. Blood Cancer J 2018;8(8):72. https://doi.org/10.1038/s41408-018-0109-0.

[102] Boddu P, Chihara D, Masarova L, et al. The co-occurrence of driver mutations in chronic myeloproliferative neoplasms. Ann Hematol 2018;97(11):2071–80. https://doi.org/10.1007/s00277-018-3402-x.

[103] Harrison C, Kiladjian JJ, Al-Ali HK, et al. JAK inhibition with ruxolitinib versus best available therapy for myelofibrosis. N Engl J Med 2012;366(9):787–98. https://doi.org/10.1056/NEJMoa1110556.

[104] Harrison CN, Vannucchi AM, Kiladjian JJ, et al. Long-term findings from COMFORT-II, a phase 3 study of ruxolitinib vs best available therapy for myelofibrosis. Leukemia 2016;30(8):1701–7. https://doi.org/10.1038/leu.2016.148.

[105] Vannucchi AM, Kiladjian JJ, Griesshammer M, et al. Ruxolitinib versus standard therapy for the treatment of polycythemia vera. N Engl J Med 2015;372(5):426–35. https://doi.org/10.1056/NEJMoa1409002.

[106] Verstovsek S, Vannucchi AM, Griesshammer M, et al. Ruxolitinib versus best available therapy in patients with polycythemia vera: 80-week follow-up from the RESPONSE trial. Haematologica 2016;101(7):821–9. https://doi.org/10.3324/haematol.2016.143644.

[107] Pardanani A, Harrison C, Cortes JE, et al. Safety and efficacy of fedratinib in patients with primary or secondary myelofibrosis: a randomized clinical trial. JAMA Oncol 2015;1(5):643–51. https://doi.org/10.1001/jamaoncol.2015.1590.

[108] Oh ST, Talpaz M, Gerds AT, et al. ACVR1/JAK1/JAK2 inhibitor momelotinib reverses transfusion dependency and suppresses hepcidin in myelofibrosis phase 2 trial. Blood Adv 2020;4(18):4282–91. https://doi.org/10.1182/bloodadvances.2020002662.

[109] Mascarenhas J, Hoffman R, Talpaz M, et al. Pacritinib vs best available therapy, including ruxolitinib, in patients with myelofibrosis: a randomized clinical trial. JAMA Oncol 2018;4(5):652–9. https://doi.org/10.1001/jamaoncol.2017.5818.

[110] Vannucchi AM, Verstovsek S, Guglielmelli P, et al. Ruxolitinib reduces JAK2 p.V617F allele burden in patients with polycythemia vera enrolled in the RESPONSE study. Ann Hematol 2017;96(7):1113–20. https://doi.org/10.1007/s00277-017-2994-x.

[111] Masarova L, Verstovsek S, Hidalgo-Lopez JE, et al. A phase 2 study of ruxolitinib in combination with azacitidine in patients with myelofibrosis. Blood 2018;

132(16):1664–74. https://doi.org/10.1182/blood-2018-04-846626.

[112] Harrison CN, Kiladjian J-J, Heidel FH, et al. Efficacy, safety, and confirmation of the recommended phase 2 starting dose of the combination of ruxolitinib (RUX) and panobinostat (PAN) in patients (Pts) with myelofibrosis (MF). Blood 2015;126(23):4060. https://doi.org/10.1182/blood.V126.23.4060.4060.

[113] Patel AA, Cahill K, Charnot-Katsikas A, et al. Clinical outcomes of IDH2-mutated advanced-phase Ph-negative myeloproliferative neoplasms treated with enasidenib. Br J Haematol 2020;190(1):e48–51. https://doi.org/10.1111/bjh.16709.

[114] Li B, Rampal RK, Xiao Z. Targeted therapies for myeloproliferative neoplasms. Biomark Res 2019;7:15. https://doi.org/10.1186/s40364-019-0166-y.

Infectious Disease

Advances in Molecular Pathology 4 (2021) 81–91
ADVANCES IN MOLECULAR PATHOLOGY

Engineering Consideration for Emerging Essential Nucleic Acid Tests for Point-of-Care Diagnostics

Ethan P.M. LaRochelle, PhD[a,b,*], Amogha Tadimety, PhD[c]
[a]Laboratory of Clinical Genomics and Advanced Technology, Department of Pathology and Laboratory Medicine, Dartmouth Hitchcock Medical Center, 1 Medical Center Drive, Lebanon, NH 03756, USA; [b]Geisel School of Medicine, Dartmouth College, Hanover, NH 03755, USA; [c]Nanopath Inc., 700 Main St North, Cambridge, MA 02139, USA

KEYWORDS
• Nucleic acid test • Point-of-care • Microfluidics • Isothermal amplification • Lateral flow
• World Health Organization

KEY POINTS

- The World Health Organization (WHO) has convened experts annually to develop and revise global recommendations and strategies for implementing essential diagnostic assays.
- All 3 stages of nucleic acid test: sample preparation, amplification, and detection should address the WHO ASSURED criteria to be considered appropriate for point-of-care.
- Microfluidics can be designed to perform much of the sample manipulation needed for nucleic acid tests.
- Lateral flow assays are inexpensive and have been demonstrated as a simple method to detect amplified DNA.

INTRODUCTION

The World Health Organization's (WHO) Strategic Advisory Group of Experts in In Vitro Diagnostics (SAGE IVD) has convened annually to develop and revise global recommendations and strategies for implementing essential diagnostic assays. The primary output of these meetings is a publication containing the WHO Essential List of In Vitro Diagnostics [1–3]. This list is categorized into 2 tiers based on the care setting: (1) community settings and health facilities without laboratories, and (2) clinical laboratories. Each year since 2019, the recommendations of the previous year's meeting have been published, and the most recent revision was published in March 2021. Although the recommendations span all forms of diagnostic assays, this article focuses solely on nucleic acid tests (NATs).

The SAGE IVD defines essential diagnostic tests (EDT) based on a number of criteria including public health and clinical need/utility, commercial availability, cost, diagnostic accuracy, and infrastructure requirements for the given setting. The publication from the first meeting of SAGE IVD recommends only a single NAT for the community health tier where dedicated laboratory equipment is not available. Subsequent meetings have added 2 assays to this tier and removed the recommendation of the first meeting. The essential list of NAT with a dedicated clinical laboratory has grown from 6 assays in the first 2019 publication to 11 by 2021. A summary of nucleic acid–based EDT recommendations is provided in Table 1. The vast majority of these tests aim to accurately diagnose communicable diseases.

*Corresponding author, *E-mail address:* ethan.phillip.m.larochelle.th@dartmouth.edu

https://doi.org/10.1016/j.yamp.2021.07.003
2589-4080/21/

TABLE 1
WHO Strategic Advisory Group of Experts in In Vitro Diagnostics Recommendations for Nucleic Acid Tests

Disease	Diagnostic Test	Test Purpose	Specimen Type	2019	2020	2021
Community and Health Settings Without Laboratories						
HIV infection	Qualitative HIV NAT	To diagnose HIV in infants <18 mo of age	Capillary whole blood, venous whole blood, dried blood spot		X	X
Influenza	Influenza A & B NAT	To diagnose seasonal influenza infection	Nasal swab, nasopharyngeal swab, nasopharyngeal aspirate or wash		X	X
Tuberculosis (TB)	Loop-mediated isothermal amplification (TB-LAMP)	For diagnosis of active TB	Sputum	X		
Health care facilities with clinical laboratories						
Cancer	BCR-ABL1 and ABL-1 transcripts	To diagnose and monitor therapy of chronic myelocytic leukemia (CML) and CML variants and prognosis of acute lymphoblastic leukemia	Venous whole blood, bone marrow		X	X
Cancer	Epidermal growth factor receptor gene mutation	To aid in the diagnosis and treatment of nonsquamous non–small-cell lung carcinoma	Formalin-fixed paraffin-embedded tissue and buffered lung tumor specimen			X
Coronavirus disease (COVID-19)	SARS-CoV-2 NAT	To diagnose infection by severe acute respiratory syndrome coronavirus 2 (SARS-CoV-2) in symptomatic and asymptomatic individuals suspected of having been exposed; for surveillance and confirmation of outbreaks	Upper respiratory specimen (eg, nasopharyngeal and oropharyngeal) and lower respiratory specimens (eg, BAL)			X

Hepatitis B	Quantitative HBV NAT	To stage chronic HBV infection, to determine the needed treatment (including use of antivirals in mother to prevent mother-to-child transmission), and to monitor response to treatment	Serum, plasma	X	X	X
Hepatitis C	Qualitative or quantitative HCV NAT	To diagnose viremic HCV and to monitor response to treatment, and as a test of cure	Capillary whole blood, venous whole blood, serum, plasma, dried blood spot	X	X	X
HIV	Qualitative HIV NAT	To Diagnose HIV infections in infants <18 mo of age	Capillary whole blood, venous whole blood, dried blood spots, plasma	X	X	X
HIV	Quantitative HIV NAT	To monitor response to antiretroviral treatment, To diagnose HIV infection in infants <18 mo of age (only if validated by the manufacturer)	Dried blood spots (whole blood or plasma), serum, plasma	X	X	X
Human papillomavirus (HPV)	HPV NAT	For cervical cancer screening	Cervical cells collected in test-specific transport fluid/vessel	X	X	X
Influenza	Influenza A and B NAT	To diagnose seasonal influenza	Nasal swab, nasopharyngeal swab, nasopharyngeal aspirate or wash			X
Neglected tropical diseases	Qualitative dengue virus NAT	For surveillance (serotype differentiation) and confirmation of outbreaks	Serum, plasma, dried blood spot		X	X
Pneumocystis pneumonia	*Pneumocystis jirovecii* NAT	To aid in the diagnosis of *Pneumocystis* pneumonia	Respiratory specimens (sputum, BAL fluid)			X

(*continued on next page*)

TABLE 1
(continued)

Disease	Diagnostic Test	Test Purpose	Specimen Type	2019	2020	2021
Sexually transmitted infection	Qualitative test for *Chlamydia trachomati* and *Neisseria gonorrhea* infections	For the diagnosis and screening of symptomatic or asymptomatic chlamydial and/or gonorrheal urogenital disease and extragenital infection	Urine, urethral swabs, endocervical swabs, vaginal swabs, rectal swabs, oropharyngeal swabs, liquid cytology		X	X
Tuberculosis (TB)	TB-LAMP	For diagnosis of active TB	Sputum		X	X
TB	*Mycobacterium tuberculosis* DNA	To diagnose active TB and simultaneously or sequentially detect rifampicin resistance	Sputum, BAL, or extrapulmonary	X	X	X
Vaccine-preventable diseases	Measles NAT	To diagnose clinically suspected measles infection	Oral fluid, throat swab, nasopharyngeal aspirates or swabs, urine			X
Zika virus	Zika virus NAT	To diagnose acute Zika virus infection	Venous whole blood, serum, plasma, urine, CSF		X	X

Abbreviations: BAL, bronchoalveolar lavage; CSF, cerebrospinal fluid; HBV, hepatitis B virus; HCV, hepatitis C virus; HIV, human immunodeficiency virus; NAT, nucleic acid test; SAGE IVD, Strategic Advisory Group of Experts in In Vitro Diagnostics; WHO, World Health Organization.

Data from Refs. [1–3].

SIGNIFICANCE

There is growing support in research to further simplify NATs toward their use in point-of-care and community health settings. A common set of criteria to assess whether an assay is appropriate for a rapid point-of-care setting has also been published by the WHO [4]. The proposed metrics evaluate whether the test is Affordable, Sensitive, Specific, User-friendly, Rapid and robust, Equipment-free and Deliverable to end-users (ASSURED). In the realm of NAT there are generally 3 stages required to move from sample to result: sample preparation, amplification, and detection. The following sections focus on a number of technological and engineering approaches in development to reduce the clinical burden of performing these tests.

THREE STAGES OF NUCLEIC ACID TEST

Sample Preparation

As can be observed in Table 1, the recommended EDTs are performed on a variety of bio-specimens. Although cell lysis is a common extraction technique suitable for certain types of downstream amplification [5–7], other more complex samples like sputum and whole blood often require additional purification and concentration steps [8]. Sample preparation steps are a key bottleneck to NATs being performed outside of a clinical laboratory due to the infrastructure and skill requirements. The dependence on laboratory infrastructure is the reason the tuberculosis loop-mediated isothermal amplification (TB-LAMP) assay was removed from the recommended community-based EDTs [2].

Amplification

Many of the amplification strategies used in clinical practice today are based on polymerase chain reaction (PCR), which relies on thermal cycling the sample to repeatedly denature DNA, anneal with primers, and then extend. The rate at which these distinct steps occur depends on the ramp rate of the heating block where the efficiency of the thermal transfer to and from the sample can be impacted by the container material and sample volume. Although methods have been investigated to address the strict thermal requirements of PCR [9,10], these design constraints are also the driving force to develop isothermal amplification techniques.

Isothermal protocols do not require repetitive thermal ramping and instead hold the sample at a constant temperature during amplification. Nucleic acid sequence-based amplification (NASBA) was one of the first described isothermal amplification methods [11]. Loop-mediated isothermal amplification (LAMP) was introduced about a decade later, and a recent literate review shows LAMP now accounts for nearly two-thirds of publications in the isothermal amplification field [12,13]. Both helicase-dependent amplification (HDA) [14] and recombinase polymerase amplification (RPA) [15] were proposed in subsequent years and have been growing in adoption [16]. Although more exhaustive lists and details have been published elsewhere [7,13,16,17], this work summarizes select isothermal methods in Table 2 as a means to discuss design criteria for point-of-care assay development.

First demonstrated for gene editing in 2013 [18,19], clustered regularly interspaced short palindromic repeats (CRISPR) and associated effector proteins (Cas) are showing increased adoption in the field of rapid diagnostics [20–22]. The amplification methods summarized in Table 2 can be paired with CRISPR/Cas procedures to perform selective diagnostic detection. This combination was first reported with the integration of Cas9 and NASBA amplification for the detection of Zika [20]. The numerous combinations of recently developed CRISPR/Cas diagnostics have been reviewed by others [23], and there is a clear trend demonstrating improved sensitivity and selectivity using these methods.

Detection

Sensitive detection often requires dedicated hardware that has traditionally been complicated and costly. Considering the ASSURED criteria, lateral flow colorimetric tests are the best match for point-of-care applications, yet, there are generally antigen tests that lack the sensitivity of NATs [24,25]. Although other detection mechanisms have been demonstrated based on electrochemical transduction, surface-enhanced Ramen scattering, or magnetic sensing, the most widely adopted method in clinical practice is optical detection, specifically fluorescence sensing [26]. Although other sensing techniques may provide high sensitivity, the ubiquitous adoption of smartphones with integrated cameras and computing power present an opportunity to leverage optical detection modalities. To reduce cost and complexity, smartphone imaging has been demonstrated for both colorimetric and fluorescence detection for NATs with the aim of transitioning clinical tests to point-of-care [25,27,28].

Engineering Considerations

Sample preparation and handling in clinical molecular pathology laboratories generally require trained technicians to aliquot microliter quantities of patient samples

TABLE 2
Overview of Select Isothermal Methods

Isothermal Method	Enzymes	Target	Primers	Initial Heating	Incubation Temperature (C°)	Amplification Time (min)	Limit of Detection (Copies)	Lyophilized Reagents
NASBA	2–3: Reverse-transcriptase, RNA polymerase	RNA	2	No	~41	60–180	1	Yes
LAMP	1: DNA polymerase	DNA	4–6	Yes	60–65	60	~5	No
HDA	2: DNA polymerase, helicase	DNA	2	No	37–65	30–120	1	No
RPA	2: DNA polymerase, recombinase	DNA/ RNA	2	No	37–42	20–90	1	Yes

Abbreviations: HDA, helicase-dependent amplification; LAMP, loop-mediated isothermal amplification; NASBA, nucleic acid sequence-based amplification; RPA, recombinase polymerase amplification.

Data from Zhao, Y., Chen, F., Li, Q., Wang, L. & Fan, C. Isothermal Amplification of Nucleic Acids. *Chem. Rev.* **115**, 12491–12545 (2015) and Lobato, I. M. & O'Sullivan, C. K. Recombinase polymerase amplification: Basics, applications and recent advances. Trends Anal. Chem. 98, 19–35 (2018).

and follow multistep protocols to combine reagents, purifying target nucleic acid. In high-throughput laboratories, autonomous pipetting instrumentation has been introduced, but these systems are optimized for high-volume testing, are expensive, and still require supervision and routine maintenance.

Two platforms used to simplify this process, but at lower throughput, are microfluidic and lateral flow assays. Microfluidic devices are generally manufactured by forming channels in soft polydimethylsiloxane (PDMS) layers [29], whereas lateral flow tests are layered sample pads and nitrocellulose membrane [30]. These modalities aim to remove some degree of sample handling because they automate fluid flow and can store reagents onboard at ambient temperatures, but require a disposable single-use microfluidic chip or lateral flow strip.

Microfluidics

An interesting benefit of microfluidics is the ability to form microwells with volumes less than 40 nL [31], which are multiple orders of magnitude smaller than the volume of microtubes (20–100 μL) [32]. The small volume increases the target concentration, which is defined in terms of molecules per volume, thus improving sensitivity. In addition, reducing the reaction chamber volume reduces the required reagents by a proportional amount, and the reaction rate increases 10:1 relative to the chamber volume [33]. The microfluidic microwell platform can be used to multiplex reactions or increase throughput. Another huge advantage of the smaller size is faster reagent diffusion or heat transfer in the event of a PCR.

The design of the microchannel can be used to perform operations on the input sample. For example, a number of microfluidic designs have been developed for mixing input fluids, including the serpentine channel, implementing staggered grooves or herringbone patterns, or placing obstacles in the channel (Fig. 1). Particle size can also be used as a filtering mechanism in which an H filter can be used to extract smaller particles with higher diffusivity. To further compartmentalize small volumes for analysis, a different carrier medium, such as oil, can be used to create discrete units of sample material, often called microfluidic droplets. These principles of laminar flow are just some of many mechanisms by which microfluidic channels can be designed to automate sample manipulation. There exist a realm of more complicated designs that use electrical, magnetic, or acoustic transducers to act on the material flowing in the channels [34].

Microfluidic devices require that samples flow through multistage channels to mimic the complex sample preparation workflow performed by

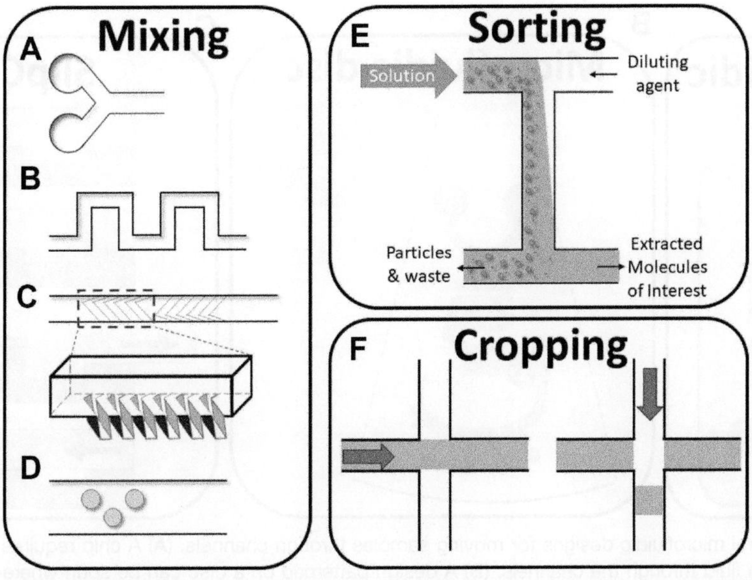

FIG. 1 Example diagrams of microfluidic designs for manipulating samples. **(A)** Two or more input ports can be mixed using different designs including **(B)** a serpentine channel, **(C)** a positive or negative herringbone design to induce chaotic mixing, or **(D)** randomly placed pillars within the channel. **(E)** Particle sorting can be implemented with an H filter, which filters based on particle size and viscosity [35]. **(F)** Cropping can be implemented to separate liquid flow, as is done in digital amplification and detection discussed in later sections.

technicians. This requires forces to act on the sample material to move it between stages of the microfluidic device. Three of the commonly reported methods for manipulating flow include the use of pressure-driven pumps [36,37], centrifugal microfluidic discs [38,39], or SlipChip [40,41] designs (Fig. 2). Each of these designs provides the ability to add both the sample and reagents, or for additional simplification, preloaded lyophilized reagents can be used [42,43].

Because commonly used laboratory external pumps are generally bulky and not appropriate for point-of-care applications, there has been considerable work to incorporate miniaturized pumps into microfluidic devices. There has been development on both mechanical and nonmechanical micropumps. Mechanical micropumps rely on electrical, pneumatic, or thermopneumatic changes to actuate, whereas nonmechanical pumps have no moving parts and instead use properties of electric and magnetic field or capillary forces to move samples [44]. Disc-based microfluidics use the angular velocity to manipulate liquid flow, where inward flow can also be achieved through rapid changes in acceleration and deceleration [39]. Although power consumption has been a critique of the disc method for point-of-care applications, recent work has aimed to address these issues by addressing the overall power budget in the design [45]. SlipChip designs use multiple layers of channels that can be translated relative to each other to perform mixing operations. This design concept relies heavily on the wettability and surface tension properties of the 2 channel materials that can be dominant when the surface-to-volume ratios are high.

Lateral Flow

Unlike microfluidics, which generally relies on actuated liquid manipulation, lateral flow techniques rely on capillary force to wick the sample toward a reaction membrane. The liquid sample is placed on a sample pad made of cellulose acetate or glass fiber, then through capillary force travels to the conjugate pad where it is labeled with an optically tagged conjugate biomolecule. The flow continues to one or more test lines and control containing DNA-probes for hybridization and optical detection [30]. This testing format is often used for low-cost point-of-care antigen-antibody detection, as this generally requires less sample preparation. When a lateral flow assay is used for nucleic acid detection, pre-amplification is often required. A range of successful development has involved combining microfluidic sample preparation and amplification

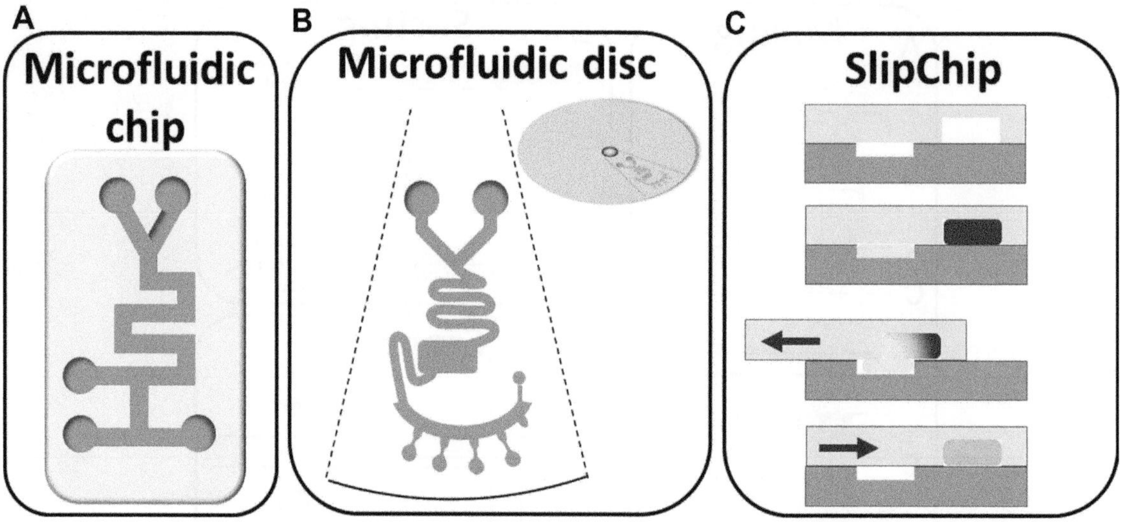

FIG. 2 General microfluidic designs for moving samples through channels. (**A**) A chip requires an external pump to push fluid through the channels. (**B**) A design patterned on a disc can be spun where the angular velocity and changes in acceleration can move liquid. This design can be combined with a strobe light and camera for optical detection. (**C**) SlipChip designs use multiple layers that are translated relative to each other. Lyophilized reagents (*yellow*) can be placed in compartments, which can then be mixed with the sample (*red*).

followed by lateral flow colorimetric of fluorescent readout [10,22].

More advanced paper-based designs incorporating sample preparation and amplification have also been demonstrated. One approach uses multiple layers and a sliding strip for sample manipulation, which is then combined with LAMP amplification [46,47]. Other approaches use paper folding to mix samples and reagents before LAMP amplification [48,49]. A third approach uses printed QR code structure to detect volatiles in the gas phase atop a bacterial sample, which can then be readout on a smartphone [50]. In these and other examples, wax printing has been demonstrated as a method to better control the liquid flow on the membrane and allow for more complicated testing protocols [51]. Although paper-based tests do not have the same level of control over sample volume and flow, they are easy and inexpensive to manufacture.

Optical Sensing

Point-of-care testing requires a simple detection mechanism, leading to the rapid uptake of colorimetric lateral flow assays due to their simplicity. However, this method of detection requires subjective judgment of a color change in which illumination conditions and difference in color perception between individuals can lead to uncertainties [52,53]. In colorimetric detection, conjugated gold nanoparticles (AuNP) are often used to collect at the detection strip. As the density of AuNP increases, the optical absorption and scattering properties are altered, resulting in a color change. The shape and size of these particles can be used to tune the optical interactions and thus the expected color change. These gold nanoparticles have the advantage of being robust to photobleaching and angle of incidence, while remaining shelf stable.

Alternatively, fluorescent molecules can be used in a similar manner for lateral flow assays and are also commonly used in microfluidic applications. Fluorescence signals occur when light at a specific wavelength excites a fluorescent molecule and on relaxation emits light at a longer wavelength. A quencher can be cleaved on detection, resulting in an increase in fluorescent signal. This phenomena is generally difficult to detect by eye, but sensitive cameras equipped with appropriate filters are commonly used. More recently, with the ubiquitous adoption of smartphones and improvements in image sensor technology, smartphone-based fluorescence detection has been demonstrated [28,54–56].

During laboratory quantitative PCR amplification, the fluorescence intensity for each thermal cycle is recorded and can be used as quantitative metric to estimate the initial target nucleic acid concentration. However, with isothermal amplification, thermal cycling is not used, so other means must be used for quantification. One method to overcome this limitation is digital

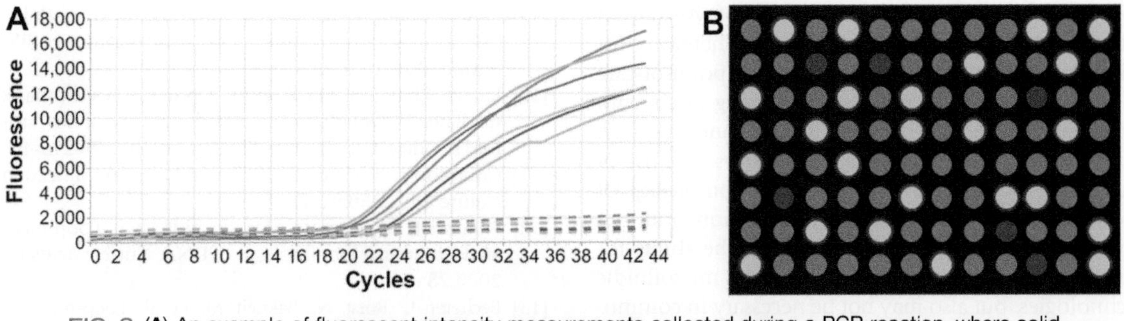

FIG. 3 (**A**) An example of fluorescent intensity measurements collected during a PCR reaction, where solid lines are positive samples and dashed lines are controls. (**B**) Digital amplification separates the sample into many smaller reaction chambers and the count of positive reactions (*bright green*) can be used as a quantitative metric.

amplification, in which microfluidics can be used to compartmentalize sample material into numerous smaller volumes, similar to the method shown in Fig. 1F [41,57,58]. A single sample can be split into individual droplets with volumes as low as 100 fL [57], and amplification is performed in parallel but independently for each well. Any fluorescence intensity above a threshold is counted and the percentage can be used for quantification (Fig. 3). This compartmentalization of the sample can also improve counting accuracy for nucleic acid quantification.

DISCUSSION AND SUMMARY

From the recommended tests for nonlaboratory settings listed in Table 1, the m-PIMA HIV-1/2 Detect (formerly Alere I, Abbott Rapid Diagnostics, Abbott Park, IL) and the Xpert HIV-1 Qual Assay (Cepheid AB, Solna, Sweden) were the first to be preapproved by WHO [59]. Both of these systems use a benchtop device to perform real-time reverse-transcriptase PCR on a microfluidic cartridge using kits that do not need to be frozen [60,61]. The Abbott and Cepheid systems report turnaround times of 52 minutes and 93 minutes, respectively. Both benchtop platforms can also be used to run other types of tests like the recommended Influenza A & B tests. As an example of the potential improvements possible with isothermal amplification, Influenza A & B assays were compared for the Cepheid platform and Abbott's ID NOW benchtop system. The ID NOW, which implements isothermal amplification, had a time to result of 33 minutes, compared with the 97 minutes for the PCR-based GeneXpert [62]. The point-of-care systems described here require minimal sample preparation, where blood is loaded directly into a cartridge, or a nasal swab is mixed in solution for 10 seconds. This simplicity in sample preparation is crucial for operation in the nonlaboratory setting, and is the reason the TB-LAMP test is no longer recommended in this care setting [2].

There continue to be a number of advancements in the field of molecular diagnostics, with a large emphasis on infectious disease detection. The Coronavirus Disease 2019 pandemic has further catalyzed development in this field and has brought a number of point-of-care and at-home diagnostic tests to the market. Many of these devices that rely on nucleic acid detection use the engineering building blocks discussed previously.

In the coming years, many of these advancements can be translated to new targets, but it is important to consider the ASSURED criteria when developing any new point-of-care diagnostic test. WHO also provides target product profiles for a range of high-importance conditions. In many cases, tests are first developed based on sensitivity and specificity, but remain inaccessible to many of the world's populations. A continued push to use combinations of these new technologies may help address the affordability and usability of diagnostic tests.

SUMMARY AND FUTURE DIRECTIONS

WHO provides a yearly list of EDTs that should be available in various health care settings. The recommended point-of-care NATs remain relatively short, but technological innovations that address the ASSURED criteria continue to drive more tests toward this care setting. As future assays are developed, it is important to consider these criteria if the goal is to make the test widely accessible. Instrument complexity increases the initial capital costs and then relies on expensive service contracts to maintain performance, both of which limit adoption in many parts of the world. Therefore, for widespread adoption, systems targeting point-of-care should avoid these components; replacing lasers with light-emitting diodes, robotic liquid handling with microfluidics, or, ideally, lateral flow strips. The use of isothermal amplification reduces the complexity of the heat blocks required for amplification and can lower turnaround time, but also reduces the ability for quantification. This can be overcome with microfluidic technologies, but also may not be necessary in community health care settings. CRISPR/Cas methodologies combined with isothermal amplification and lateral flow detection show great promise in this area. Future work should focus on minimizing sample preparation and handling, while increasing system sensitivity and specificity.

ACKNOWLEDGEMENTS

Funding for E.P.M.L. was provided by the DHMC Pathology Department Latham French Fund as part of the Emerging Diagnostic and Investigative Technologies fellowship program.

REFERENCES

[1] WHO. First WHO model list of essential in vitro diagnostics. World Health Organization; 2019.
[2] WHO. Report of the second meeting of the strategic advisory group of experts on in vitro diagnostics. Geneva, Switzerland: World Health Organization; 2019.
[3] WHO. The selection and use of essential in vitro diagnostics - TRS 1031. World Health Organization; 2021.
[4] Kosack CS, Page A-L, Klaster PR. WHO | A guide to aid the selection of diagnostic tests. Bull World Health Organ 2017;95(9):639–45.
[5] Curtis KA, Rudolph DL, Owen SM. Rapid detection of HIV-1 by reverse-transcription, loop-mediated isothermal amplification (RT-LAMP). J Virol Methods 2008;151:264–70.
[6] Turner SA, Deharvengt SJ, Lyons KD, et al. Implementation of multicolor melt curve analysis for high-risk human papilloma virus detection in low- and middle-income countries: a pilot study for expanded cervical cancer screening in Honduras. J Glob Oncol 2017;1–8.
[7] Walker FM, Hsieh K. Advances in directly amplifying nucleic acids from complex samples. Biosensors 2019;9: 117.
[8] Paul R, Ostermann E, Wei Q. Advances in point-of-care nucleic acid extraction technologies for rapid diagnosis of human and plant diseases. Biosens Bioelectron 2020;169:112592.
[9] Park S, Zhang Y, Lin S, et al. Advances in microfluidic PCR for point-of-care infectious disease diagnostics. Biotechnol Adv 2011;29:830–9.
[10] Liu W, Zhang M, Liu X, et al. A point-of-need infrared mediated PCR platform with compatible lateral flow strip for HPV detection. Biosens Bioelectron 2017;96:213–9.
[11] Compton J. Nucleic acid sequence-based amplification. Nature 1991;350:91–2.
[12] Notomi T, Okayama H, Masubuchi H, et al. Loop-mediated isothermal amplification of DNA. Nucleic Acids Res 2000;28:e63.
[13] Becherer L, Borst N, Bakheit M, et al. Loop-mediated isothermal amplification (LAMP) – review and classification of methods for sequence-specific detection. Anal Methods 2020;12:717–46.
[14] Vincent M, Xu Y, Kong H. Helicase-dependent isothermal DNA amplification. EMBO Rep 2004;5:795–800.
[15] Piepenburg O, Williams CH, Stemple DL, et al. DNA detection using recombination proteins. PLoS Biol 2006;4:e204.
[16] Li J, Macdonald J, Stetten F. Review: a comprehensive summary of a decade development of the recombinase polymerase amplification. Analyst 2018;144:31–67.
[17] Li J, Macdonald J. Advances in isothermal amplification: novel strategies inspired by biological processes. Biosens Bioelectron 2015;64:196–211.
[18] Cong L, Ran FA, Cox D, et al. Multiplex genome engineering using CRISPR/Cas systems. Science 2013;339:819–23.
[19] Mali P, Yang L, Esvelt KM, et al. RNA-guided human genome engineering via cas9. Science 2013;339:823–6.
[20] Pardee K, Green AA, Takahashi MK, et al. Rapid, low-cost detection of zika virus using programmable biomolecular components. Cell 2016;165:1255–66.
[21] Huang M, Zhou X, Wang H, et al. Clustered regularly interspaced short palindromic repeats/Cas9 triggered isothermal amplification for site-specific nucleic acid detection. Anal Chem 2018;90:2193–200.
[22] Gootenberg JS, Abudayyeh O, Kellner MJ, et al. Multiplexed and portable nucleic acid detection platform with Cas13, Cas12a, and Csm6. Science 2018;360:439–44.
[23] Li Y, Li S, Wang J, et al. CRISPR/Cas systems towards next-generation biosensing. Trends Biotechnol 2019;37:730–43.
[24] Yager P, Edwards T, Fu E, et al. Microfluidic diagnostic technologies for global public health. Nature 2006;442: 412–8.
[25] Rodriguez-Manzano J, Karymov MA, Begolo S, et al. Reading out single-molecule digital RNA and DNA isothermal amplification in nanoliter volumes with unmodified camera phones. ACS Nano 2016;10:3102–13.
[26] Wang C, Liu M, Wang Z, et al. Point-of-care diagnostics for infectious diseases: from methods to devices. Nano Today 2021;37:101092.
[27] Yoo SM, Lee SY. Optical biosensors for the detection of pathogenic microorganisms. Trends Biotechnol 2016;34:7–25.
[28] McCracken E, Yoon J-Y. Recent approaches for optical smartphone sensing in resource-limited settings: a brief review. Anal Methods 2016;8:6591–601.

[29] Chen L, Manz A, Day R, et al. Total nucleic acid analysis integrated on microfluidic devices. Lab Chip 2007;7:1413–23.

[30] Bahadır EB, Sezgintürk MK. Lateral flow assays: principles, designs and labels. Trac Trends Anal Chem 2016; 82:286–306.

[31] Jang Y-H, Kwon CH, Kim SB, et al. Deep wells integrated with microfluidic valves for stable docking and storage of cells. Biotechnol J 2011;6:156–64.

[32] Kathrada AI, Wei S-C, Xu Y, et al. Microfluidic compartmentalization to identify gene biomarkers of infection. Biomicrofluidics 2020;14:061502.

[33] Zhang J, Hoshino K. Molecular sensors and nanodevices. Oxford, UK: Elsevier; 2014. https://doi.org/10.1016/C2012-0-07668-5.

[34] Burklund A, Tadimety A, Nie Y, et al. Chapter one - advances in diagnostic microfluidics. In: Makowski GS, editor. Advances in clinical chemistry, vol. 95. Oxford, UK: Elsevier; 2020. p. 1–72.

[35] Brody JP, Yager P. Diffusion-based extraction in a microfabricated device. Sens Actuators Phys 1997;58:13–8.

[36] Munyan W, Fuentes V, Draper M, et al. Electrically actuated, pressure-driven microfluidic pumps. Lab Chip 2003;3:217–20.

[37] Monolithic microfabricated valves and pumps by multilayer soft lithography | Science. Available at: https://science.sciencemag.org/content/288/5463/113.full.

[38] Lutz S, Weber P, Focke M, et al. Microfluidic lab-on-a-foil for nucleic acid analysis based on isothermal recombinase polymerase amplification (RPA). Lab Chip 2010; 10:887–93.

[39] Clime L, Daoud J, Brassard D, et al. Active pumping and control of flows in centrifugal microfluidics. Microfluid Nanofluidics 2019;23:29.

[40] Zhukov V, Khorosheva EM, Khazaei T, et al. Microfluidic SlipChip device for multistep multiplexed biochemistry on a nanoliter scale. Lab Chip 2019;19:3200–11.

[41] Yu Z, Lyu W, Yu M, et al. Self-partitioning SlipChip for slip-induced droplet formation and human papillomavirus viral load quantification with digital LAMP. Biosens Bioelectron 2020;155:112107.

[42] Ghosh S, Aggarwal K, Vinitha TU, et al. A new microchannel capillary flow assay (MCFA) platform with lyophilized chemiluminescence reagents for a smartphone-based POCT detecting malaria. Microsyst Nanoeng 2020;6:1–18.

[43] Mauk MG, Song J, Liu C, et al. Simple approaches to minimally-instrumented, microfluidic-based point-of-care nucleic acid amplification tests. Biosensors 2018;8:17.

[44] Zhang C, Xing D, Li Y. Micropumps, microvalves, and micromixers within PCR microfluidic chips: advances and trends. Biotechnol Adv 2007;25:483–514.

[45] Smith S, Mager D, Perebikovsky A, et al. CD-based microfluidics for primary care in extreme point-of-care settings. Micromachines 2016;7(2):22.

[46] Connelly JT, Rolland JP, Whitesides GM. "Paper machine" for molecular diagnostics. Anal Chem 2015;87: 7595–601.

[47] Ru Choi J, Hu J, Tang R, et al. An integrated paper-based sample-to-answer biosensor for nucleic acid testing at the point of care. Lab Chip 2016;16:611–21.

[48] Fang X, Guan M, Kong J. Rapid nucleic acid detection of Zaire ebolavirus on paper fluidics. RSC Adv 2015;5: 64614–6.

[49] Trieu PT, Lee NY. Paper-based all-in-one origami microdevice for nucleic acid amplification testing for rapid colorimetric identification of live cells for point-of-care testing. Anal Chem 2019;91:11013–22.

[50] Burklund A, Saturley-Hall HK, Franchina FA, et al. Printable QR code paper microfluidic colorimetric assay for screening volatile biomarkers. Biosens Bioelectron 2019;128:97–103.

[51] Magro L, Escadafal C, Garneret P, et al. Paper microfluidics for nucleic acid amplification testing (NAAT) of infectious diseases. Lab Chip 2017;17:2347–71.

[52] Hu J, Wang S, Wang L, et al. Advances in paper-based point-of-care diagnostics. Biosens Bioelectron 2014;54: 585–97.

[53] Eltzov E, Guttel S, Low Yuen Kei A, et al. Lateral flow immunoassays – from paper strip to smartphone technology. Electroanalysis 2015;27:2116–30.

[54] Hernández-Neuta I, Neumann F, Brightmeyer J, et al. Smartphone-based clinical diagnostics: towards democratization of evidence-based health care. J Intern Med 2019;285:19–39.

[55] Priye A, Wong S, Bi Y, et al. Lab-on-a-drone: toward pinpoint deployment of smartphone-enabled nucleic acid-based diagnostics for mobile health care. Anal Chem 2016;88:4651–60.

[56] Wu X, Pan J, Zhu X, et al. MS 2 device: smartphone-facilitated mobile nucleic acid analysis on microfluidic device. Analyst 2021. https://doi.org/10.1039/D1AN00367D.

[57] Yang H, Chen Z, Cao X, et al. A sample-in-digital-answer-out system for rapid detection and quantitation of infectious pathogens in bodily fluids. Anal Bioanal Chem 2018;410:7019–30.

[58] Rolando JC, Jue E, Schoepp NG, et al. Real-time, digital LAMP with commercial microfluidic chips reveals the interplay of efficiency, speed, and background amplification as a function of reaction temperature and time. Anal Chem 2019;91:1034–42.

[59] Agutu CA, Ngetsa CJ, Price MA, et al. Systematic review of the performance and clinical utility of point of care HIV-1 RNA testing for diagnosis and care. PLoS One 2019;14:e0218369.

[60] Cepheid | HIV-1 molecular test - Xpert HIV-1 qual. Available at: https://www.cepheid.com/en/tests/Virology/Xpert-HIV-1-Qual. Accessed April 30, 2021.

[61] m-PIMATM HIV-1/2 detect. Available at: https://www.globalpointofcare.abbott/en/product-details/m-pima-hiv-12-detect.html. Accessed April 30, 2021.

[62] Farfour E, Roux A, Ballester M, et al. Improved performances of the second generation of the ID NOW influenza A&B 2® and comparison with the GeneXpert®. Eur J Clin Microbiol Infect Dis 2020;39:1681–6.

Advances in Molecular Pathology 4 (2021) 93–101
ADVANCES IN MOLECULAR PATHOLOGY

Emerging Molecular Diagnostic Methods for Prosthetic Joint Infections

Robert Hamilton, MD, Samantha Stephen, DO*
Department of Pathology and Laboratory Medicine, Dartmouth-Hitchcock Medical Center, One Medical Center Drive, Lebanon, NH 03756, USA

KEYWORDS
• Prosthetic joint infection • Nanopore sequencing • 16S • NGS

KEY POINTS

- Prosthetic joint infection (PJI) is a challenging diagnostic space with critical, time-sensitive clinical outcomes.
- Molecular testing has good agreement with gold-standard methods, and offers potential advantages in turnaround time and in diagnosis of patients recently treated with antibiotics.
- Nanopore sequencing is an emerging molecular diagnostic method with numerous applications, including infectious disease diagnosis.
- Molecular genetic testing can help identify pathogens involved in PJIs swiftly, which can facilitate treatment and reduce complications.

INTRODUCTION

Prosthetic joints afford patients with painful and often debilitating joint disease the opportunity to regain mobility, independence, and comfort. Complications involving arthroplasties can be devastating to a patient and their prosthetic joint.

Prosthetic joint infection (PJI) is a well-known and recognized complication of joint replacement surgery in which bacteria or other microorganisms proliferate in the synovial cavity and/or on the surface of a prosthesis itself. If infection occurs less than 3 months postoperatively it is considered to be early-onset; if between 3 months and 1 to 2 years, it is "delayed." Subsequent infections are considered "late" onset, and are occasionally due to hematogenous spread [1]. Most PJIs occur within 2 years of joint replacement [2].

PJIs can result from bacteria introduced during the surgical procedure and contiguous spread from nearby tissue. Hematogenous seeding is also a potential infectious source, although less common [1]. PJIs are caused by a wide variety of microbial pathogens, and the most common organisms vary by the site, timing of infection relative to surgery, patient age, and source of infection. Many of the pathogens involved are found on the surface of the skin or as colonizing organisms in one or more typical ecosystems of the body [1], creating a significant challenge in differentiating clinically significant organisms from contaminants and/or nonpathogenic components of a polymicrobial infection. Although the problem of distinguishing contaminants and colonizers from an organism causing disease is a universal problem of microbiology, it is made more difficult in PJI because many of the most common pathogens in PJI (*Staphylococcus aureus, Staphylococcus epidermidis, Cutibacterium acnes, Streptococcus agalactiae*) frequently colonize human skin and mucosa. This challenge

*Corresponding author, *E-mail address:* Samantha.A.Stephen@hitchcock.org

https://doi.org/10.1016/j.yamp.2021.07.004
2589-4080/21/

remains regardless of the method used to assess the PJI; the various sequencing approaches and culture are all susceptible to this issue. Further diagnostic pitfalls can occur in culture-negative situations, as aseptic joint failures, or "aseptic loosening," should be distinguished from culture-negative PJIs.

Many bacteria that cause PJIs, including some of the most common offenders, form biofilms. Biofilms, or extracellular structural matrices, can be formed by a variety of bacteria on many medical implants, including prosthetic joints and play a critical role in PJIs. Monomicrobial or polymicrobial colonies of bacteria can aggregate on the artificial joint surface in a biofilm. Biofilms allow bacteria to evade the host immune system and can make traditional routes of diagnosis challenging [1].

Hematogenous PJIs are generally monomicrobial and caused by the same organism causing the patient's bacteremia. Other PJIs are more variable, although the measured prevalence of polymicrobial infections varies widely between different studies; values from 15% [3] to 64% [4] are attested. The degree to which these other PJIs are polymicrobial or monomicrobial is still actively being characterized by both traditional and emerging methods. The composition of communities implicated in polymicrobial PJI is also an area of active study [4].

Several diagnostic standards exist for PJI, including criteria from the Infectious Disease Society of America (IDSA), the Musculoskeletal Infection Society (MSIS), and the European Bone and Joint Infection Society. Although it is impractical to fully discuss the clinical diagnosis of PJI here, there are several critical points that should be mentioned before proceeding with a discussion of laboratory diagnostics for PJI.

1. PJI is clinically heterogeneous; patients can have very alarming presentations with obvious infection or inflammation, or relatively minimal and nonspecific symptoms [1].
2. A number of clinical factors can play a role in the diagnosis of PJI, with a draining sinus tract or the presence of the same organism in 2 or more cultures from the joint being the major criteria of the MSIS classification in both the original [5] and updated versions [6].
3. Various additional tests, including inflammatory markers, the presence of a given number of polymorphonuclear cells or gross purulence in the joint cavity, and others may also influence the diagnosis [6].
4. PJI can range from a straightforward to an extremely challenging clinical diagnosis, so there is a strong need for reliable laboratory testing.
    a. There exists a potential role for molecular testing in ambiguous or unclear cases [6].

Proper and timely diagnosis of PJI is imperative: potential consequences can be severe, and can include costly and morbid revision surgeries[1], prolonged antibiotic treatment and permanent disability [7]. Current diagnostic testing methods include a variety of cultures performed on tissue, joint fluid, or sonication fluid from the explanted prosthesis, synovial fluid white blood cell counts, neutrophil percentage, leukocyte esterase tests and various genetic studies including polymerase chain reaction (PCR) and next generation sequencing (NGS).

From the perspective of the clinical laboratory, several traits are desirable for diagnostic studies. The ideal study would provide results within hours. It would be largely hands-off, safe to perform, specific, sensitive, robust to the presence of contaminants or other issues with the specimen, and economical for patients. It would not require tissue, sonication fluid from an explanted prosthesis, or other specimens acquired using invasive surgical procedures. The ideal study would provide a species-level identification of the pathogen and inform providers about the antibiotic resistance profile and any clinically or prognostically relevant virulence factors the pathogen might possess. Needless to say, there is no currently available methodology that performs ideally across all of these categories.

The current gold-standard study for organism identification is culture. Culture is a well-studied methodology with numerous useful features. It is not only a test of organism presence, but a proof of viability. If an isolate is grown, gold-standard phenotypic antibiotic susceptibility testing can be performed. The means of identification are quite flexible; identification can proceed via phenotypic biochemical reactions, proteomic means (Matrix-Assisted Laser Desorption/Ionization-Time Of Flight [MALDI-TOF]), or genetic sequencing of the isolate. Culture can be a very economical diagnostic method if identification by MALDI-TOF or biochemical phenotype is used.

Culture also has several notable disadvantages, however. Cultures need to be incubated for 7 days in most circumstances, and potentially up to 14 days for some organisms (*C acnes*, *Peptostreptococcus*, and *Corynebacterium* spp in particular) [7]. A variety of specimens, including tissue samples, synovial fluid, and sonication fluid are useful in diagnosis [1], but obtaining tissue or sonication fluid requires an arthrotomy rather than an arthrocentesis. Two positive cultures are needed to diagnose PJI; a single positive culture may be accepted for an organism of known pathogenicity or in the presence of compatible ancillary testing [5,6]. Like all studies in the microbiology laboratory, cultures may be contaminated, a particular problem in PJI due to overlap between common culture contaminants (*S epidermidis*, for instance) and common causes of PJI. Long incubation times may increase the risk of contamination as well; in one study in which cultures were held for 14 days, most organisms grown after 7 days of incubation were contaminants [7]. Finally, many suspected cases of PJI are culture-negative, particularly following antimicrobial treatment [1]. Effective antimicrobial therapy can eliminate any viable pathogen available for culture, or reduce the available inoculum size to the point where growth in culture is not observable. Other causes of culture-negative PJI can be due to infection with fastidious organisms that fail to grow under the conditions or in the amount of time for which they are cultured. Culture-negative PJIs present a particular diagnostic conundrum; depending on definitions, 7% to 42% of suspected PJIs will fail to grow organisms in culture [8].

One additional approach to diagnosis by culture involves directly sampling the prosthetic surface by sonication [9]. Sonication, typically performed on the explanted prosthesis itself, assists in the removal of bacteria and their biofilms from the prosthetic implant [10]. During sonication, the biofilm is disrupted and bacteria are released into a diluent, which can subsequently be centrifuged to concentrate bacteria. Following sonication, the sonication fluid can be cultured and analyzed as usual [10,11]. Although tissue culture and synovial fluid analysis are currently the standard of care [11], compared with synovial fluid analysis, sonication fluid analysis can provide more sensitive results from culture [1].

Presumably, some culture-negative PJIs could be identified though using sonication to release bacteria from adherent biofilms after attempted identification through synovial fluid analysis fails. However, even with sonication, culture-negative PJIs persist in both antibiotic-treated and untreated patients. Other microbial organisms, such as fungi or fastidious bacteria, are often culprits as well [11].

At present, with limited exceptions, genetic studies are advantageous for yielding a presumptive organism identification in cases of culture-negative PJI. Many molecular diagnostic methods have the potential to prove useful in identifying causative organisms in PJIs. Notably, multiplex PCR, broad-spectrum 16S RNA PCR, NGS, and long-read sequencing are technologies that could help better identify pathogens and assist in determining the best treatment for the patient. In this article, we review several available and emerging molecular diagnostic methodologies for PJI. We consider how these tests function and discuss the potential place of each methodology in the testing ecosystem.

DISCUSSION

NGS offers a variety of genetic analysis techniques that have been studied as an alternative to traditional culturing for pathogen identification. NGS encompasses targeted 16S and ITS (Internal Transcribed Spacers) gene sequencing, whole genome, and metagenomics. There are a handful of sequencing platforms available, with a few different sequencing methodologies. Broadly speaking, NGS studies proceed through a multistage process including isolation of genetic material, purification, preparation of a library, sequencing the genetic material, and bioinformatics analysis of the sequencing results. NGS can offer information about a wide range of microbes present in samples. However, despite recent improvements in both speed and expense, NGS remains relatively time-consuming and costly to run. Between library preparation and actual sample analysis, some NGS tests offer results after a week to 10 days. This turnaround time is particularly concerning in the setting of microbiology diagnostics, which are often time-sensitive.

However, NGS platforms do have a number of advantages worth considering. The technology is, compared with emerging methods, mature and well understood. There are established workflows and pipelines with which many laboratories have substantial clinical experience. Although there are many steps in the process, some of these conduce to additional flexibility. Library preparation allows for selective enrichment and/or removal of DNA fragments matching many different characteristics. Bioinformatics methods can provide an additional level of filtration for fragments of interest. Finally, NGS platforms have a distinct accuracy advantage over long-read sequencing.

One NGS approach of interest for microbiology is "shotgun" metagenomics. These methods involve the nonspecific sequencing of all genomic DNA in the specimen. By sequencing the entirety of the genomic DNA in the specimen, it is possible to identify theoretically arbitrary organisms and resistance genes. Clinical application of shotgun sequencing in general is limited at present relative to 16S sequencing, but the potential is easy to appreciate: a single test, suited to a wide variety of specimens, with the capacity to simultaneously report species/strain-level identifications and numerous potential sources of resistance. Fungi, viruses, and bacteria are all encompassed, in theory, by this one test. In addition, in settings of abundant microbial DNA, shotgun sequencing may actually be more able to identify low-prevalence organisms, although results differ between studies with respect to this question [12]. In theory, it may be possible to identify markers of biofilm formation, potentially helping to resolve the question of contamination [13].

Hypothesis agnosticism is to some extent both a bug and a feature of shotgun metagenomic by sequencing all of the genomic DNA of a specimen, one introduces the risk of large-scale host DNA contamination and loses some coverage depth, but in the event of a positive result, gains a great deal of additional information about the pathogen.

There are some drawbacks to metagenomic sequencing. First, if measures are not taken to deplete host DNA, host DNA contamination may become a significant issue. In one metagenomic study, 98% of all sequencing reads mapped to the human host, whereas for most specimens, bacterial reads made up less than 1% of the total [14]. Although that particular study nevertheless demonstrated 93% sensitivity of shotgun sequencing relative to sonication culture, high levels of host DNA likely result in a corresponding decrease in coverage of other fragments, which in turn would result in reduced sensitivity for organisms and resistance-causing mutations. Second and relatedly, a robust bioinformatics pipeline is required for analysis of the large volume of incoming data. Depending on the pipeline and hardware, this step can substantially increase the time to diagnosis. Finally, although shotgun sequencing performs well when microbial DNA is abundant, it may be less sensitive to low levels of microbial DNA than PCR-amplified methods [12].

The literature contains numerous well-written examples of shotgun sequencing for NGS diagnosis. One good example of the use of metagenomics NGS for diagnosis of PJI is found in Street and colleagues [14], cited previously. Another study using these methods was carried out by Thoendel and colleagues [15], which demonstrated sensitivity of 95% relative to sonicate fluid culture, with 86% overall agreement between the 2 methodologies. Thoendel and colleagues [15] reported a relatively high rate of organism identification in culture-negative PJI compared with other studies, identifying a potentially pathogenic organism in roughly 30% of culture-negative PJIs. Thoendel and colleagues [15] caution about the presence of numerous short, low-complexity microbial reads in specimens from aseptic joint failures they examined, emphasizing the need for robust bioinformatics analysis to avoid false positives.

PCR is another well-established technology used for microbiologic diagnosis, which involves the use of DNA polymerases to amplify nucleic acid sequences of interest. Melting curves, labeled probes, or primers can be used to directly render diagnosis on the basis of a PCR result, often in real time. The turnaround time is considerably faster than NGS, and the cost is often more affordable; however, PCR, unlike sequencing methods, usually requires some kind of knowledge of the target DNA sought, even if it is as broad as "a bacterium" or "a fungal organism." PCR primers can be very specific, in some cases even to the level of an individual species, or very broad, on the level of the genus. PCR can serve as either a primary diagnostic study or as part of the library preparation for NGS.

Although in focused studies, species and genus-specific PCR studies are available for clinical use, we discuss PCR as a multiplex study and in the context of the 16S ribosomal subunit.

Multiplex PCR is a method incorporating many different primers for different organisms or families. A prototypical example of multiplex PCR relevant to PJI is the Unyvero ITI cartridge, used in several European studies to identify pathogens in joint fluid and sonicate specimens [16–18]. The cartridge-based system offers a quick turnaround time (~5 hours) and sensitivity overall comparable to culture over the organisms included in its panel, with sensitivity for *Cutibacterium* spp and coagulase-negative staphylococci notably variable among the 3 studies [16–18]. It has the additional ability to detect a subset of known resistance genes. Naturally, a PCR system is not able to detect any organism or genetic alteration not included in its primer set, which constitutes a significant limitation. The Unyvero ITI does include a universal bacterial primer; in theory, this may be able to provide information on whether an otherwise unidentified bacterial organism is present. As far as we know, there is no Food and Drug Administration–approved PCR system for PJI available for use in the United States at this time.

The other major approach to PCR diagnosis involves the use of the 16S ribosomal subunit. PCR is incorporated, almost by definition, into 16S sequencing studies. There are numerous examples of 16S sequencing in both the research literature and current clinical practice; a significant number of national reference laboratories now perform them on a wide variety of specimen types. In a major study of 16S PCR, Bémer and colleagues [3] found good specificity for 16S PCR and sequencing, although sensitivity was limited; there were a total of 40 culture-confirmed PJI cases (of a total of 215 PJI cases) for which PCR was negative. The sensitivity overall was 73% for PJI as diagnosed by the IDSA criteria. Of note, in a group of 23 culture-negative PJIs, Bémer and colleagues [3] reported successful identification of an organism by 16S PCR and sequencing in 8 of these cases, all of which had recently undergone antibiotic treatment, underscoring a potential area of utility for molecular diagnostics. A number of other studies have reported roughly comparable results for 16S sequencing [19].

Contrariwise, the use of 16S PCR enables higher-sensitivity examinations through better sequencing coverage of a region of interest, but provides data on a limited subset of the genome that may not be informative for some problems of organism identification or mechanisms of resistance. Relative to culture, both methods may be able to identify organisms in any given culture-negative specimen, but do not provide the test of viability inherent in culture. Although agreement between culture and NGS was generally good in the studies we read, numerous culture-positive/NGS-negative and culture-negative/NGS-positive cases are seen throughout the literature. Antimicrobial therapy, small inoculum size, or fastidious organisms can often explain the latter. A multitude of diverse concerns can affect NGS reactions, and it is not always possible to infer the probable cause of NGS reaction failure when reading a finished study. In any case, the meaning of a single isolated NGS or culture positive is not always clear, particularly if the organism identified is not a known pathogen at the relevant body site.

In contrast to NGS ("short-read") sequencing approaches, there are several long-read platforms available as well. Pacific Biosciences ("PacBio") SMRTbell and Oxford Nanopore are the 2 most prominent methods.

Nanopore sequencing, developed by Oxford Nanopore Technologies (ONT), is a method of sequencing DNA that uses alterations in electrical current as DNA passes through a small pore to determine base sequence. Initially suffering from a low accuracy rate (approximately 85%) [20], subsequent innovations have increased the accuracy of the system to approximately 95% [21], while maintaining an economic cost profile and rapid turnaround time. Nanopore sequencing continues to struggle with homopolymers and low-complexity material; the current generation of pore (R10.3) can accurately resolve homopolymers approximately 10 bases long [21]. It should be noted that sequencing-by-synthesis approaches may also struggle to accurately determine the length of homopolymers.

PacBio single-molecule, real-time (SMRT) is a long-read platform that, like Illumina and Ion Torrent devices, performs sequencing by synthesis. Nucleotide incorporation is monitored through the emission of fluorescent light. The template is circular, which allows the polymerase to pass over the template and sequence in multiple passes. Circular consensus sequencing results in impressively accurate long reads, with accuracies of greater than 99%, or "HiFi reads." Continuous long-read sequencing produces the longest possible reads the machine has to offer [10]. We were not able to locate any prior papers specifically applying SMRT sequencing in clinical PJIs.

Long-read sequencing can pose technical challenges due to the large amount of data generated. In their efforts to make Nanopore sequencing accessible, ONT has developed a variety of user-friendly tools for laboratories with limited bioinformatics experience to help facilitate the process of converting data files and analyzing them. Their open-source platform, "EPI2ME," has multiple different apps to help with each step of the data processing. Other long-read sequencing platforms, such as SMRT, generally require more hands-on data processing. For those with bioinformatics experience, there are a number of free resources for both SMRT and Nanopore sequencing on GitHub [22].

In the setting of the microbiology laboratory, Nanopore sequencing is an appealing potential diagnostic tool. It is a quick, efficient, and cost-effective way to identify pathogens rapidly. Nanopore sequencing can produce data on the microorganism within as little as 4 hours [23]. Nanopore sequencing can be followed in real time, which allows progress of the sequencing reaction to be monitored throughout the process. There is potential for extremely rapid identification if the results are processed as the reaction runs. Generally, Nanopore sequencing is suitable for many of the same applications as NGS, including, potentially, organism detection in culture-negative PJIs.

One fascinating capability of the Nanopore technology arising from being able to receive data in real time is the Read Until method. Using this method, first implemented by Loose and colleagues [24], Nanopore is able to expel unwanted nucleotide sequences from the pore and thereby concentrate read coverage on sequences of interest. As noted by Kovaka and colleagues [25], this effectively allows for a targeted sequencing protocol that does not interfere with Nanopore's capacity to produce long reads or eliminate epigenetic changes present in the material to be sequenced. By contrast, PCR is generally limited to producing shorter transcripts than a Nanopore unit can accommodate (wasting some of the capacity of the method) and does not transcribe epigenetic changes. Other methods relying on depleting unwanted genetic material (Hybrid Capture, CRISPR/CAS 9) are not subject to these particular limitations, but like PCR, they require additional overheads in terms of preparation time and reagents. In principle, Read Until could enable a targeted sequencing study on a direct patient specimen with minimal library preparation. Using software-based mapping techniques, such as UNCALLED, signals can be matched rapidly to reference sequences. If the sequence aligns to the human host genome, or other undesirable target (a bacterial genome if fungal sequences are being sought, for instance), the undesirable sequence can be ejected from the pore. This enables the pore to be used for a different sequence later [25].

Kovaka and colleagues [25] provided a proof-of-concept of this exciting possibility. Although use of this method could result in the same forms of bias as other enrichment methods, Kovaka and colleagues [25] reported running a second flow cell with a regular base-calling algorithm [25] in parallel, so the bias introduced could presumably be eliminated by a full sequencing run, which would result sometime after the "enriched" procedure.

Considering these characteristics, it is not surprising that clinical proof-of-concept testing of the Nanopore platform has begun to emerge in the microbiology laboratory. It has been successfully used for nonclinical influenza testing [26], identification of resistance-conferring plasmids [23,27], and PJI.

Schmidt and colleagues [23] applied Nanopore sequencing to clinical urine specimens, and achieved rapid and accurate identification from both clinical and spiked specimens. They also identified antimicrobial resistance elements with excellent concordance with NGS from the same organism. Of note, they were able to deplete host DNA content to between 2% and 12% of the total reads [23]. Other studies have reported still more complete depletion of host DNA in the metagenomics setting; the most promising figure we encountered was 0.1% of total reads [28].

To date, a few small studies have specifically put Nanopore sequencing to use in the diagnosis of PJIs. Both Sanderson and colleagues [29] and Wang and colleagues [30] compared Nanopore-based metagenomics to NGS metagenomics and culture; they each report rapid and accurate identification of bacterial pathogens in 9 samples, with good concordance with culture and NGS data. Wang and colleagues [30] also evaluated the presence of various genetic elements known to cause antimicrobial resistance. Although they detected a number of possible candidates, there was no concordance between NGS and Nanopore in the actual resistance elements detected [30]. Wang and colleagues [30] further noted a dissimilarity with local patterns of resistance, and commented that the actual presence of antimicrobial resistance elements within the genome is one of many genotypic factors influencing the expression of resistance.

We would add that there are many nongenetic variables affecting the expression of resistance as well. One potential explanation for the differential resistance testing results between Schmidt and colleagues [23] and Wang and colleagues [30] is a striking difference in coverage: Wang and colleagues [30] reported that there was only a single NGS read for each of the resistance elements identified by NGS, whereas they reported from 3 to 330,931 reads for the elements identified by Nanopore. Schmidt and colleagues [23] reported greater than 10,000 "pass" reads for each of 3 runs of their MDRO-spiked specimen.

We are fortunate to be living and practicing during an efflorescence of new diagnostic studies and techniques in microbiology, and genetic methods show great promise. Nanopore sequencing is a technique of particular interest due to its favorable turnaround time and cost characteristics. However, it has yet to be operationalized on any scale in the clinical laboratory. In our judgment, this is partially due to Nanopore-specific factors (it is relatively new and unstudied, and there remain some lingering questions about sequencing accuracy) and in part due to larger questions around the use of sequencing for diagnosis in the microbiology laboratory in general. Larger issues around the use of genetic testing in microbiology include an uncertain relationship to gold-standard studies such as culture, a lack of consensus on how to consider low-prevalence organisms and/or organisms not known to cause human disease, and the inability to perform gold-standard antimicrobial susceptibility testing without a culture isolate. Finally, PJI and especially culture-negative PJI are a complex diagnostic space with many challenges, and the difficulty of establishing the "ground truth" in many of the cases for which molecular diagnostic studies would in theory be most helpful is likely a contributing factor to the slow uptake of molecular studies.

Technical issues surrounding molecular genetic studies, although still undergoing optimization, are overall proving tractable. Bacterial DNA contamination is a continual risk, and careful practice at every stage is required to mitigate the danger of false-positive diagnoses [15]. Host DNA levels vary widely; it appears that preparatory methodologies may have a major impact, although ReadUntil-using approaches may ultimately

TABLE 1
Comparison of Traditional Culture to Next Generation Sequencing (NGS)

Characteristic	Culture	NGS
Ease of use	Requires significant technical expertise and staffing.	Additional informatics infrastructure required; otherwise requires significant technical expertise and staffing.
Cost	Usually lower.	High; current applications limited as a result.
Turnaround time	Long; most, but not all, PJI-relevant organisms will grow within 3 d. Sensitivity testing and ancillary studies will add more time.	Variable; can be more or less than 3 days depending on workflow. Send out testing almost always longer than 3 d due to logistics.
Inhibitors	Antibiotics, organism may be fastidious, slow growing, or wrong culture type ordered.	Variable, but frequently different from culture.
Specimen	Requires fresh specimen; viability declines over time.	Amenable to a wide variety of specimens, including formalin-fixed tissues.
Other Benefits	A positive culture serves as proof of organism viability.	May provide additional information about drug resistance, relationship to epidemic strains, or other characteristics of interest.

prove able to mitigate high levels of unwanted DNA in the specimen.

Current studies of the Nanopore methodology, although promising, have a limited number of patients on which they base their data, especially in the context of PJI. In future research we hope to see significantly larger studies. Another potentially beneficial study would be a prospective trial of one or more novel diagnostic techniques in culture-negative PJI, including longitudinal data on patient courses and treatment success or failure based on combined molecular and culture findings. Such a trial would be valuable because it would provide a look at the functional utility of these novel diagnostic assays in actual patient care, something not clearly reported in the literature we perused in writing this article.

Overall, the findings of the studies we perused are quite heterogeneous with respect to the efficacy of molecular diagnostics. In general, they tended to demonstrate a pattern of overlapping identification by NGS and culture, with some organisms detected by only one methodology or the other (Table 1). Sensitivity and specificity tended to be roughly comparable across the board. We would therefore suggest an ancillary role for molecular genetic studies in general in the diagnosis of PJI, particularly where clinical suspicion is strong but culture results are unhelpful. Areas in which genetic studies show particular promise are cases in which antibiotics have been recently used [1] and cases that have been previously culture-negative [15]. The significance of the additional organism identifications sometimes made by molecular genetic studies in otherwise culture-positive cases appears to be less well understood.

SUMMARY

PJIs are a serious complication of artificial joint replacement that require prompt diagnosis and treatment. Accurate and timely diagnosis of any bacterial pathogen is crucial to mitigate potential damage. The current gold-standard diagnostic method is culture, which can take up to a week to result, and sometimes fails to identify a causative pathogen. Emerging molecular diagnostic methods have the potential to provide critical information accurately and rapidly. Methods, such as Nanopore sequencing, PacBio SMRT sequencing, and 16S, are promising alternative methods to diagnosis. Ideally, these methods would be quick, affordable, and accessible more so than the current gold standard of culture. Methods, such as Nanopore sequencing, have been examined in various studies that illuminate the potential benefits of these sequencing methods. Future studies need to be performed with larger patient populations to better compare these methods to the well-established gold standard of culture. It would also be beneficial to see more studies analyzing the utility and ease of use in the setting of diagnosing PJI.

CLINICS CARE POINTS

- Molecular genetic studies have potential utility in cases of suspected PJI where cultures are unhelpful, particularly if antibiotics were administered before culture.
- A helpful role for molecular diagnostics in already culture-positive cases is not currently established.
- For both culture and molecular diagnostics, positive results may be of unclear significance if only a single submitted specimen is positive, particularly if the organism is a common contaminant in the medical setting.
- Coagulase-negative staphylococci and *C acnes* are examples of organisms that are both common contaminants and capable of causing PJI.

DISCLOSURE

The authors have nothing to disclose.

REFERENCES

[1] Tande AJ, Patel R. Prosthetic joint infection. Clin Microbiol Rev 2014;27(2):302–45.

[2] Beam E, Osmon D. Prosthetic joint infection update. Infect Dis Clin North Am 2018;32(Issue 4). https://doi.org/10.1016/j.idc.2018.06.005.

[3] Bémer P, Plouzeau C, Tande D, et al. Evaluation of 16S rRNA gene PCR sensitivity and specificity for diagnosis of prosthetic joint infection: a prospective multicenter cross-sectional study. J Clin Microbiol 2014;52(10): 3583–9.

[4] Xu Y, Rudkjøbing VB, Simonsen O, et al. Bacterial diversity in suspected prosthetic joint infections: an exploratory study using 16S rRNA gene analysis. FEMS Immunol Med Microbiol 2012;65(Issue 2):291–304.

[5] Parvizi J, Zmistowski B, Berbari EF, et al. New definition for periprosthetic joint infection: from the Workgroup of the Musculoskeletal Infection Society. Clin Orthop Relat Res 2011;469(11):2992–4.

[6] Parvizi J, Tan TL, Goswami K, et al. The 2018 definition of periprosthetic hip and knee infection: an evidence-based and validated criteria. J Arthroplasty 2018;33(5): 1309–14.e2.

[7] Schwotzer N, Wahl P, Fracheboud D, et al. Optimal culture incubation time in orthopedic device-associated infections: a retrospective analysis of prolonged 14-day incubation. J Clin Microbiol 2014;52(1):61–6.

[8] Yoon HK, Cho SH, Lee DY, et al. A review of the literature on culture-negative periprosthetic joint infection: epidemiology, diagnosis and treatment. Knee Surg Relat Res 2017;29(3):155–64.

[9] Tzeng A, Tzeng TH, Vasdev S, et al. Treating periprosthetic joint infections as biofilms: key diagnosis and management strategies. Diagn Microbiol Infect Dis 2015;81(3):192–200.

[10] Eid J, Fehr A, Gray J, et al. Real-time DNA sequencing from single polymerase molecules. Science 2009; 323(5910):133–8.

[11] Palan J, Nolan C, Sarantos K, et al. Culture-negative periprosthetic joint infections. EFORT Open Rev 2019;4(10): 585–94.

[12] Durazzi F, Sala C, Castellani G, et al. Comparison between 16S rRNA and shotgun sequencing data for the taxonomic characterization of the gut microbiota. Sci Rep 2021;11:3030.

[13] Unverdorben L, Goswami K, Wright, et al. Synovial fluid sequencing: a look into the future of prosthetic joint infection detection. FASEB J 2020;34:1.

[14] Street TL, Sanderson ND, Atkins BL, et al. Molecular diagnosis of orthopedic-device-related infection directly from sonication fluid by metagenomic sequencing. J Clin Microbiol Jul 2017;55(8):2334–47.

[15] Thoendel MJ, Jeraldo PR, Greenwood-Quaintance KE, et al. Identification of prosthetic joint infection pathogens using a shotgun metagenomics approach. Clin Infect Dis 2018;67(9):1333–8.

[16] Renz N, Feihl S, Cabric S, et al. Performance of automated multiplex PCR using sonication fluid for diagnosis of periprosthetic joint infection: a prospective cohort. Infection 2017;45:877–84.

[17] Morgenstern C, Cabric S, Perka C, et al. Synovial fluid multiplex PCR is superior to culture for detection of low-virulent pathogens causing periprosthetic joint infection. Diagn Microbiol Infect Dis 2018;90(Issue 2): 115–9.

[18] Sigmund IK, Windhager R, Sevelda F, et al. Multiplex PCR Unyvero i60 ITI application improves detection of low-virulent microorganisms in periprosthetic joint infections. Int Orthop 2019;43(8):1891–8.

[19] Zhang Y, Feng S, Chen W, et al. Advantages of 16S rRNA PCR for the diagnosis of prosthetic joint infection. Exp Ther Med 2020;20(4):3104–13.

[20] Sahlin K, Medvedev P. Error correction enables use of Oxford Nanopore technology for reference-free transcriptome analysis. Nat Commun 2021;12:2.

[21] Sheka D, Alabi N, Gordon PMK. Oxford nanopore sequencing in clinical microbiology and infection diagnostics. Brief Bioinform 2021. https://doi.org/10.1093/bib/bbaa403 bbaa403.

[22] Petersen LM, Martin IW, Moschetti WE, et al. Third-generation sequencing in the clinical laboratory: exploring the advantages and challenges of nanopore sequencing. J Clin Microbiol 2020;58e:01315–9.

[23] Schmidt K, Mwaigwisya S, Crossman LC, et al. Identification of bacterial pathogens and antimicrobial resistance directly from clinical urines by nanopore-based metagenomic sequencing. J Antimicrob Chemother 2017; 72(1):104–14.

[24] Loose M, Malla S, Stout M. Real-time selective sequencing using nanopore technology. Nat Methods 2016;13:751–4.
[25] Kovaka S, Fan Y, Ni B, et al. Targeted nanopore sequencing by real-time mapping of raw electrical signal with UNCALLED. Nat Biotechnol 2021;39:431–41.
[26] Lewandowski K, Xu Y, Pullan ST, et al. Metagenomic nanopore sequencing of influenza virus direct from clinical respiratory samples. J Clin Microbiol 2019;58(1): e00963-19.
[27] Lemon JK, Khil PP, Frank KM, et al. Rapid nanopore sequencing of plasmids and resistance gene detection in clinical isolates. J Clin Microbiol 2017;55(12): 3530–43.
[28] Sanabria A, Hjerde E, Johannessen M, et al. Shotgun-metagenomics on positive blood culture bottles inoculated with prosthetic joint tissue: a proof of concept study. Front Microbiol 2020;11:1687.
[29] Sanderson ND, Street TL, Foster D, et al. Real-time analysis of nanopore-based metagenomic sequencing from infected orthopaedic devices. BMC Genomics 2018;19: 714.
[30] Wang C xin, Huang Z, Fang W, et al. Preliminary assessment of nanopore-based metagenomic sequencing for the diagnosis of prosthetic joint infection. Int J Infect Dis 2020;97:54–9.

Pharmacogenomics

Advances in Molecular Pathology 4 (2021) 103–116
ADVANCES IN MOLECULAR PATHOLOGY

The Role of the Human Gutome on Chronic Disease

A Review of the Microbiome and Nutrigenomics

Carrie C. Hoefer, PhD, MBA[a,*], Leah K. Hollon, ND, MPH[b,1], Jennifer A. Campbell, PharmD[c]
[a]James L. Winkle College of Pharmacy, University of Cincinnati, 231 Albert Sabin Way, MSB 3005, Cincinnati, OH 45267, USA; [b]Richmond Natural Medicine, National University of Natural Medicine Residency, 9211 Forest Hill Avenue, Richmond, VA 23235, USA; [c]Manchester University, College of Pharmacy, Natural, and Health Sciences, 10627 Diebold Road, Fort Wayne, IN 46845, USA

KEYWORDS
- Nutrigenomics • Microbiome • Nutrition • Diabetes • Cardiovascular • Obesity • Breast cancer • Colon cancer

KEY POINTS
- The microbiome and optimal nutrition vary among individuals and may be used along with pharmacogenomics to further improve individualized treatment strategies.
- Common genetic variants associated with chronic disease and the therapeutic effects of nutrition and human microbiome are summarized.
- The gut microbiome and nutrigenomics modify chronic disease and acute disease progression and outcomes.
- The gut microbiome and nutrigenomics influence obesity, diabetes, cardiovascular disease, and cancer treatment.

INTRODUCTION

The human gutome is a mosaic of nutrients, gut flora/bacteria, and genomic biomarkers that play a role in human health and disease [1,2]. One can look at the gutome in 2 distinct ways: the human gut microbiome and nutrigenomics. Nutrigenomics studies the influence and interaction of nutrition and genes and can facilitate understanding of nutrient consumption and genomic biomarkers that may lead to the development of nutrition-related diseases and metabolic syndromes [1,3]. The human gut microbiome is defined as the totality of microorganisms, bacteria, viruses, protozoa, and fungi, including their collective genetic material inhabiting the gastrointestinal system [4]. Therefore, the gut microbiome is a notably diverse habitat that provides a collective and historical picture of the environmental exposures throughout one's life. Although it is colonized throughout life, it is initially seeded during fetal development and thus imprinted from our ancestors. It has been noted that "Homeostasis of the intestinal microbial environment is likely to be affected multiple times across the lifespan of the average individual due to antibiotic usage, inflammation, aging, psychological stress, nutrition and lifestyle choices, as well as other environmental factors" [5].

The gut microbiome plays a significant role in health as well as the development of chronic disease owing to its ability to regulate the immune, endocrine, and neurologic

C.C. Hoefer and L.K. Hollon: contributing first author.
[1] Present address: 9211 Forest Hill Avenue, Richmond, VA 23235.

*Corresponding author. 128 Burbank Drive, Amherst, NY 14226. *E-mail address:* hoefercc@ucmail.uc.edu

https://doi.org/10.1016/j.yamp.2021.06.003
2589-4080/21/

systems [5,6]. This role of the human gut microbiome is a more recently recognized determinant in human disease; little research has assessed the interaction of the gut microbiome and genomic biomarkers in disease [1]. Furthermore, the gut microbiome, which varies throughout the lifetime, may begin to metabolize orally administered medications and lead to variability in medication response. Additionally, this collaborative community of organisms is constantly communicating within the microbiome and requires key nutrients for effective function [7]. Deficiencies of certain nutrients including vitamins A, D, and E, calcium, and magnesium are associated with fewer healthy bacterial populations and can also promote harmful populations within the microbiome [8]. The purpose of this review is to bring together the 2 concepts of the human gut microbiome and nutrigenomic factors that impact nutrition related diseases.

SIGNIFICANCE

Gut Microbiome

The human gut microbiome has been an evolving source of information in the quest to understand ongoing health and disease. Similarities as well as differences exist from person to person relating to microbiome diversity. Yet, within each individual, these organisms can be symbiotic, commensal, therapeutic, and even pathogenic. Inherently, some species are pathogenic and others are beneficial. Certain species that are inherently commensal or neutral can become pathogenic. In these cases, the role of the organism can be based on the amount found within the gut and the balance of other flora. In general, the greater the diversity of flora the more protective against chronic disease. This diversity of flora leads to greater stability of the mucosal barrier facilitating appropriate production of carbohydrate and protein fuel for the gut. Yet, if only a few species are found in excess and are inherently pathogenic or excess of commensal bacteria exist, microbial metabolism of intestinal contents is altered because these species have the ability to hijack the functions at the mucosal lining, altering the carbohydrates made to promote their own food for consumption and leading to overpopulation [9]. This influence on the health and variability of the gut have led some investigators to believe that the human gut microbiome should be considered its own organ system, in addition to seeing it as a collection of our external environmental experiences over life.

This variability begins in utero and continues into childbirth where genetic and nongenetic material are passed from mother to child [10,11]. As such, some individuals are seeded early with pathogenic microbes or may lack commensal flora owing to determinants of their mother's health, including her diet, pharmacotherapy, immune (infections), and endocrine functions [12,13]. Throughout life, this variability compounds; some individuals are more likely to retain beneficial microbes fostering health, whereas others may adopt pathogenic growth. The human gut microbiome changes throughout one's life as well as throughout various times of the year [14]. This demonstrates the microbiome is modifiable and can therefore be altered to improve or worsen health.

If the microbiome contains overpopulated dysbiosis, there can be an increased risk of chronic disease, specifically autoimmune disease. One of the earliest and most notable findings within the literature demonstrated *Klebsiella* fostered the development of rheumatoid arthritis and inflammatory bowel disease (IBD) [13,15]. In some cases, bacteria had been laid years before their presentation of autoimmune disease. This knowledge of autoimmune disease now extends to include *Bifidobacterium, Staphylococcus, Enterococcus, Salmonella, Lactobacillus, Pseudomonas,* and *Proteus* [5]. Additionally, deficient amounts of *Faecalibacterium* and *Roseburia* lead to an increased risk of rheumatoid arthritis and IBD [16,17]. As discussed elsewhere in this article, gut flora balance is a significant determinant of whether or not disease presents itself. In cases where pathogenic bacteria play a role, a key mechanism remains at the lining of the gut. Secretory IgA serves as a protective lining, but can be altered under stress, poor food choices (eg, inflammatory foods), and even pharmacotherapy. This factor impacts the permeability of the lining, leading pathogens and food particulates to cross over outside of the gut. At this point, immune proteins including IL-23 alert additional inflammatory pathways including tumor necrosis factor-alpha, which become systemic and cross-reactive with other parts of the body, causing peripheral symptoms such as pain [17]. Thus, excessive, or insufficient microbes can contribute to autoimmune disease.

Nutrigenomics and Disease

To fully understand the human gutome, one must be able to identify the molecular level at which metabolic syndromes can be exacerbated. As much as diet can have beneficial effects on overall health, there is a wide range of interindividual variability in response to specific diets [3]. Just as pharmacogenomics can be used to predict drug response, nutrigenomics assesses the genetic predictability in diseases relevant to diet and nutrition [2]. The intestinal tract in which drug and food absorption occurs contains numerous phase

I and II drug-metabolizing enzymes. The alteration of pharmacokinetics via microbial activity is an additional level of interindividual drug response altering the disposition and toxicity of drugs and their metabolites [18,19]. With both enzymes and microbial activity altering drug therapy and nutrition, it should be concerning that obesity has increased by more than 10% in the last 20 years, because obesity is linked to poor gut health [20]. Obesity is one of the leading risk factors in developing metabolic syndromes, which can lead to diseases such as type 2 diabetes (T2DM) and cardiovascular disease (CVD) [21]. Table 1 is a representative example of genes linked to obesity that frequently appear in the literature.

The World Health Organization estimates that 422 million people worldwide have diabetes. Diabetes is considered one of the largest health burdens globally, especially those in low- and middle-income countries [22]. T2DM is a complex disease owing to the numerous biomarkers, such as insulin secretion and resistance, environmental factors including diet and nutrition, and genes associated with T2DM. Gene–nutrient interactions play a crucial role in the pathogenesis of T2DM; therefore, a better understanding of the nutrigenomics of diabetes is essential to the development of prevention, detection, and treatment of the disease [23]. Table 2 is a representative example of genes linked to T2DM that frequently appear in the literature.

CVD encompasses numerous disorders such as heart disease, heart attack, stroke, congenital heart disease, and heart failure [3]. As of 2019 CVD had a prevalence of about 18.6 million people and was the leading global cause of death [24]. The American Heart Association has seven health factors to gauge the risk of CVD known as Life's Simple 7. Included in Life's Simple 7 are smoking, physical inactivity, nutrition, obesity, cholesterol, diabetes, and high blood pressure. Therefore, lifestyle, especially diet, impacts CVD risk both directly and indirectly [24,25]. As with obesity and T2DM, there is a large amount of interindividual variability with diet and CVD risk/mortality; thus, it is prudent to determine which genetic factors are linked with CVD and nutrition. Table 3 is a representative example of genes linked to CVD that frequently appear in the literature.

As seen in the tables in this article, the same gene and polymorphism show up across diseases related to the metabolic syndrome. This connection is also seen in the disease states; obesity can lead to T2DM and CVD. For example, *FTO* is said to impact both obesity and T2DM. *FTO* is associated with higher body mass index and a higher body mass index can lead to T2DM. Additionally, *MTHFR* is associated with obesity and modest changes in homocysteine levels [3]. Of note, although common *MTHFR* variants were historically thought to be associated with mild hyperhomocysteinemia, leading to increased risk for thrombophilia, coronary heart disease, and recurrent miscarriage, currently, *MTHFR* genetic testing is thought to have limited clinical usefulness alone [26]. Interestingly, each of these genes may have a different impact depending on a person's diet. For example, the *APOE* gene harbors 3 different alleles that carry different probabilities of developing CVD and differing responses to environmental factors such as fat included in the diet [27].

Furthermore, many common cancers, such as breast cancer and colorectal cancer have been linked in part to metabolic syndromes [28]. The American Cancer Society notes that one in 3 individuals will be diagnosed with cancer within their lifetime [29]. Foods including processed meats are associated with several cancers and can alter gut microbiome forming a hospitable environment for tumorigenesis with 1 study showing 50 g of processed meat increasing colon cancer by 20% [30,31]. Similarly, high glycemic index foods present a risk for developing colon, breast, and endometrial cancers [32]. Previously discussed genes of *FTO*, *MTHFR*, *APOA*, and *APOE* have been implicated in cancer risk. Specifically, polymorphisms of *FTO* along with obesity increase cancer risk and thus play an active role in adipogenesis and tumorigenesis [33]. Table 4 is a representative example of nutrigenomic genes linked to cancer that frequently appear in the literature.

Diet and the Gutome

The importance of nutrigenomics has been well-demonstrated through certain lineage diets. One such lineage diet, known as the Mediterranean diet, has been useful in enhancing the human gut microbiome. The Mediterranean diet consists of using olive oil as the principal source of fat for cooking, and choosing white meats, such as chicken or fish, over red meats [34]. Some studies have found red meat to be of increased risk of cancer owing to many being processed with nitrates and nitrites. These nitroso compounds can become beneficial S-nitroso compounds or carcinogenic, but it depends on dietary and environmental factors including food macronutrients such as fats and fiber, gastric acidity, and microbial flora [35]. Additionally, one reason that the Mediterranean diet is effective is that it alters the microbiome by increasing the levels of short-chain fatty acids and certain gut flora, including *Prevotella* and some fiber-degrading *Firmicutes* [36]. Meslier and colleagues [37] demonstrated that those adopting a Mediterranean diet for 2 months decreased

TABLE 1
Genes and Polymorphisms Related to Obesity and/or Fat Gain

Gene	Prominent SNPs (Minor Allele; Frequency)	Evidence Associations	References
APOA Family	rs5082 (MA:G; 0.24)	Associated with higher intake of PUFAs (T-allele), and BMI (C-allele)	[3,62]
	rs662799 (MA:G; 0.16)	Associated with HDL and intake of PUFAs (TT-genotype)	[3,63]
	rs3135506 (MA:C; 0.06)	Associated with high saturated fats and total fat consumption (GG-genotype)	[3,63]
APOE	rs429358 (MA:C; 0.15)	Associated with lipid metabolism disturbances	[34,64]
	rs7412 (MA:T; 0.08)	Associated with lipid metabolism disturbances	[34,64]
CLOCK	rs4580704 (MA:G; 0.28)	Associated with C-reactive protein levels and HDL/ApoA1 ratios (CC-genotype)	[34,65]
	rs1801260 (MA:G; 0.23)	Associated with body weight reduction (A-allele)	[34,65]
FTO	rs9930506 (MA:G; 0.29)	Associated with higher BMI and weight (G-allele)	[3,66]
	rs9939609 (MA:A; 0.34)	Associated with BMI, fat mass, weight, c-reactive protein, and leptin levels (A-allele)	[3,63,67]
	rs17817449 (MA:G; 0.31)	Associated with higher weight, BMI, waist-hip circumference, cholesterol, triglycerides, adiponectin and fasting glucose (GG-genotype)	[3,68]
INSIG2	rs12464355 (MA:G; 0.03)	Associated with LDL levels (G-allele)	[3,69]
	rs17047757 (MA:G; 0.12)	Associated with weight	[3,69]
	rs7566605 (MA:C; 0.29)	Associated with obesity (CC-genotype)	[3,70]
MC4R	rs2229616 (MA:T; 0.02)	Associated with features of metabolic syndrome and lower risk of obesity, and appetite control (I103 allele)	[3,71,72]
	rs17782313 (MA:C; 0.24)	Associated with obesity, and appetite control (C-allele)	[34,71]
MTHFR	rs1801133 (0.25)	Associated with obesity, high homocysteine and low folate	[26,34,72]
PPARA	rs1800206 (MA:G; 0.02)	Associated with lipid metabolism disturbances	[34,71]
PPARG	rs1801282 (MA:G; 0.07)	Associated with obesity and lipid parameters	[34,71]
TCF7L2	rs7903146 (MA:T; 0.23)	Associated with fat intake, and dietary components, nuclear and cytoplasm regulatory machinery for fat gain	[34,71]

Minor allele frequency was determined using the minor allele frequency from phase III populations: https://useast.ensembl.org/index.html.

Abbreviations: BMI, body mass index; HDL, high-density lipoproteins; LDL, low-density lipoproteins; PUFA, polyunsaturated fatty acids; SNP, single nucleotide polymorphism.

TABLE 2
Genes and Polymorphisms Related to T2DM

Gene	Prominent SNPs (Minor Allele Frequency)	Evidence Associations	References
ADIPOQ	rs1501299 (MA:T; 0.30)	Associated with higher fasting blood glucose and HbA1C, and insulin signaling (T-allele)	[23,73]
	rs2241766 (MA:G; 0.15)	Associated with decreased risk of T2DM, and insulin signaling (G-allele)	[23,73]
CAV2	rs2270188 (MA:G; 0.45)	Associated with higher risk of T2DM and insulin signaling (T-allele)	[23,73]
CLOCK	rs4580704 (MA:G; 0.28)	Associated with decreased risk of T2DM (G-allele)	[23]
	rs1801260 (MA:G; 0.23)	Associated with fasting insulin levels (C-allele)	[73,74]
CRY1	rs2287161 (MA:C; 0.46)	Associated with fasting insulin, an increase in HOMA-IR index, and a decrease in QUICK1 (C-allele)	[23,73]
FTO	rs9939609 (MA:A; 0.34)	Associated with lower risk of T2DM (A-allele)	[23,73]
	rs8050136 (MA:A; 0.32)	Associated with lower risk of T2DM (A-allele)	[23]
IRS1	rs7578326 (MA:G; 0.29)	Associated with decreased resistance to (plasma) insulin (G-allele)	[23,63,71]
	rs2943641 (MA: T; 0.25)	Associated with decreased resistance to (plasma) insulin, hyperinsulinemia, dyslipidemia and with HOMA-IR index (T-allele)	[23,73,75,76]
PLIN1	rs894160 (MA:T; 0.33)	Associated for HOMA-IR index in woman, and intake of fat and carbohydrates (A-allele)	[23,77]
	rs1052700 (MA:T; 0.28)	Associated with HOMA-IR and intake of fat and carbohydrates (A-allele)	[23,73,77]
PPARG	rs180282 (MA:C; 0.19)	Associated with higher risk of T2DM, and HOMA-IR index (G-allele)	[23,73,75,76]
SLC30A8	rs11558471 (MA:G; 0.26)	Associated with smaller levels of fasting plasma glucose (A-allele)	[23,73,76]
	rs13266634 (MA:T; 0.26)	Associated with T2DM risk (C-allele)	[23,73,76]

(continued on next page)

TABLE 2
(*continued*)

Gene	Prominent SNPs (Minor Allele Frequency)	Evidence Associations	References
TCF7L2	rs7903146 (MA:T; 0.23)	Associated with T2DM risk (T-allele)	[23,62,76]
	rs12255372 (MA:G; 0.21)	Associated with T2DM risk (T-allele)	[23,73,75,76]
	rs12573128 (MA:G; 0.43)	Associated with HOMA-IR index and oral glucose tolerance (G-allele)	[73,75,76]
TRPM6	rs3750425 (MA:T; 0.18)	Associated for T2DM risk in woman (T-allele)	[23]
	rs2274924 (MA:C; 0.29)	Associated for T2DM risk in woman, and fasting glucose levels (T-allele)	[23,73]

Minor allele frequency was determined using the minor allele frequency from phase III populations: https://useast.ensembl.org/index.html.
Abbreviations: HbA1C, hemoglobin A1C; HOMA-IR, insulin resistance calculator; QUICK1, quantitative insulin sensitivity check index; SNP, single nucleotide polymorphism.

their cholesterol, increased bile acid elimination, and improved insulin sensitivity; and there was enhanced diversity and increased amounts of microbiota species [32]. Additionally, the microbiome was enhanced to further house fiber-degrading *Faecalibacterium prausnitzii*, and there was also an increase of genes degrading microbial carbohydrates within the gut. Specifically, one gene upregulated to increase butyrate metabolism [37]. This is notable as butyrate is one of the most protective compounds known to reduce the risk of nonalcoholic steatohepatitis, atherosclerosis, IBD [38], and various cancers [39]. One study found the Mediterranean diet to be protective against the development of colon cancer through mediating DNA methylation of the CpG site cg-20674490-RUNX3 that prevents the onset of the disease [40].

Similarly, the Mediterranean diet also has clinical relevance for those with HER2+ breast cancers and carriers of *BRCA1*/*BRCA2* mutations owing to its ability to impact glucose regulation and insulin sensitivity, both of which are imperative in *BRCA1* and *BRCA2* mutation carriers [35,41,42]. Bruno and colleagues [43] found that in BRCA mutation carriers, the Mediterranean diet improved insulin sensitivity through insulin-like growth factor protein 1. Additionally, women observed a decrease in weight, a slimmer waistline and hips, and lowered cholesterol and triglycerides [43]. Thus, the nutrigenomics of some of the most concerning forms of breast cancer showed improved endocrine and immune balance through implementation of the Mediterranean diet.

In addition to the Mediterranean diet, certain religious diets including fasting have nutrigenomic effects on the microbiome. A small study conducted during the month of Ramadan by Özkul and colleagues [44] showed fasting improved the microbiome. Fasting increased bacteria known as *Akkermansia muciniphila* and *Bacteroides fragilis*. This finding is significant, because a deficiency in *A muciniphila* can be associated with chronic diseases including amyotrophic lateral sclerosis, Alzheimer's disease, and IBD, whereas the addition of *A muciniphila* to the gutome can slow the progression of amyotrophic lateral sclerosis [43–47]. A possible explanation for the benefits of fasting on the microbiome may be through by balancing nicotinamide, which is known to assist with the integrity of tissues, including skin and mucosal membranes, as well as enhancing detoxification processes through NADPH.

In contrast, an excess of *A muciniphila* has been associated with other diseases. In 1 study, a 4-fold increase of *A muciniphila* was found to be correlated with colon cancer [48,49]. As with colon cancer and other cancers, the -omics approaches may permit specific or targeted therapeutic options. These options include both diet and pharmacotherapy, including chemotherapy. Thus, therapeutic options should be based on the collaborative components of the gutome to be individualized. Nutrigenomics plays an interactive role in microbiome

TABLE 3
Genes and Polymorphisms Related to CVD

Gene	Prominent SNPs (Minor Allele Frequency)	Evidence Associations (Risk Allele)	References
APOA family	rs662799 (MA:G; 0.16)	Associated with elevated plasma triglycerides, increased risk of hypertriglyceridemia, VLDL and reduced HDL (C-allele)	[3,78–80]
	rs670 (MA:T; 0.19)	Associated with higher PUFA intake and higher HDL in woman (A-allele)	[3,78–80]
APOE	ε2/ε3/ε4	Associated with increased risk of CVD, CHD	[3]
CDKN2B	rs10757274 (MA: G; 0.40)	Associated with coronary heart disease, myocardial infarction, and atherosclerosis (C-allele)	[81–83]
	rs2383206 (MA:G; 0.49)	Associated with coronary heart disease, myocardial infarction, and atherosclerosis (G-allele)	[81–83]
	rs10757278 (MA: G; 0.41)	Associated with coronary heart disease, myocardial infarction, and atherosclerosis (C-allele	[81,83,84]
	rs1333049 (MA:C; 0.42)	Associated with coronary artery disease and myocardial infarction (C-allele)	[81,83]
MTHFR	rs1801133 (MA:A; 0.25)	Historically associated with modestly higher homocysteine levels and oxidative modification of LDL (C-allele); no longer believed to be a significant CVD factor alone.	[3,78,80]
PPARA	rs1800206 (MA:G; 0.02)	Associated with higher waist circumference, lipid oxidation, inflammation and telomere length	[3,85]

Minor allele frequency was determined using the minor allele frequency from phase III populations: https://useast.ensembl.org/index.html.
Abbreviations: CHD, congenital heart diseases; HDL, high-density lipoprotein; LDL, low-density lipoprotein; PUFA, polyunsaturated fatty acid; SNP, single nucleotide polymorphism; VLDL, very low-density lipoprotein.

stability for some of the most serious diseases by way of supporting or thwarting specific species of microbes and expanding future therapy options.

DISCUSSION AND FUTURE PERSPECTIVES

Metabolic Syndromes and the Gutome

Understanding the role of nutrigenomics and the gutome provides windows of opportunity in shifting the nature of chronic disease. As noted elsewhere in this article, chronic disease is interactive, nonstatic, and can be altered if given the appropriate materials. This factor has significant consequences related to disease management, progression, therapeutics, and minimizing the burden on individuals and society. Nutrigenomics serves as an additional tool of prevention to enhance quality of life, alter chronic disease severity, and even diminish the severity of acute illness among those with existing chronic diseases including obesity, CVD, diabetes, and cancer.

TABLE 4
Genes and Polymorphisms Related to Cancer Risk

Gene	Prominent SNPs (Minor Allele Frequency)	Evidence associations (CRC/BC)	References
APOA family	rs1799837 (MA:T; <0.01)	(BC) Inhibit growth and invasion of tumor cells, variations lead to increased risk of BC (A-allele)	[86]
	rs5069 (MA:A; 0.12)	(BC) Inhibit growth and invasion of tumor cells, variations lead to increased risk of BC (T-allele)	[86]
	rs670 (MA:T; 0.19)	(BC) Poor surgery prognosis and increase risk of disease progression (A-allele)	[87]
	Nonspecified	(CRC) Increase elimination of bile acids leading to gut carcinogenesis	[88]
APOE	Nonspecified	(CRC) Increase elimination of bile acids leading to gut carcinogenesis; absence of e3 allele may increase risk with western diet in older individuals	[88,89]
	e4/e4	(BC) higher serum triglycerides leading to increased risk of BC depending on tumor staging	[90,91]
BRCA1	Nonspecified	(BC) Associated with familial cases of breast cancer. Lower risk with coffee consumption, genistein, folate and cobalamin intake, selenium supplementation, and fruit and veggie intake. Higher risk with iron consumption.	[92,93]
BRCA2	Nonspecified	(BC) Associated with familial cases of breast cancer. Lower risk with soy, genistein, fruits and vegetable intake	[92,93]
FTO	Nonspecified	(CRC) Dysregulated in CRC and may play a significant role in progression; regulates PD-L1 expression	[94]
	rs1558902 (MA:A; 0.23) rs8050136 (MA A; 0.32) rs3751812 (MA:T; 0.22) rs9939609 (MA:A; 0.34)	(CRC) positive association with CRC (Minor Allele of each SNP associated with increased risk)	[95]

(*continued on next page*)

TABLE 4
(*continued*)

Gene	Prominent SNPs (Minor Allele Frequency)	Evidence associations (CRC/BC)	References
MTHFR	rs1801133 (MA:A; 0.25)	(CRC) decreased enzyme activity may lead to susceptibility especially with low folate intake and low vitamin B6. Additionally, increased risk of microsatellite-high tumors (T-allele) (BC) TT genotype may lead to increased risk of BC, along with intake of B-vitamins (T-allele)	[88,92,96,97]
	rs1801131 (MA:G; 0.25)	(CRC) decreased enzyme activity may lead to susceptibility (CC-genotype)	[88,98]
PPARG	Nonspecified	(CRC) expression in tumors in associated with longer survival (BC) associated with disease free survival	[99–101]

Minor allele frequency was determined using the minor allele frequency from phase III populations: https://useast.ensembl.org/index.html.
Abbreviations: BC, breast cancer; CRC, colorectal cancer; PD-L1, programmed death ligand 1; SNP, single nucleotide polymorphism.

One area of further interest related to nutrigenomics and the prevention of diabetes, metabolic disease, and CVD is to examine specific heterozygous and homozygous patterns related to the management of disease. As noted elsewhere in this article, lineage diets, including the Mediterranean diet, may serve as an additional tool in therapeutic options and management. One such study compared the Mediterranean and Central European diets, where individual carriers of *FTO* and *PPARG* were assessed in relationship to blood pressure, obesity, cholesterol, and body habitus. The study assessed postmenopausal women with central obesity [50]. Both diets over 16 weeks showed metabolic improvements in some form. Yet the study further explored *FTO* (rs9939609) and *PPARG* (rs1801282) heterozygous and homozygous status in relation to these 2 ancestral diets. Among those on the Central European Diet, *PPARG* rs1801282 G carriers had a greater reduction in weight and high-density lipoproteins than those homozygous for the C allele. Additionally, *FTO* rs9939609 T allele homozygotes showed superior outcomes in diastolic blood pressure when compared with G allele carriers. Stratifying by those on the Mediterranean diet, greater fat reduction was observed in *PPARG* rs1801282 G allele carriers [50]. Similarly, the Mediterranean Diet was also assessed in relationship to MTHFR C677 T and potential positive metabolic changes [51]. Over 12 weeks of dietary changes, both individuals who did and did not carry the T allele showed a reduction of overall weight and body fat. However, 71.4% of individuals with a C/C genotype were able to lose weight and total body fat as compared with only 28.6% of T allele carriers. Additionally, T allele carriers were more likely to lose lean body mass when compared with C/C individuals [51]. Thus, specific polymorphisms may guide diet selection as an additional therapeutic tool in the prevention and reversal of metabolic syndromes.

Another notable and timely example is seen with acute disease in those who contracted coronavirus disease 2019 (COVID-19). As observed globally, not all people share equal risk of severity or mortality. In fact, those with CVD, diabetes, and obesity had a higher risk of hospitalizations and mortality. Numerous studies found that the gut microbiome may serve as a contributor to increased COVID hospitalizations and mortality among these individuals [52]. In fact, gut dysbiosis was found in hospitalized patients with COVID-19 with a lower diversity of flora, specifically *Lactobacillus and Bifidobacterium*. These same individuals with chronic disease maintained a higher level of pathogenic bacteria of *Actinomyces*, *Rothia*, and *Streptococcus* [53]. Once again, CVD, diabetes, and obesity are not isolated diseases, but their foundation of the gut biome plays a role in morbidity and mortality even in cases of acute disease.

As noted elsewhere in this article, apolipoprotein E is correlated with obesity and CVD and more recently the apolipoprotein E e4e4 genotype is associated with a 4-fold increase in mortality from COVID-19 [54]. The ability to prevent severe acute infection for those with metabolic disease and CVD may not be random, but instead housed within the biome where epigenetics not only play a role in progression of chronic disease, but alter the immune response during times of acute disease. Therefore, nutrigenomics may be beneficial in the prevention of acute disease among those with CVD and obesity in addition to well-established hygienic practices and vaccination. It is this understanding that serves as a window of opportunity to further identify those at greatest risk and to minimize further morbidity or mortality.

The Gutome and Cancer

As noted elsewhere in this article, a more balanced microbiome yields advantageous effects on health including protection against certain diseases. One such example includes estrogen receptor-positive breast cancer [55]. The gut microbiome has a unique ability to regulate and metabolize estrogens using the same phase II detoxification reactions that metabolize medications, including glucuronidation, methylation, glutathione conjugation, and sulfation. With an unbalanced or dysbiotic biome, unmetabolized and unbound estrogens increase. Estrogen regulation of the gut may alter total body estrogen and impact the breast tissue, increasing the risk of estrogen receptor-positive breast cancer [56]. This process is so significant that it serves as its own ecosystem, known as the estrobolome, referring to the intestinal bacterial microbiome that metabolizes and regulates circulating estrogens [55]. Beta-glucuronidase serves as an important enzyme in carbohydrate degradation, but, in excess, can cleave key bonds of the intestinal lining leading to leaky gut. It also serves as a competitor to glucuronidation, thus impairing estrogen degradation. Certain microbes alter beta-glucuronidase, including bacteriodes, bifidobacterium, and lactobacillus [55]. Thus, in balance and under the best of circumstances the human microbiome can serve as a protector against cancer. Nutrients also impact estrogen receptor-positive and HER2-positive breast cancer, where fat-soluble vitamins including A, D, and E alter the flora and are correlated to more positive outcomes [57–59]. Fish oil, cod liver oil, and foods that contain essential fatty acids also show specific promise in improving the flora. Additionally, vitamins A, D, and E have shown to enhance the benefits of certain chemotherapy and aromatase inhibitors and even reduce drug resistance [60,61].

SUMMARY

Nutrigenomics is ever evolving. Owing to extensive recent research, the role of the microbiome, both in terms of impact on chronic disease and how it influences the efficacy of specialized diets and pharmacotherapies, is beginning to be better understood. Our approach to chronic disease should continue to advance in therapeutic options based on the individual. In recent years, pharmacogenomics has been increasingly incorporated into clinical practice. Perhaps in the future, the microbiome's role in drug metabolism could be used to further refine medication selection. Nutrigenetic advances may be used in the future to guide selection of specialized diets that could be used as an adjunct to pharmacotherapy, as well as to influence the composition of the microbiome. Finally, further interventions to alter the microbiome (eg, probiotics, fecal transplantation, or alteration through nutrient intake) may be used as additional approaches to improve health and treat disease. Using genetics and epigenetics in each of these contexts, a patient's therapeutic response can be maximized. These improved outcomes serve to reduce morbidity and mortality and enhance quality of life.

DISCLOSURE

The authors have nothing to disclose related to this article.

REFERENCES

[1] Dimitrov DV. The human gutome: nutrigenomics of the host–microbiome interactions. Omi A J Integr Biol 2011;15(7–8):419–30.
[2] Ferguson JF, Allayee H, Gerszten RE, et al. Nutrigenomics, the microbiome, and gene-environment interactions: new directions in cardiovascular disease research, prevention, and treatment. Circ Cardiovasc Genet 2016; 9(3):291–313. Available at: https://www.ahajournals.org/doi/10.1161/HCG.0000000000000030.
[3] Peña-Romero AC, Navas-Carrillo D, Marín F, et al. The future of nutrition: nutrigenomics and nutrigenetics in obesity and cardiovascular diseases. Crit Rev Food Sci Nutr 2018;58(17):3030–41.

[4] Cresci GAM, Izzo K. Gut microbiome. In: Adult short bowel syndrome. Elsevier; 2019. p. 45–54. https://doi.org/10.1016/B978-0-12-814330-8.00004-4.

[5] Ratsika A, Codagnone MC, O'Mahony S, et al. Priming for life: early life nutrition and the microbiota-gut-brain axis. Nutrients 2021;13(2). https://doi.org/10.3390/nu13020423.

[6] Petra AI, Panagiotidou S, Hatziagelaki E, et al. Gut-microbiota-brain axis and its effect on neuropsychiatric disorders with suspected immune dysregulation. Clin Ther 2015;37(5):984–95.

[7] Yamamoto EA, Jørgensen TN. Relationships between vitamin D, gut microbiome, and systemic autoimmunity. Front Immunol 2019;10:3141.

[8] Yang Q, Liang Q, Balakrishnan B, et al. Role of dietary nutrients in the modulation of gut microbiota: a narrative review. Nutrients 2020;12(2).

[9] Bäumler AJ, Sperandio V. Interactions between the microbiota and pathogenic bacteria in the gut. Nature 2016;535(7610):85–93.

[10] Knoop KA, Holtz LR, Newberry RD. Inherited nongenetic influences on the gut microbiome and immune system. Birth Defects Res 2018;110(20):1494–503.

[11] Prince AL, Chu DM, Seferovic MD, et al. The perinatal microbiome and pregnancy: moving beyond the vaginal microbiome. Cold Spring Harb Perspect Med 2015;5(6). https://doi.org/10.1101/cshperspect.a023051.

[12] Dunlop AL, Mulle JG, Ferranti EP, et al. Maternal microbiome and pregnancy outcomes that impact infant health: a review. Adv Neonatal Care 2015;15(6):377–85.

[13] Yao Y, Cai X, Fei W, et al. Regulating gut microbiome: therapeutic strategy for rheumatoid arthritis during pregnancy and lactation. Front Pharmacol 2020;11:594042.

[14] Gominak SC. Vitamin D deficiency changes the intestinal microbiome reducing B vitamin production in the gut. The resulting lack of pantothenic acid adversely affects the immune system, producing a "pro-inflammatory" state associated with atherosclerosis and autoimmunity. Med Hypotheses 2016;94:103–7.

[15] Marchesi JR, Adams DH, Fava F, et al. The gut microbiota and host health: a new clinical frontier. Gut 2016;65(2):330–9.

[16] Khan I, Ullah N, Zha L, et al. Alteration of gut microbiota in inflammatory bowel disease (IBD): cause or consequence? IBD treatment targeting the gut microbiome. Pathog (Basel, Switzerland) 2019;8(3). https://doi.org/10.3390/pathogens8030126.

[17] Salem F, Kindt N, Marchesi JR, et al. Gut microbiome in chronic rheumatic and inflammatory bowel diseases: Similarities and differences. United Eur Gastroenterol J 2019;7(8):1008–32.

[18] Wilson ID, Nicholson JK. Gut microbiome interactions with drug metabolism, efficacy, and toxicity. Transl Res 2017;179:204–22.

[19] Tuteja S, Ferguson JF. Gut microbiome and response to cardiovascular drugs. Circ Genomic Precis Med 2019; 12(9). https://doi.org/10.1161/CIRCGEN.119.002314.

[20] Prevention C for DC and. Adult obesity facts. Overweight and obesity. Available at: https://www.cdc.gov/obesity/data/adult.html. Accessed March 30, 2021.

[21] Saltiel AR, Olefsky JM. Inflammatory mechanisms linking obesity and metabolic disease. J Clin Invest 2017; 127(1):1–4.

[22] Organization WH. Diabetes. Health topics. 2021. Available at: https://www.who.int/health-topics/diabetes#tab=tab_1. Accessed March 30, 2021.

[23] Ortega Á, Berná G, Rojas A, et al. Gene-diet interactions in type 2 diabetes: the chicken and egg debate. Int J Mol Sci 2017;18(6). https://doi.org/10.3390/ijms18061188.

[24] Virani SS, Alonso A, Aparicio HJ, et al. Heart disease and stroke statistics—2021 update. Circulation 2021;143(8). https://doi.org/10.1161/CIR.0000000000000950.

[25] Barrea L, Annunziata G, Bordoni L, et al. Nutrigenetics—personalized nutrition in obesity and cardiovascular diseases. Int J Obes Suppl 2020;10(1):1–13.

[26] Hickey SE, Curry CJ, Toriello HV. ACMG practice guideline: lack of evidence for MTHFR polymorphism testing. Genet Med 2013;15(2):153–6.

[27] Nutrigenomics MM. The genome – food interface. Environ Health Perspect 2007;115(12):A582–9.

[28] Esposito K, Chiodini P, Colao A, et al. Metabolic syndrome and risk of cancer: a systematic review and meta-analysis. Diabetes Care 2012;35(11):2402–11.

[29] ACS. American Cancer Society. Available at: https://www.cancer.org/. Accessed March 30, 2021.

[30] Publishing HH. Cancer and diet: what's the connection? Harvard Men's Health Watch. Available at: https://www.health.harvard.edu/cancer/cancer-and-diet-whats-the-connection. Accessed March 30, 2021.

[31] Anderson JJ, Darwis NDM, Mackay DF, et al. Red and processed meat consumption and breast cancer: UK Biobank cohort study and meta-analysis. Eur J Cancer 2018;90:73–82.

[32] Sieri S, Krogh V. Dietary glycemic index, glycemic load and cancer: an overview of the literature. Nutr Metab Cardiovasc Dis 2017;27(1):18–31.

[33] Deng X, Su R, Stanford S, et al. Critical enzymatic functions of FTO in obesity and cancer. Front Endocrinol (Lausanne) 2018;9. https://doi.org/10.3389/fendo.2018.00396.

[34] de Toro-Martín J, Arsenault BJ, Després JP, et al. Precision nutrition: a review of personalized nutritional approaches for the prevention and management of metabolic syndrome. Nutrients 2017;9(8):1–28.

[35] Kobayashi J. Effect of diet and gut environment on the gastrointestinal formation of N-nitroso compounds: a review. Nitric Oxide Biol Chem 2018;73:66–73.

[36] Bruno E, Manoukian S, Venturelli E, et al. Adherence to Mediterranean diet and metabolic syndrome in BRCA mutation carriers. Integr Cancer Ther 2018;17(1):153–60.

[37] Meslier V, Laiola M, Roager HM, et al. Mediterranean diet intervention in overweight and obese subjects lowers plasma cholesterol and causes changes in the gut microbiome and metabolome independently of energy intake. Gut 2020;69(7):1258–68.

[38] Liu H, Wang J, He T, et al. Butyrate: a double-edged sword for health? Adv Nutr 2018;9(1):21–9.

[39] McNabney SM, Henagan TM. Short chain fatty acids in the colon and peripheral tissues: a focus on butyrate, colon cancer, obesity and insulin resistance. Nutrients 2017;9(12). https://doi.org/10.3390/nu9121348.

[40] Fasanelli F, Giraudo MT, Vineis P, et al. DNA methylation, colon cancer and Mediterranean diet: results from the EPIC-Italy cohort. Epigenetics 2019;14(10):977–88.

[41] Castelló A, Pollán M, Buijsse B, et al. Spanish Mediterranean diet and other dietary patterns and breast cancer risk: case–control EpiGEICAM study. Br J Cancer 2014; 111(7):1454–62.

[42] Kiechle M, Dukatz R, Yahiaoui-Doktor M, et al. Feasibility of structured endurance training and Mediterranean diet in BRCA1 and BRCA2 mutation carriers - an interventional randomized controlled multicenter trial (LIBRE-1). BMC Cancer 2017;17(1):752.

[43] Bruno E, Oliverio A, Paradiso AV, et al. A Mediterranean dietary intervention in female carriers of BRCA mutations: results from an Italian prospective randomized controlled trial. Cancers (Basel) 2020;12(12). https://doi.org/10.3390/cancers12123732.

[44] Özkul C, Yalınay M, Karakan T. Islamic fasting leads to an increased abundance of Akkermansia muciniphila and Bacteroides fragilis group: a preliminary study on intermittent fasting. Turk J Gastroenterol 2019;30(12): 1030–5.

[45] Ou Z, Deng L, Lu Z, et al. Protective effects of Akkermansia muciniphila on cognitive deficits and amyloid pathology in a mouse model of Alzheimer's disease. Nutr Diabetes 2020;10(1):12.

[46] Haran JP, Bhattarai SK, Foley SE, et al. Alzheimer's disease microbiome is associated with dysregulation of the anti-inflammatory P-glycoprotein pathway. MBio 2019; 10(3). https://doi.org/10.1128/mBio.00632-19.

[47] Inacio P. Gut microbiome may help slow ALS progression, study indicates. ALS News Today. 2019. Available at: https://alsnewstoday.com/news-posts/2019/07/25/gut-microbiome-slow-als-progression-study/. Accessed December 3, 2021.

[48] Bian X, Wu W, Yang L, et al. Administration of Akkermansia muciniphila ameliorates dextran sulfate sodium-induced ulcerative colitis in mice. Front Microbiol 2019;10:2259.

[49] Weir TL, Manter DK, Sheflin AM, et al. Stool microbiome and metabolome differences between colorectal cancer patients and healthy adults. PLoS One 2013; 8(8):e70803.

[50] Chmurzynska A, Muzsik A, Krzyżanowska-Jankowska P, et al. PPARG and FTO polymorphism can modulate the outcomes of a central European diet and a Mediterranean diet in centrally obese postmenopausal women. Nutr Res 2019;69:94–100.

[51] Di Renzo L, Rizzo M, Iacopino L, et al. Body composition phenotype: Italian Mediterranean diet and C677T MTHFR gene polymorphism interaction. Eur Rev Med Pharmacol Sci 2013;17(19):2555–65. Available at: http://www.ncbi.nlm.nih.gov/pubmed/24142599.

[52] Viana SD, Nunes S, Reis F. ACE2 imbalance as a key player for the poor outcomes in COVID-19 patients with age-related comorbidities - role of gut microbiota dysbiosis. Ageing Res Rev 2020;62:101123.

[53] Xu K, Cai H, Shen Y, et al. [Management of corona virus disease-19 (COVID-19): the Zhejiang experience]. Zhejiang Da Xue Xue Bao Yi Xue Ban 2020;49(1):147–57.

[54] Kuo C-L, Pilling LC, Atkins JL, et al. ApoE e4e4 genotype and mortality with COVID-19 in UK Biobank. J Gerontol A Biol Sci Med Sci 2020;75(9):1801–3.

[55] Kwa M, Plottel CS, Blaser MJ, et al. The intestinal microbiome and estrogen receptor-positive female breast cancer. J Natl Cancer Inst 2016;108(8). https://doi.org/10.1093/jnci/djw029.

[56] Baker JM, Al-Nakkash L, Herbst-Kralovetz MM. Estrogen–gut microbiome axis: physiological and clinical implications. Maturitas 2017;103:45–53.

[57] Miro Estruch I, de Haan LHJ, Melchers D, et al. The effects of all-trans retinoic acid on estrogen receptor signaling in the estrogen-sensitive MCF/BUS subline. J Recept Signal Transduct Res 2018;38(2):112–21.

[58] Bak MJ, Das Gupta S, Wahler J, et al. Inhibitory effects of γ- and δ-tocopherols on estrogen-stimulated breast cancer in vitro and in vivo. Cancer Prev Res (Phila) 2017;10(3):188–97.

[59] Tam K-W, Ho C-T, Lee W-J, et al. Alteration of α-tocopherol-associated protein (TAP) expression in human breast epithelial cells during breast cancer development. Food Chem 2013;138(2–3):1015–21.

[60] Koay DC, Zerillo C, Narayan M, et al. Anti-tumor effects of retinoids combined with trastuzumab or tamoxifen in breast cancer cells: induction of apoptosis by retinoid/trastuzumab combinations. Breast Cancer Res 2010;12(4):R62.

[61] Tiwary R, Yu W, Sanders BG, et al. α-TEA cooperates with chemotherapeutic agents to induce apoptosis of p53 mutant, triple-negative human breast cancer cells via activating p73. Breast Cancer Res 2011;13(1):R1.

[62] Corella D, Peloso G, Arnett DK, et al. APOA2, dietary fat, and body mass index: replication of a gene-diet interaction in 3 independent populations. Arch Intern Med 2009;169(20):1897–906.

[63] Domínguez-Reyes T, Astudillo-López CC, Salgado-Goytia L, et al. Interaction of dietary fat intake with APOA2, APOA5 and LEPR polymorphisms and its relationship with obesity and dyslipidemia in young subjects. Lipids Health Dis 2015;14:106.

[64] Koopal C, Van Der Graaf Y, Asselbergs FW, et al. Influence of APOE-2 genotype on the relation between adiposity and plasma lipid levels in patients with vascular disease. Int J Obes 2015;39(2):265–9.

[65] Garaulet M, Corbalán MD, Madrid JA, et al. CLOCK gene is implicated in weight reduction in obese patients participating in a dietary programme based on the Mediterranean diet. Int J Obes (Lond) 2010;34(3):516–23.

[66] Scuteri A, Sanna S, Chen W-M, et al. Genome-wide association scan shows genetic variants in the FTO gene are associated with obesity-related traits. Plos Genet 2007;3(7):e115.
[67] Qi Q, Kilpeläinen TO, Downer MK, et al. FTO genetic variants, dietary intake and body mass index: insights from 177,330 individuals. Hum Mol Genet 2014; 23(25):6961–72.
[68] Duicu C, Mărginean CO, Voidăzan S, et al. FTO rs 9939609 SNP is associated with adiponectin and leptin levels and the risk of obesity in a cohort of Romanian children population. Medicine (Baltimore) 2016; 95(20):e3709.
[69] Kaulfers A-M, Deka R, Dolan L, et al. Association of INSIG2 polymorphism with overweight and LDL in children. PLoS One 2015;10(1):e0116340.
[70] Heid IM, Huth C, Loos RJF, et al. Meta-analysis of the INSIG2 association with obesity including 74,345 individuals: does heterogeneity of estimates relate to study design? Plos Genet 2009;5(10):e1000694.
[71] Martínez JA. Perspectives on personalized nutrition for obesity. J Nutrigenet Nutrigenomics 2014;7(1):6–8.
[72] Di Renzo L, Gualtieri P, Romano L, et al. Role of personalized nutrition in chronic-degenerative diseases. Nutrients 2019;11(8):1–24.
[73] Berná G, Oliveras-López MJ, Jurado-Ruíz E, et al. Nutrigenetics and nutrigenomics insights into diabetes etiopathogenesis. Nutrients 2014;6(11):5338–69.
[74] Corella D, Asensio EM, Coltell O, et al. CLOCK gene variation is associated with incidence of type-2 diabetes and cardiovascular diseases in type-2 diabetic subjects: dietary modulation in the PREDIMED randomized trial. Cardiovasc Diabetol 2016;15:4.
[75] Dedoussis GVZ, Kaliora AC, Panagiotakos DB. Genes, diet and type 2 diabetes mellitus: a review. Rev Diabet Stud 2007;4(1):13–24.
[76] Ali O. Genetics of type 2 diabetes. World J Diabetes 2013;4(4):114–23.
[77] Corella D, Qi L, Sorlí JV, et al. Obese subjects carrying the 11482G>A polymorphism at the perilipin locus are resistant to weight loss after dietary energy restriction. J Clin Endocrinol Metab 2005;90(9):5121–6.
[78] Engler MB. Nutrigenomics in cardiovascular disease: implications for the future. Prog Cardiovasc Nurs 2009;24(4):190–5.
[79] Iacoviello L, Santimone I, Latella MC, et al. Nutrigenomics: a case for the common soil between cardiovascular disease and cancer. Genes Nutr 2008;3(1):19–24.
[80] Ordovas JM, Kaput J, Corella D. Nutrition in the genomics era: cardiovascular disease risk and the Mediterranean diet. Mol Nutr Food Res 2007;51(10): 1293–9.
[81] Do R, Xie C, Zhang X, et al. The effect of chromosome 9p21 variants on cardiovascular disease may be modified by dietary intake: evidence from a case/control and a prospective study. Plos Med 2011;8(10). https://doi.org/10.1371/journal.pmed.1001106.
[82] Aleyasin SA, Navidi T, Davoudi S. Association between rs10757274 and rs2383206 SNPs as genetic risk factors in Iranian patients with coronary artery disease. J Tehran Heart Cent 2017;12(3):114–8. Available at: http://www.ncbi.nlm.nih.gov/pubmed/29062378.
[83] Hannou SA, Wouters K, Paumelle R, et al. Functional genomics of the CDKN2A/B locus in cardiovascular and metabolic disease: what have we learned from GWASs? Trends Endocrinol Metab 2015;26(4):176–84.
[84] Niemiec P, Gorczynska-Kosiorz S, Iwanicki T, et al. The rs10757278 polymorphism of the 9p21.3 locus is associated with premature coronary artery disease in Polish patients. Genet Test Mol Biomarkers 2012;16(9): 1080–5.
[85] Aberle J, Hopfer I, Beil FU, et al. Association of peroxisome proliferator-activated receptor delta +294T/C with body mass index and interaction with peroxisome proliferator-activated receptor alpha L162V. Int J Obes (Lond) 2006;30(12):1709–13.
[86] Zhou Y, Luo G. Apolipoproteins, as the carrier proteins for lipids, are involved in the development of breast cancer. Clin Transl Oncol 2020;22(11):1952–62.
[87] Pirro M, Ricciuti B, Rader DJ, et al. High density lipoprotein cholesterol and cancer: marker or causative? Prog Lipid Res 2018;71:54–69.
[88] Caramujo-Balseiro S, Faro C, Carvalho L. Metabolic pathways in sporadic colorectal carcinogenesis: a new proposal. Med Hypotheses 2021;148:110512.
[89] Slattery ML, Sweeney C, Murtaugh M, et al. Associations between apoE genotype and colon and rectal cancer. Carcinogenesis 2005;26(8):1422–9.
[90] Moysich KB, Freudenheim JL, Baker JA, et al. Apolipoprotein E genetic polymorphism, serum lipoproteins, and breast cancer risk. Mol Carcinog 2000;27(1):2–9.
[91] Porrata-Doria T, Matta JL, Acevedo SF. Apolipoprotein E allelic frequency altered in women with early-onset breast cancer. Breast Cancer (Auckl) 2010;4:43–8. Available at: http://www.ncbi.nlm.nih.gov/pubmed/20697532.
[92] Riscuta G, Dumitrescu RG. Nutrigenomics: implications for breast and colon cancer prevention. Methods Mol Biol 2012;343–58. https://doi.org/10.1007/978-1-61779-612-8_22.
[93] Sellami M, Bragazzi NL. Nutrigenomics and breast cancer: state-of-art, future perspectives and insights for prevention. Nutrients 2020;12(2):512.
[94] Liu X, Liu L, Dong Z, et al. Expression patterns and prognostic value of m6A-related genes in colorectal cancer. Am J Transl Res 2019;11(7):3972–91. Available at: http://www.ncbi.nlm.nih.gov/pubmed/31396313.
[95] Yamaji T, Iwasaki M, Sawada N, et al. Fat mass and obesity-associated gene polymorphisms, pre-diagnostic plasma adipokine levels and the risk of colorectal cancer: the Japan Public Health Center-based Prospective Study. PLoS One 2020;15(2):e0229005.
[96] Davis CD. Nutrigenomics and the prevention of colon cancer. Pharmacogenomics 2007;8(2):121–4.

[97] Levine AJ, Figueiredo JC, Lee W, et al. Genetic variability in the MTHFR gene and colorectal cancer risk using the Colorectal Cancer Family Registry. Cancer Epidemiol Biomarkers Prev 2010;19(1):89–100.

[98] Cecchin E, Perrone G, Nobili S, et al. MTHFR-1298 A>C (rs1801131) is a predictor of survival in two cohorts of stage II/III colorectal cancer patients treated with adjuvant fluoropyrimidine chemotherapy with or without oxaliplatin. Pharmacogenomics J 2015; 15(3):219–25.

[99] Ogino S, Shima K, Baba Y, et al. Colorectal cancer expression of peroxisome proliferator-activated receptor γ (PPARG, PPARgamma) is associated with good prognosis. Gastroenterology 2009;136(4):1242–50.

[100] Girnun G. PPARG: a new independent marker for colorectal cancer survival. Gastroenterology 2009;136(4): 1157–60.

[101] Papadaki I, Mylona E, Giannopoulou I, et al. PPARgamma expression in breast cancer: clinical value and correlation with ERbeta. Histopathology 2005;46(1):37–42.

Advances in Molecular Pathology 4 (2021) 117–125
ADVANCES IN MOLECULAR PATHOLOGY

The Importance of Use of Genetics to Guide Hypertension Therapy

Using β-Blockade as an Example

Eric M. Snyder, PhD[a,*], Ryan Sprissler, PhD[a,b], Thomas P. Olson, PhD[a,c]
[a]Geneticure, Inc., 4 3rd Street Southwest Suite 305 1/2 B, Rochester, MN 55902, USA; [b]Genomics Core Facility, University of Arizona, 1657 E Helen St, Rm 106, Tucson, AZ 85721, USA; [c]Department of Cardiovascular Diseases, Mayo Clinic, 200 1st St SW, Rochester, MN 55901, USA

KEYWORDS
• Hypertension • Pharmacogenetics • Adrenergic receptor

KEY POINTS

- Hypertension control rates are poor, even in patients who take their medication as prescribed.
- Hypertension control rates have decreased by 10% from 2014 to 2018.
- Each of the common anti-hypertensive therapies have a well-studied bell-curve response in the population.
- Iterative administration of monotherapy (giving one pharmacotherapy, removing in place of another, if not successful) increases blood pressure control with monotherapy from 50% to ~75%.
- Genotypes of the β-adrenergic receptors differentially affect blood pressure control and clinical outcomes.

INTRODUCTION

Hypertension has repeatedly been shown to be the largest modifiable risk factor for morbidity and mortality worldwide [1–3]. Target organ damage occurs at the onset of hypertension and, as such, rapid control rates are critical. Control rates for hypertension had been steadily increasing from 2000 until 2014, when they increased from 31.8% control to 53.8% control [4]. However, unlike many other chronic disease conditions, control rates from 2014 to 2018 decreased by 10% to 43.7%. This decrease in control rates occurred during a time when the number of hypertension medications used per patient has increased, with most patients now on multiple pharmacotherapies [5]. A major hypothesis for this decrease in control rates is that the major guidelines given in 2013 to 2014 included a lower cut-off to establish a standard for high blood pressure. 2017 to 2018 guidelines generally suggest 130/90 mm Hg for hypertension (while patients who are considered "normotensive" have a blood pressure (BP) below 120/80 mm Hg), whereas the 2013 to 2014 guidelines focused on 140/90 mm Hg as a cut off for hypertension [6]. There are likely other contributing factors to this reduction in control rates and we hypothesize that one may be due to the relegation of β-blockers to second-line therapy without attention to genotypes that may differentially influence β-blockade.

Significance

Previous work has demonstrated a significant heritable component to hypertension that has been elucidated using twin studies and studies with a focus on BP and

*Corresponding author, *E-mail address:* eric@geneticure.com

https://doi.org/10.1016/j.yamp.2021.06.005
2589-4080/21/

Na^+ reabsorption patterns in sons of normotensive versus sons of hypertensive individuals, among others [7–9]. Given that the development of hypertension has a significant heritable contribution, it is logical that the treatment for hypertension may be better guided by genetics as well. Previous studies have demonstrated associations, or improvements, in BP for each of the major drug classes: angiotensin-converting enzyme (ACE)-inhibition, angiotensin-receptor blockade, diuretic responsiveness, Ca^+ channel inhibition, and β-blockade when genetics are used as an independent variable [10–15]. Some of the most consistent data on genetics and response to pharmacotherapy in hypertension is that which has examined β_1 and β_2 adrenergic receptor (AR) genotypes and β-blockade [12,13].

There are currently more than 500 genotypes that have been shown to be associated with the risk of developing hypertension, although very few of these have been demonstrated to be functional in hypothesis-driven clinical trials and detailed phenotypic follow-up studies are needed [16]. The response to pharmacotherapy in hypertension for each drug class is far from uniform. In fact, studies from as far back as the late 1980s have demonstrated a consistent bell-curve response to pharmacologic treatment in which some individuals demonstrate a drop in BP, some demonstrate no change, and some demonstrate an increase in BP after the initiation of a pharmacotherapy [11,17,18]. The average drop in BP, beyond the placebo effect, is approximately 7-8 mm Hg [17,19,20]. A systematic review with a focus on the cessation of antihypertensive treatments has demonstrated that approximately 40% of patients maintain BP control after discontinuation of treatment, suggesting the potential use of ineffective BP pharmacotherapy [21]. Furthermore, when focused on monotherapy, previous work has demonstrated that a patient is approximately 50% likely to achieve BP control when prescribed a given monotherapy at random. Even more dramatic pharmacotherapies, such as the sympathetic nervous system inhibition with clonidine, reduce BP in approximately 50% of patients when used as a monotherapy [22]. However, if a hypertensive patient is given one monotherapy, removed from that monotherapy, and then given another until one works, they are 75% likely to achieve BP control with monotherapy [23,24]. This highlights the fact that not all pharmacotherapies work for all patients and that monotherapy can be highly effective, if guided toward a drug class that works for that patient. This is an important point because the use of multiple, sometimes ineffective, therapies may be detrimental to the patient in terms of side effects and cardiovascular clinical outcomes, particularly in older individuals. Specifically, the administration of two or more antihypertensive medications, resulting in low systolic BP (SBP), has been shown to be associated with increased mortality in older patients [25]. In addition, the layering of medications has been shown to decrease medication adherence more than 70% [26].

When race is used to assess the BP response to pharmacotherapy, large differences between the response to various hypertension classes begin to emerge. In a 2005 summary analysis, the authors noted that African American patients responded worse than non–African American subjects when taking an ACE inhibitor or a β-blocker, but responded significantly better when taking a diuretic, a difference that ranged from 4-8 mm Hg, depending on the drug class [27]. Of note, there are significant differences in the functional genotypes of the βARs, and genotypes important in Na^+ reabsorption, between black and white individuals (Table 1). Although it would, therefore, seem tempting to use race as a surrogate to guide treatment, the bell-curve response to hypertensive therapy is well-established even within racial groupings, with some patients responding well to the drug class that has been shown to be less effective to their racial group overall [11,18].

Despite the evidence that hypertension is heritable, that the correct monotherapy can lead to 75% control rates if an iterative process of monotherapy prescribing is used, and that the use of genetics leads to differential treatment outcomes in hypertensive patients, very few clinicians use genetics to guide hypertension in practice. Although the reasons for the lack of clinical adoption are multifactorial (and like other diseases and clinical conditions), it includes a lack of awareness of the trials demonstrating how genotyping can guide treatment in hypertension and inadequate randomized control trial data on pharmacogenetic panels that have been commercialized with a need to demonstrate an improvement above the standard of care. Therefore, in this manuscript, we review one area of hypertension treatment that has a good deal of strong (and consistent) research behind it, that of the adrenergic receptor genotypes and β-blockade.

The Beta-Adrenergic Receptors and β-Blockade in Hypertension

The βARs are G-protein coupled receptors that are important within the sympathetic nervous system. There are three known classes of the β-adrenergic receptors: the β_1-adrenergic receptors (β_1AR), the β_2-adrenergic receptors (β_2AR), and the β_3-adrenergic receptors (β_3AR). The β_1AR are found throughout the heart and

TABLE 1
Minor Allele Frequency for Common Variants Impacting the Heart and Kidneys

	Gene/Variant	rs#	White MAF	Black MAF
Heart	***ADRB2_16***	1042713	0.66	0.51
	ADRB2_27	1042714	0.35	0.21
	ADRB1_49	1801252	0.11–0.13	0.13–0.29
	ADRB1_389	1801253	0.24–0.28	0.42–0.44
Kidneys	***ADD1***	4961	0.20	0.05
	SCNN1A	2228576	0.31	0.05
	SLC12A3	1529927	0.96	1.00
	WNK1	1159744	0.74	0.73
	WNK1	2107614	0.32	0.58
	WNK1	2277869	0.81	0.83

Abbreviations: ADRB1, β_1-adrenergic receptor genotype at amino acids 49 and 389; *ADRB2*, β_2-adrenergic receptor genotype at amino acids 16 and 27; *ADD1*, alpha adducin genotype; MAF, minor allele frequency; *SCNN1A*, alpha subunit of the epithelial Na^+ channel; *WNK*, with no lysine/k serine-threonine kinase.

comprise ~95% of the sinoatrial node and 70% to 80% of the ventricular wall. Therefore, the β_1AR are the primary adrenergic receptor that regulates both heart rate and ventricular contractility at rest and under conditions of stress [28]. The β_2AR are located throughout the body including the heart, blood vessels, and kidneys. Classically, β_1AR have been shown to primarily influence cardiac function (heart rate and stroke volume), whereas the β_2AR have been shown to primarily influence vascular function. In the heart, the β_2AR are located in the ventricular walls, atria, and to a lesser extent, the sinoatrial node [29,30]. The ratio of β_1AR to β_2AR in the ventricular walls in healthy humans is thought to be ~80:20, and in the atria, this ratio is thought to increase to ~70:30 [31,32].

Following stimulation with an endogenous agonist, epinephrine or norepinephrine, the 7-transmembrane spanning βAR undergo a conformational change, which results in an internal signal that results in an exchange of guanosine diphosphate (GDP) to guanosine triphosphate (GTP). This exchange then leads to the separation of the Gα from the Gβɣ internal signaling units. The activation of the $G_{\alpha s}$ (stimulatory) subunit results in the activation of adenylyl cyclase, which then converts adenosine triphosphate (ATP) to cyclic adenosine monophosphate (cAMP). Protein kinase A (PKA) and cAMP are then associated with a multitude of downstream events that can result in a variety of cellular events, including those that can stimulate cardiac cellular function [31]. Interestingly, all βAR can stimulate the $G_{\alpha s}$ pathway, but the β_2AR and β_3AR are known to influence the $G_{\alpha i}$ (inhibitory pathway) and the β_3AR are not widely present in the cardiac tissue. This delineation may be important for genotype-specific differences in β-blockade between genetic variants of the *ADRB1* and *ADRB2*. Knockout of the β_2AR leads to an increase in heart rate (HR) and BP during exercise, potentially due to differences in $G_{\alpha s}$ versus $G_{\alpha i}$ internal signaling and a relative increase in $G_{\alpha s}$, whereas deletion of the β_1 and β_2AR leads to decreases in stroke volume when compared with wild-type mice [33]. Overexpression of the β_2AR can act to reduce the cardiac dysfunction that is associated with heart failure in animal models, which is consistent internal $G_{\alpha i}$ pathway activation through these receptors [34,35].

β-blockers are thought to primarily reduce BP through an inhibition of the chronotropic effects of the β_1AR and the inotropic effects of both β_1AR and β_2AR. Beyond the regulation of cardiac function, heart rate, and cardiac output, the β_1AR are also associated with renin release [36]. Stimulation of the β_1AR increases renin release in humans and can, therefore, increase BP through additional noncardiac means. β-blockers have been shown to be effective for BP reduction, when compared with placebo, as well as for improvements in clinical outcomes in a significant portion of patients with hypertension.

β-blockers have an interesting history in cardiovascular disease in which β-agonists were initially used in the failing heart (in an attempt to compensate for the reduction in cardiac function). This agonism of the β-AR served only to cause additional cellular damage and was replaced with inhibition of the β-AR, which led to improvements in cardiac function, left-ventricular ejection fraction, ventricular mass, and heart failure class. Before 2012, β-blockade was included as a first-line therapy in hypertension as well. The stated relegation of β-blockers to second-line therapy in the 2013 guidelines was based primarily on an increased risk of stroke in one trial comparing β-blockade to valsartan, which the authors' note was not demonstrated in other trials comparing β-blockers to other classes of pharmacotherapy [37]. The conclusion that β-blockers are not effective is also limited by the inclusion of randomized clinical trials that used β-blockers that have been shown to be inferior in the reduction of CV events [38,39]. Detailed work has demonstrated that there is no difference in either BP or clinical outcomes between Ca^+ channel blockade and β-blockade in patients with hypertension within 2 years of initiation of treatment [40]. Furthermore, β-blockade has been shown to lead to improvements in clinical outcomes, although this is most specific to stroke, when compared with placebo [41]. On average, and without consideration for genetic differences, the effect of β-blockers on hypertension and morbidity has been mixed but, again, many of these trials used older β-blockers that are less effective at reductions in cardiovascular disease (CVD) incident rates. As we will describe further, even within the large INVEST trial (which compared β-blockade to valsartan use), there was a genotype by risk effect in follow-up trials in the valsartan versus β-blockade trial. Therefore, using β-blockers as only one example within the many genotypes that can be used to guide hypertension treatment, it is evident that some of the previous mixed results may be improved upon when genetics are considered.

Genetic Variation of the β_1AR and β_2AR and β-Blocker Responsiveness in Hypertension

Like all pharmacologic treatments for hypertension, β-blockade has a well-demonstrated bell-curve response that shows many patients with a drop in BP, some with no change, and a small portion with an increase in BP after β-blockade. Although white individuals tend to respond significantly better than black individuals to β-blockade (likely due to differences in minor allele frequency of the functional genotypes of the adrenergic receptors), this is only true when considering population means. Within a racial group there remains a bell-curve response to treatment, although there is a rightward shift to β-blockade of the bell curve with fewer black individuals showing a response (drop in BP), but some patients do respond to the less functional therapy.

The β_1AR have two commonly studied and functional genotypes at sites 49 and 389. At position 49, humans present with either serine (Ser49) or glycine (Gly49), in which the Ser49 genotype has demonstrated enhanced functionality. At position 389, humans present with either arginine (Arg389) or glycine (Gly389), in which Arg389 has demonstrated enhanced functionality. Early work in mice and human cardiac tissue demonstrated that the Arg389 genotype of *ADRB1* had greater receptor function, cardiac contractility, and response to β-antagonism when compared with Gly389 animals or tissue [42,43]. With respect to hypertension, previous work has demonstrated that the Ser49 and Arg389 (the functional genotypes of *ADRB1*) demonstrated an enhanced response to β-blockade [13,44].

The β_2AR have been shown to have multiple common and functional polymorphisms in humans. Overexpression of the β_2AR can act to reduce the cardiac dysfunction that is associated with heart failure in animal models [34,35], potentially due to the internal $G_{\alpha i}$ pathway activation through these receptors. Specifically, an arginine for glycine substitution at codon 16 (Arg16 and Gly16, respectively) and a glutamine for glutamic acid substitution at amino acid 27 (Gln27 and Glu27, respectively) have been described [45–47]. Significant linkage disequilibrium exists between these sites so that typically when Arg is present at position 16 only Gln is found at position 27 [48–50]. We have previously demonstrated that individuals with the Gly16 genotype had enhanced ventricular function at rest and during exercise, when compared with subjects with the Arg genotype at this position [51]. We have also demonstrated altered cardiac function in patients with heart failure, according to genetic variation of the *ADRB2* gene [52]. Also of interest, Arg16 patients who are prescribed a β-blocker after hospital discharge with acute coronary syndrome were at a higher risk for mortality, when compared with Gly16 patients [53]. We have previously hypothesized that this may be due to differences in cardiac receptor reserve between the genotypes because the Gly16 polymorphism is associated with greater β_2AR density and, as mentioned, the β_2AR tend to have cardioprotective effects in times of cardiac stress [54].

In addition to these logical influences of *ADRB2* on the cardiac system, the β_2AR are also found within the kidney and control renal Na^+ handling. There is an important relationship between the cardiac and renal systems with the intention of maintaining BP in humans. To highlight this, we have previously demonstrated that the Arg16 genotype had an enhanced natriuretic response to Na^+ loading, along with a significant increase in BP [55]. In addition, a prolonged Na^+ restriction diet led to a reduction in cardiac output and an increase in total peripheral resistance in Gly16 subjects, when compared with Arg16 subjects [56]. Taken together, it is possible that variants of the *ADRB2* influence the BP response to β-blockade, beyond the well-established effect on cardiac function.

Although it is clear that the β_2AR are present in the cardiac tissue, and that the genotypes influence cardiac function and clinical outcomes, the data on the BP response to β-blockade according to genotypes of the β_2AR are less clear. This is likely a function of the high prevalence of the use of selective β-blockers in the previous clinical trials. When assessing verapamil versus β-blockade, previous work has demonstrated that the Gly16 and Glu27 genotypes were associated with increased risk of CV event when treated with atenolol when compared with verapamil [57]. Although the data on *ADRB2* genotypes and BP is not as strong as those for *ADRB1* in clinical trials that primarily focus on selective β-blockade, they seem to impact clinical outcomes, which may be due to differences in receptor density, receptor function, or differential internal signaling mechanisms.

Although β-blockers have been relegated to second-line therapeutics in the two most recent guideline statements, it is possible that the consideration of *ADRB1* and *ADRB2* genotypes may improve association with clinical outcomes in hypertension with β-blockade, even beyond BP control. For instance, with β-blocker use, the Gly49 genotype (nonfunctional genotype) is

TABLE 2
Examples of Other Genotypes that Have Been Shown to Be Important in the Blood Pressure Response to Pharmacotherapy

Gene	ID	Average MAP Difference: Fx Genotype on Target Therapy vs Not (Current Literature)	Haplotype Difference
ADRB1_49	rs1801252	5.3 mm Hg	
ADRB1_389	rs1801253	8.7 mm Hg	>15 mm Hg when combined
ADRB2_16	rs1042713	5.7 mm Hg	
ADRB2_27	rs1042714	7 mm Hg (SBP only)	>9 mm Hg when combined
*CYP2D6 *4*	rs3892097	0 mm Hg	>10 mm Hg when target also fx
WNK1	rs1159744	3.7 mm Hg	
WNK1	rs2107614	5.0 mm Hg	
WNK1	rs2277869	7.0 mm Hg	>10 mm Hg when combined
SCL12A3	rs13306673	~5 mm Hg	
SCNN1A	rs2228576	~5 mm Hg	
ADD1	rs4961	10 mm Hg	
REN	rs12750834	~5 mm Hg	
AGT	rs5051	8 mm Hg	
AGT	rs699	8.3 mm Hg	
AGT	rs7079	5.3 mm Hg	If 2 of 3, >10 mm Hg for ACE/ARB
ACE	rs1799752	5.7 mm Hg	
AGTR1	rs5186	6.3 mm Hg	

Abbreviations: ACE, angiotensin-converting enzyme genotype; *ADD1*, alpha adducin genotype; *ADRB1*, β_1-adrenergic receptor at amino acids 49 and 389, respectively; *ADRB2*, β_2-adrenergic receptor at amino acids 16 and 27, respectively; *AGT*, angiotensinogen genotype; *AGTR1*, angiotensin type-1 receptor genotype; *CYP2D6*, cytochrome P450 2D6; MAP, mean arterial blood pressure; *SCNN1A*, alpha subunit of the epithelial Na^+ channel; *SLC12A3*, Na+/Cl-co-transporter; *REN*, renin genotype; *WNK*, with no lysine/k serine-threonine kinase.

associated with an increased risk of major adverse cardiovascular events (hazard ratio = 2.03), when compared with the Ser49 genotype [58]. Patients with the functional genotype of *ADRB1* at position 389 (Arg389) have a 40% reduction in mortality when using a β-blocker, when compared with other medications [42]. These genotype-related differences in clinical outcomes, beyond BP control, are similar to other genotype by treatment effects such as that demonstrated with alpha-adducin. Previous work has demonstrated that the risk of myocardial infarction and stroke were cut in half when patients with the functional variant of alpha-adducin achieved BP control with a thiazide-like diuretic, when compared with achieving BP control with other pharmacotherapies [59]. Findings such as these highlight the need for incorporation of genetics in guiding hypertension pharmacotherapy.

Present Relevance and Future Directions

There is clearly a relationship between genotypes of *ADRB1* (and some data on genotypes of *ADRB2*) and both BP and clinical outcomes with β-blockade in patients with hypertension. It is possible that the previous research that has shown an increase in CV events in hypertensive patients using β-blockers oversampled nonfunctional genotypes (that have previously been shown to have poorer survival with β-blockade compared with the functional genotype) and that these guidelines would be altered if genetically guided treatment, or at least an understanding of the genotype distribution of the β-adrenergic receptors within their population were assessed. Nevertheless, the global data for β-blockade, that which does not consider genetic variants, tend to support the relegation of β-blockers to second-line therapy, for now. However, when β-blockers are used, the current data support the use of genotyping for the βAR before prescribing to improve morbidity and mortality.

SUMMARY

Unlike most chronic diseases, hypertension control rates have gone down over the past half of a decade. This has occurred during a time where the average number of antihypertensive medications used per patient has increased and most hypertensive patients are on more than one medication per day. Approximately, 40% of hypertensive patients who are taking their medications as prescribed do not have their BP under control [60]. In addition, more recent studies have demonstrated that smartphone medication management assist devices improve medication adherence in hypertension, but do not impact BP values [61]. Similarly, at home BP monitoring with electronic clinical intervention and medication titration only slightly lowered BP in the intervention group (SBP = −3.4 mm Hg and DBP = −0.5 mm Hg) [62]. Based on these data, along with studies on the population variability to hypertension treatment from decades ago, it is clear that not only adherence, but adherence to a pharmacotherapy that actually works for the patient, is important.

Here, we describe a small number of genotypes within the cardiac system that have been shown to influence the BP and clinical outcomes of β-blockade. While we discuss β-blockers, there is a great deal of work showing that different genotype groups differentially respond to BP treatment for most hypertensive medication classes using hypothesis-driven trials (Table 2). Despite this, there has been little push to use genetics to guide treatment of hypertension, outside of drug metabolizing enzyme genotypes. Driving adoption for the use of genetic testing to improve pharmacotherapy has been a challenge. A portion of this is that clinicians have not been made widely aware of the promising data and potential importance of genetics to guide treatment (such as the example of β_1AR genotypes and the differential response to β-blockade), and that genetic data have not yet been included in clinical guidelines of the American Heart Association or American College of Cardiology. Importantly, much of this challenge is due to self-inflicted wounds within the field of pharmacogenetics and lies on the responsibility of an industry that did not generally lead with an "evidence first" philosophy. Clinicians have been promised for more than 20 years that genetics will be used to guide therapy; however, clinicians need evidence, and they need a demonstration that a genetic/pharmacogenetic test is superior to the standard of care. This clinical need is very appropriate, given that these tests are developed to treat patients and it is the responsibility of those developing the tests to demonstrate that they have a clinical benefit and, more importantly, that they will not harm the patient.

CLINICS CARE POINTS

- Using genetics to guide treatment in blood pressure with monotherapy has been shown to be effective in previous trials.
- With a simple focus on genetics of the beta-adrenergic receptors, patients with the functional genotype

can demonstrate a 2-3-fold greater reduction in BP than the average reduction for any given pharmacotherapy.

- The use of monotherapy has been shown to be highly effective if clinicians use an iterative (rather than layering) approach, suggesting patients may benefit from genetically-guided treatment to the monotherapy that is effective.
- To make genetically-guided treatment a reality in hypertension randomized-controlled trials are needed to assess genetically-guided treatment across drug classes against the standard of care.

AUTHOR CONTRIBUTIONS

E.M. Snyder, R. Sprissler, and T.P. Olson have contributed significantly to the composition, review, and submission of this manuscript.

DISCLOSURE

E.M. Snyder, T.P. Olson, and R. Sprissler have financial interest in Geneticure Inc., which has developed multigene panels for pharmacotherapy prescribing using pharmacogenetics.

REFERENCES

[1] Chobanian AV, Bakris GL, Black HR, et al. The Seventh Report of the Joint National Committee on Prevention, Detection, Evaluation, and Treatment of High Blood Pressure: the JNC 7 report. J Am Med Assoc 2003; 289(19):2560–72.

[2] Forouzanfar MH, Liu P, Roth GA, et al. Global burden of hypertension and systolic blood pressure of at least 110 to 115 mm hg, 1990-2015. J Am Med Assoc 2017; 317(2):165–82.

[3] Kearney PM, Whelton M, Reynolds K, et al. Global burden of hypertension: analysis of worldwide data. Lancet 2005;365(9455):217–23.

[4] Muntner P, Hardy ST, Fine LJ, et al. Trends in Blood Pressure Control Among US Adults With Hypertension, 1999-2000 to 2017-2018. J Am Med Assoc 2020; 324(12):1190–200.

[5] Jarari N, Rao N, Peela JR, et al. A review on prescribing patterns of antihypertensive drugs. Clin Hypertens 2015;22:7.

[6] Whelton PK, Carey RM, AronowWS, et al. 2017 ACC/AHA/AAPA/ABC/ACPM/AGS/APhA/ASH/ASPC/NMA/PCNA Guideline for the Prevention, Detection, Evaluation, and Management of High Blood Pressure in Adults: A Report of the American College of Cardiology/American Heart Association Task Force on Clinical Practice Guidelines. Hypertension 2018;71(6):e13–115.

[7] Schwartz GL, Turner ST, Sing CF. Twenty-four-hour blood pressure profiles in normotensive sons of hypertensive parents. Hypertension 1992;20(6):834–40.

[8] Kupper N, et al, Willemsen G, Riese H. Heritability of daytime ambulatory blood pressure in an extended twin design. Hypertension 2005;45(1):80–5.

[9] Snieder H, et al, Hayward CS, Perks U. Heritability of central systolic pressure augmentation: a twin study. Hypertension 2000;35(2):574–9.

[10] Gong Y, McDonough CW, Wang Z, et al. Hypertension susceptibility loci and blood pressure response to antihypertensives: results from the pharmacogenomic evaluation of antihypertensive responses study. Circ Cardiovasc Genet 2012;5(6):686–91.

[11] Gong Y, Wang Z, Beitelshees AL, et al. Pharmacogenomic Genome-Wide Meta-Analysis of Blood Pressure Response to beta-Blockers in Hypertensive African Americans. Hypertension 2016;67(3):556–63.

[12] Johnson JA, Turner ST. Hypertension pharmacogenomics: current status and future directions. Curr Opin Mol Ther 2005;7(3):218–25.

[13] Johnson JA, Zineh I, Puckett BJ, et al. Beta 1-adrenergic receptor polymorphisms and antihypertensive response to metoprolol. Clin Pharmacol Ther 2003;74(1):44–52.

[14] Turner ST, Schwartz GL, Boerwinkle E. Personalized medicine for high blood pressure. Hypertension 2007; 50(1):1–5.

[15] Turner ST, Schwartz GL, Chapman AB, et al. WNK1 kinase polymorphism and blood pressure response to a thiazide diuretic. Hypertension 2005;46(4):758–65.

[16] Evangelou E, Warren HR, Mosen-Ansorena D, et al. Genetic analysis of over 1 million people identifies 535 new loci associated with blood pressure traits. Nat Genet 2018;50(10):1412–25.

[17] Chapman AB, Schwartz GL, Boerwinkle E, et al. Predictors of antihypertensive response to a standard dose of hydrochlorothiazide for essential hypertension. Kidney Int 2002;61(3):1047–55.

[18] Smith SM, et al. Blood pressure responses and metabolic effects of hydrochlorothiazide and atenolol. Am J Hypertens 2012;25(3):359–65.

[19] Neaton JD, Gong Y, Turner ST, et al. Treatment of Mild Hypertension Study. Final results. Treatment of Mild Hypertension Study Research Group. J Am Med Assoc 1993; 270(6):713–24.

[20] Hiltunen TP, Donner KM, Sarin AP, et al. Pharmacogenomics of hypertension: a genome-wide, placebo-controlled cross-over study, using four classes of antihypertensive drugs. J Am Heart Assoc 2015; 4(1):e001521.

[21] van der Wardt V, Harrison JK, Welsh T, et al. Withdrawal of antihypertensive medication: a systematic review. J Hypertens 2017;35(9):1742–9.

[22] Onesti G, Schwartz AB, Kim KE, et al. Antihypertensive effect of clonidine. Circ Res 1971;28(5 Suppl 2):53–69.

[23] Materson BJ, Reda DJ, Cushman WC, et al. Single-drug therapy for hypertension in men. A comparison of six

antihypertensive agents with placebo. The Department of Veterans Affairs Cooperative Study Group on Antihypertensive Agents. N Engl J Med 1993;328(13):914–21.
[24] Dickerson JE, Hingorani AD, Ashby MJ, et al. Optimisation of antihypertensive treatment by crossover rotation of four major classes. Lancet 1999;353(9169):2008–13.
[25] Benetos A, Labat C, Rossignol P, et al. Treatment With Multiple Blood Pressure Medications, Achieved Blood Pressure, and Mortality in Older Nursing Home Residents: The PARTAGE Study. JAMA Intern Med 2015; 175(6):989–95.
[26] Gupta P, Patel P, Strauch B, et al. Risk Factors for Nonadherence to Antihypertensive Treatment. Hypertension 2017;69(6):1113–20.
[27] Wu J, Kraja AT, Oberman A, et al. A summary of the effects of antihypertensive medications on measured blood pressure. Am J Hypertens 2005;18(7):935–42.
[28] Lefkowitz RJ, Rockman HA, Koch WJ. Catecholamines, cardiac beta-adrenergic receptors, and heart failure. Circulation 2000;101(14):1634–7.
[29] Friedman DB, Musch TI, Williams RS, et al. Beta adrenergic blockade with propranolol and atenolol in the exercising dog: evidence for beta 2 adrenoceptors in the sinoatrial node. Cardiovasc Res 1987;21(2):124–9.
[30] Rodefeld MD, Beau SL, Schuessler RB, et al. Beta-adrenergic and muscarinic cholinergic receptor densities in the human sinoatrial node: identification of a high beta 2-adrenergic receptor density. J Cardiovasc Electrophysiol 1996;7(11):1039–49.
[31] Bristow MR, Hershberger RE, Port JD, et al. Beta 1- and beta 2-adrenergic receptor-mediated adenylate cyclase stimulation in nonfailing and failing human ventricular myocardium. Mol Pharmacol 1989;35(3):295–303.
[32] Brodde OE. Beta 1- and beta 2-adrenoceptors in the human heart: properties, function, and alterations in chronic heart failure. Pharmacol Rev 1991;43(2):203–42.
[33] Bernstein D. Cardiovascular and Metabolic Alterations in Mice Lacking [beta]1- and [beta]2-Adrenergic Receptors. Trends Cardiovasc Med 2002;12(7):287–94.
[34] Dorn GW 2nd, Tepe NM, Lorenz JN, et al. Low- and high-level transgenic expression of beta2-adrenergic receptors differentially affect cardiac hypertrophy and function in Galphaq-overexpressing mice. Proc Natl Acad Sci U S A 1999;96(11):6400–5.
[35] Tevaearai HT, Eckhart AD, Walton GB, et al. Myocardial gene transfer and overexpression of beta2-adrenergic receptors potentiates the functional recovery of unloaded failing hearts. Circulation 2002;106(1):124–9.
[36] Kopp U, Aurell M, Nilsson IM, et al. The role of beta-1-adrenoceptors in the renin release response to graded renal sympathetic nerve stimulation. Pflugers Arch 1980;387(2):107–13.
[37] James PA, Oparil S, Carter BL, et al. 2014 evidence-based guideline for the management of high blood pressure in adults: report from the panel members appointed to the Eighth Joint National Committee (JNC 8). J Am Med Assoc 2014;311(5):507–20.
[38] Zhang Y, Sun N, Jiang X, et al. Comparative efficacy of beta-blockers on mortality and cardiovascular outcomes in patients with hypertension: a systematic review and network meta-analysis. J Am Soc Hypertens 2017; 11(7):394–401.
[39] Larochelle P, Tobe SW, Lacourciere Y. beta-Blockers in hypertension: studies and meta-analyses over the years. Can J Cardiol 2014;30(5 Suppl):S16–22.
[40] Pepine CJ, Handberg EM, Cooper-DeHoff RM, et al. A calcium antagonist vs a non-calcium antagonist hypertension treatment strategy for patients with coronary artery disease. The International Verapamil-Trandolapril Study (INVEST): a randomized controlled trial. J Am Med Assoc 2003;290(21):2805–16.
[41] Bangalore S, Gong Y, Cooper-DeHoff RM, et al. 2014 Eighth Joint National Committee panel recommendation for blood pressure targets revisited: results from the INVEST study. J Am Coll Cardiol 2014;64(8):784–93.
[42] Liggett SB, Mialet-Perez J, Thaneemit-Chen S, et al. A polymorphism within a conserved beta(1)-adrenergic receptor motif alters cardiac function and beta-blocker response in human heart failure. Proc Natl Acad Sci U S A 2006;103(30):11288–93.
[43] Small KM, Brown KM, Seman CA, et al. Complex haplotypes derived from noncoding polymorphisms of the intronless alpha2A-adrenergic gene diversify receptor expression. Proc Natl Acad Sci U S A 2006;103(14): 5472–7.
[44] Liu Z, Barnes SA, Sokolnicki LA, et al. Beta-2 adrenergic receptor polymorphisms and the forearm blood flow response to mental stress. Clin Auton Res 2006;16(2): 105–12.
[45] Green SA, Cole AG, Jacinto M, et al. A polymorphism of the human beta 2-adrenergic receptor within the fourth transmembrane domain alters ligand binding and functional properties of the receptor. J Biol Chem 1993; 268(31):23116–21.
[46] Green SA, Turki J, InnisM, et al. Amino-terminal polymorphisms of the human beta 2-adrenergic receptor impart distinct agonist-promoted regulatory properties. Biochemistry 1994;33(32):9414–9.
[47] Green SA, Turki J, Hall IP, et al. Implications of genetic variability of human beta 2-adrenergic receptor structure. Pulm Pharmacol 1995;8(1):1–10.
[48] Taylor DR, Kennedy MA. Genetic variation of the beta(2)-adrenoceptor: its functional and clinical importance in bronchial asthma. Am J Pharmacogenomics 2001;1(3):165–74.
[49] Bray MS, Krushkal J, Li L, et al. Positional genomic analysis identifies the beta(2)-adrenergic receptor gene as a susceptibility locus for human hypertension. Circulation 2000;101(25):2877–82.
[50] Drysdale CM, McGraw DW, Stack CB, et al. Complex promoter and coding region beta 2-adrenergic receptor haplotypes alter receptor expression and predict in vivo responsiveness. Proc Natl Acad Sci U S A 2000;97(19): 10483–8.

[51] Snyder EM, Beck KC, Dietz NM, et al. Arg16Gly polymorphism of the beta2-adrenergic receptor is associated with differences in cardiovascular function at rest and during exercise in humans. J Physiol 2006;571(Pt 1):121–30.

[52] Wolk R, Snyder EM, Somers VK, et al. Arginine 16 glycine beta2-adrenoceptor polymorphism and cardiovascular structure and function in patients with heart failure. J Am Soc Echocardiogr 2007;20(3):290–7.

[53] Lanfear DE, Jones PG, Marsh S, et al. Beta2-adrenergic receptor genotype and survival among patients receiving beta-blocker therapy after an acute coronary syndrome. J Am Med Assoc 2005;294(12):1526–33.

[54] Snyder EM, Johnson BD. Beta2-adrenergic receptor genotype and survival after acute coronary syndrome. J Am Med Assoc 2006;295(7):756–7, author reply 757-8.

[55] Snyder EM, Turner ST, Joyner MJ, et al. The Arg16Gly polymorphism of the beta2-adrenergic receptor and the natriuretic response to rapid saline infusion in humans. J Physiol 2006;574(Pt 3):947–54.

[56] Eisenach JH, Schroeder DR, Pike TL, et al. Dietary sodium restriction and beta2-adrenergic receptor polymorphism modulate cardiovascular function in humans. J Physiol 2006;574(Pt 3):955–65.

[57] Pacanowski MA, Gong Y, Cooper-Dehoff RM, et al. beta-adrenergic receptor gene polymorphisms and beta-blocker treatment outcomes in hypertension. Clin Pharmacol Ther 2008;84(6):715–21.

[58] Magvanjav O, McDonough CW, Gong Y, et al. Pharmacogenetic Associations of beta1-Adrenergic Receptor Polymorphisms With Cardiovascular Outcomes in the SPS3 Trial (Secondary Prevention of Small Subcortical Strokes). Stroke 2017;48(5):1337–43.

[59] Psaty BM, Smith NL, Heckbert SR, et al. Diuretic therapy, the alpha-adducin gene variant, and the risk of myocardial infarction or stroke in persons with treated hypertension. J Am Med Assoc 2002;287(13):1680–9.

[60] Gu Q, Burt VL, Dillon CF, et al. Trends in antihypertensive medication use and blood pressure control among United States adults with hypertension: the National Health And Nutrition Examination Survey, 2001 to 2010. Circulation 2012;126(17):2105–14.

[61] Morawski K, Ghazinouri R, Krumme A, et al. Association of a Smartphone Application With Medication Adherence and Blood Pressure Control: The MedISAFE-BP Randomized Clinical Trial. JAMA Intern Med 2018;178(6):802–9.

[62] McManus RJ, Little P, Stuart B, et al. Home and Online Management and Evaluation of Blood Pressure (HOME BP) using a digital intervention in poorly controlled hypertension: randomised controlled trial. BMJ 2021;372:m4858.

Informatics

Advances in Molecular Pathology 4 (2021) 127–143
ADVANCES IN MOLECULAR PATHOLOGY

Blood Group Genotyping

Jensyn K. Cone Sullivan, MD[a,b], Nicholas Gleadall, PhD[c], William J. Lane, MD, PhD[d,e,*]
[a]Department of Pathology, The Neely Cell Therapy Center, Tufts Medical Center, 800 Washington Street, #826, Boston, MA 02111, USA; [b]Tufts University School of Medicine, Boston, MA, USA; [c]Department of Haematology, University of Cambridge, University of Cambridge Biomedical Campus, Long Road, Cambridge, CB2 0PT, UK; [d]Department of Pathology, Brigham and Women's Hospital, Hale Building for Transformative Medicine, Room 8002L, 60 Fenwood Road, Boston, MA 02115, USA; [e]Harvard Medical School, Boston, MA, USA

KEYWORDS
• Next generation sequencing • Red blood cells • Erythrocyte antigens • Blood groups • Blood group antigens • Array • Genomics

KEY POINTS

- Erythrocyte antigens-surface structures capable of eliciting specific, humoral immune responses-were historically characterized by antibody-based methodologies, occasionally precluding accurate phenotyping and compatible blood transfusion.
- Single-nucleotide variants (SNVs) code for most blood group antigens, although there are also many well-characterized indels, structural variants, copy number variants, or regulatory region variants.
- Next Generation Sequencing (NGS) accurately calls SNV erythrocyte phenotypes. Adding long-, paired-end, and split reads and copy number analysis accurately calls more challenging blood group systems.
- NGS aids analysis of challenging serologic cases, phenotypes without requiring blood samples, identifies rare blood donors and prevents alloimmunization via improved blood product matching.
- Similarly, array technology advances allow rapid, inexpensive, and nearly exhaustive identification of known (and predicted) variants.

Red blood cell (RBC) antigens are inherited, intrinsic or adsorbed surface structures provoking specific humoral immune response. Historically, serologic—antibody-based and relatively unchanged since the early 20th century—assays imperfectly defined these antigens, at times hindering accurate phenotyping and compatible RBC transfusion and solid organ transplantation. Single-nucleotide variants (SNV), and less frequently structural variants, copy number variants or regulatory region variants encode RBC antigens. Whole genome, whole exome, and targeted next-generation sequencing (NGS) characterize these antigens more reliably and specifically than serology. Furthermore, long-reads, paired-end reads, split reads, and copy number analysis allow accurate prediction of challenging blood group systems including ABO, Rh, and MNS. NGS enriches analysis of challenging serologic cases by producing accurate phenotype data when blood samples are unobtainable, by screening the existing donor pool for rare blood identifying compatible blood for recipients via more rigorous standards and by preventing alloimmunization and hemolytic transfusion reactions. Similarly, recent array technology rapidly, accurately, inexpensively, and nearly exhaustively identifies known (and predicted) variants. Owing to significant time, cost, and clinical and research benefits, utilization of molecular RBC typing is expanding rapidly.

*Corresponding author. Department of Pathology, Brigham and Women's Hospital, Hale Building for Transformative Medicine, Room 8002L, 60 Fenwood Road, Boston, MA 02115. *E-mail address:* wlane@bwh.harvard.edu; Twitter: @bloodantigens

https://doi.org/10.1016/j.yamp.2021.07.009
2589-4080/21/

INTRODUCTION

Red Blood Cell Antigen Phenotypes and Blood Groups

Red blood cell antigens

Red blood cell (RBC) antigens are inherited, polymorphic, intrinsic or adsorbed cell-surface protein or carbohydrate structures capable of eliciting a specific, humoral immune response (Fig. 1A). RBC phenotyping, performed serologically with a spectrum of monoclonal reagents, deems antigens present on the RBC surfaces "positive" and those absent "negative". Antigen variants include weak, el, mod, and partial antigens. Weak antigens are present lower in number than expected, while mod and el are present in such low numbers that sensitive serologic methods (ie, absorption-elution) must be used to identify them. Partial variants lack portions of the antigen structure and may produce alloantibodies targeting the absent portions.

Blood groups

Blood groups consist of one or multiple related antigens coded by a single gene or by closely linked genes (Table 1; Fig. 1B). The International Society for Blood Transfusion (ISBT) recognizes 43 blood group systems [1].

Blood group systems must

- Possess an erythrocyte surface structure
- Have known genetic basis
- Be targeted by a specific antibody

Functionally, the gene products that define RBC antigen expression fill many cellular roles, acting as

- Enzymes (ABO, *ABO*, glycosyltransferases)
- Surface receptors (Duffy, *DARC*, chemokine receptors)
- Cell adhesion molecules (Lutheran, *BCAM*, B-cell adhesion molecule)
- Channels (Colton, *AQP1*, aquaporin)
- Bacterial and parasite receptors (MNS, *GYPA/GYPB*, glycophorins)
- Complement defense (Cromer, *CD55*, decay-inhibiting factor).

Historical blood group testing (serology) and transfusion

RBC transfusion, a form of an allotransplantation, exposes recipients to nonself donor antigens and leads to development of specific antibodies targeting nonself antigens. Chronically transfused patients of African ancestry form alloantibodies more frequently than transfusion recipients broadly (>50% vs approximately 3%, respectively) [2]. Sensitization increases the risk of hemolytic transfusion reaction, hemolytic disease of the fetus and newborn (HDFN) [3], further alloimmunization [4], and the difficulty of finding compatible donor blood. Compatible units must contain RBCs that are negative for antigens targeted by the recipient's alloantibodies to prevent acute hemolysis (Fig. 1C). Posttransfusion complications in sensitized patients range from minor hemolysis to death and follow 3% to 30% [5] of transfusions.

Pretransfusion testing includes serologic ABO and Rh donor and recipient typing and recipient alloantibody identification. Notwithstanding the gold standard status, serologic studies are labor- and time-intensive and may be erroneous, particularly in the case of variant Rh antigens which are more common in individuals of African ancestry.

Serologic studies

- Require fresh recipient RBCs (potentially challenging or dangerous to obtain from fetuses, neonates, children, and severely anemic patients)
- Cannot identify rare antigens (ie, no Dombrock antisera widely exist [6])
- Inconsistently type variants
- Require separate testing for identification of each RBC antigen [7].

In contrast, genotyping rapidly and increasingly inexpensively analyzes DNA from any cell source (and some acellular sources), accurately characterizes rare antigens, and exhaustively types both blood and platelet antigens [8].

Call out 1: Blood group terms

Blood Group Genetic Changes

Terminology

Alleles—alternate nucleotide sequences inhabiting specific genomic locations (loci) within coding sequences (CDS)—produce alternate gene products. The Genome Reference Consortium maintains a widely used, composite, idealized human reference genome (HRG), hg38 [9]. Comparing next-generation sequencing (NGS) sequences against hg38 allows variant allele calling. Genomic coordinates denote specific loci, such as genes, by chromosome number (chr7) and positional base number along the chromosome for locus start and end (eg, chr9:133233278-133276024 denotes the *ABO* gene in the GRCh38 reference genome).

Variant databases

Various resources compile blood group antigens, their variants, and their alleles (Table 2). Blood Group Antigen FactsBook [14], initially published in 1997, provides a clinically relevant summary. BGMUT [10,11]

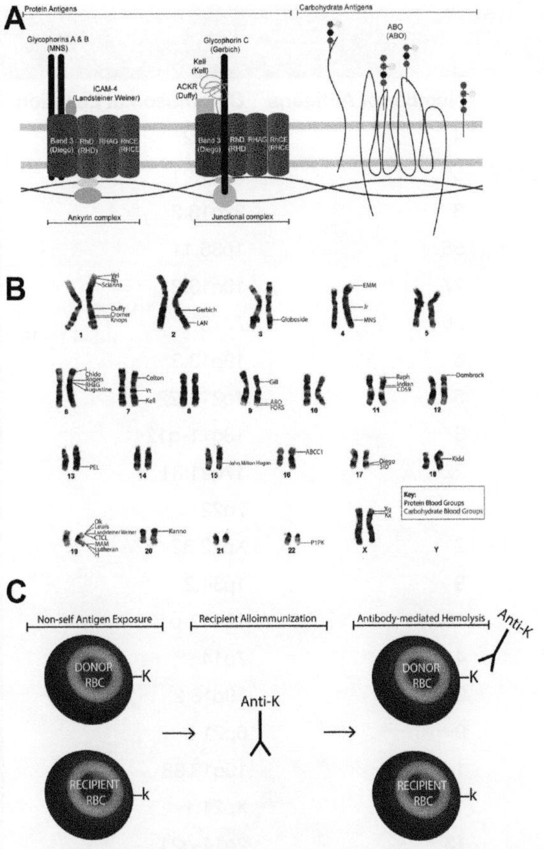

FIG. 1 **(A)** Schematic of selected protein and carbohydrate RBC antigens, including protein antigens housed within structural complexes and carbohydrate antigens located on surface glycoproteins. Structures names are listed, with corresponding blood group in parentheses. Black or white typeface denotes protein antigens and associated structures. Red typeface denotes carbohydrate antigens. **(B)** Blood group antigen coding genes by chromosomal location. Black typeface denotes blood groups with protein antigens. Red typeface denotes blood groups with carbohydrate antigens. **(C)** Schematic representation of the process of alloimmunization: A recipient encounters a nonself antigen and produces a specific alloantibody targeting the nonself antigen. The alloantibody is capable of producing hemolysis.

and drRBC [12] databases, merged in 1999 and closed in 2017, listed common antigens and rare variants. RheususBase [13] and Erythrogene [13,15] (both 2014-present) contain similar information. The ISBT updates and curates portable document format (PDF) allele tables for each blood group system [17], describing broadly, not exhaustively, antigen variants' genetic bases. No centralized resource unites all known data, although a *recent compilation* united the aforementioned resources, providing one of the most exhaustive known databases at the time of publication [5]. Algorithms seeking to accurately identify antigens via genetic sequence must use such pools of variant data.

Variant types

Multiple variant types affect antigen expression on RBCs. One or multiple single-nucleotide variants (SNVs) (and single-nucleotide polymorphisms [SNPs], SNVs present in less than 1% of a given population) account for well-documented structures and the cell-surface density of most antigens.

SNVs alter antigen expression through

- Nonsense mutations
- Missense mutations
- Regulatory region alterations [18]
- Structural alterations.

Structural variants (SVs)—gene conversions, large insertions, deletions, copy number variants, and translocations—also alter antigen expression. Glycosyltransferases (ABO, *ABO;* Lewis, *FUT2, FUT3*) transfer immunodominant sugars A, B, and H onto the RBC surface, creating carbohydrate antigens. SNV and SV in *ABO* and *FUT* genes alter enzyme action, decreasing or obliterating sugar installation. Homologous genes (Rh's *RHD* and *RHCE,* or MNS' *GYPA, GYPB,* and *GYPE*) undergo gene conversion: recombination of homologous regions, producing hybrid genes and altered gene products. Additionally, RBC structural changes such as South Asian ovalocytosis (variant *SLC4A1* coding variant band 3 protein) depress numerous antigens' surface expression [19]. Algorithms inferring antigens from genetic sequence must recognize all variant types.

Weak

Weak variants decrease surface antigen expression, although residual expression prevents alloantibody formation. For example,

- A_{weak}: variants encode weak enzymatic forms of ABO glycosyltransferases including single or multiple SNVs [20,21], minisatellite repeats [22], deletions [23], and splice-site-mutation-produced hybrid genes [24].
- $Fy(b + _w)$: Variants encode for forms of the ACKR1 protein with weaker serologic reactivity of the Fy^b antigen often due to missense variants [6].
- Del: Significantly decreases surface antigen expression of D antigen; due to many types of variants—splice site mutations, intronic SNVs [25], or exon 8 deletions [26].

TABLE 1
Blood Group Antigen Systems

System Number	System Name	Gene(s)	Number of Antigens	Chromosomal Location
1	ABO	*ABO*	4	9q34.2
2	MNS	*GYPA, GYPB, GYPE*	50	4q31.21
3	P1PK	*A4GALT*	3	22q13.2
4	Rh	*RHD, RHCE*	55	1p36.11
5	Lutheran	*BCAM*	27	19q13.2
6	Kell	*KEL*	36	7q33
7	Lewis	*FUT3*	6	19p13.3
8	Duffy	*ACKR1*	5	1q21-q22
9	Kidd	*SLC14A1*	3	18q11-q12
10	Diego	*SCL4A1*	22	17q21.31
11	Yt	*ACHE*	5	7q22
12	Xg	*XG, MIC2*	2	Xp22.32
13	Scianna	*ERMAP*	9	1p34.2
14	Dombrock	*ART4*	10	12p13-p12
15	Colton	*AQP1*	4	7p14
16	Landsteiner-Wiener	*ICAM4*	3	19p13.2
17	Chido/Rogers	*C4A, C4B*	9	6p21.3
18	H	*FUT1*	1	19q13.33
19	Kx	*XK*	1	Xp21.1
20	Gerbich	*GYPC*	13	2q14-q21
21	Cromer	*CD55*	20	1q32
22	Knops	*CR1*	12	1q32.2
23	Indian	*CD44*	6	11p13
24	Ok	*BSG*	3	19p13.3
25	Raph	*CD151*	1	11p15.5
26	John Milton Hagan	*SEMA7A*	8	15q22.3-q23
27	I	*GCNT2*	1	6p24.2
28	Globoside	*B3GALNT1*	2	3q25
29	Gill	*AQP3*	1	9p13
30	Rh-associated glycoprotein	*RHAG*	4	6p12.3
31	FORS	*GBGT1*	1	9q34.13-q34.3
32	JR	*ABCG2*	1	4q22.1
33	LAN	*ABCB6*	1	2q36
34	Vel	*SMIM1*	1	1p36.32
35	CD59	*CD59*	1	11p13
36	Augustine	*SLC29A1*	4	6p21.1

(*continued on next page*)

TABLE 1
(continued)

System Number	System Name	Gene(s)	Number of Antigens	Chromosomal Location
37	Kanno	*PRNP*	1	20p13
38	SID	*BGALNT2*	1	17q21.32
39	CTL2	*SCL44A2*	2	19p13.2
40	PEL	*ABCC4*	1	13q32.1
41	MAM	*EMP3*	1	19q13.33
42	EMM	*PIGG*	1	4p16.3
43	ABCC1	*ABCC1*	1	16p13.11

Adapted from Table of Blood Group Systems. International Society of Blood Transfusion (ISBT) Working Party on Red Cell Immunogenetics and Blood Group Terminology; 2021. https://www.isbtweb.org/fileadmin/user_upload/Table_of_blood_group_systems_v._9.0_03-FEB-2021.pdf; with permission.

- K_{mod}: Variants encode for forms of the Kel protein with altered and weaker serologic reactivity of the K antigen often due to missense variants [6].

Null. Null allele-coding variants obliterate antigen expression, potentially resulting in alloantibodies targeting the missing structure.

Common ABO null variants:

- NM_020469.2:c.261delG truncates the glycosyltransferase, preventing group A's immunodominant sugar from being transferred to RBCs.

Common RHD Null Variants

- Complete *RHD* deletion with fusion of upstream and downstream Rhesus boxes (most common in all ethnicities)
- Pseudogene *RHD**Ψ [27], an intron 3-exon 4 duplication producing a premature stop codon (common among Africans)

Combined RhD and RhCE null variants (Rh_{null})

- Amorph
- Regulator

Other null mutations decrease expression of all Rh gene products in both *RHD* and *RHCE* (Rh_{null}). The "amorph"-type Rh_{null} variant is caused by mutations (*RHCE* frameshift, deletion frameshift, or intronic splice site [6]) producing truncated or misfolded structures either unstable after membrane insertion or never inserted into the membrane. "Regulator"-type variants follow mutations (SNVs, SNV leading to partial exon skipping, frameshift or intronic splice site [6]) preventing surface expression of the Rh-stabilizing integral surface protein RhAG. U-(null) RBCs commonly follow complete deletions of *GYPB* [28].

Partial. Partial allele-coding variants lack epitopes, portions of the antigen structure. Partial variants may test serologically antigen positive, but similar to null variants, they may provoke alloantibodies which target lacking epitopes. Partial Rh variants DIIIa, DAR, and DIV and DVI result from multiple SNVs.

Other. Hybrid alleles alter antigen expression by changing enzyme activity (A hybrid B-O gene produced a product with group A transferase activity [29]), altering antigen expression (Hybrid RHD-CE-Ds have only partial C expression.) or by creating new antigens (low-frequency antigens HIL, MINY, Dantu follow *GYPA-GYPB* hybrid recombination). Conversely, variants in one blood group system may alter expression of a dependent blood group system: Gerbich-negative variants may decrease Kell expression, Kpa-antigen trans (on the opposite chromosome to) K antigen decreases K expression, and variation in the Xk protein destabilizes Kell, significantly decreasing expression, producing the McLeod phenotype [6].

Call out 2: Allele terminology

Call out 3: Blood group governance

SIGNIFICANCE

Next-Generation Sequencing

Many advances undergird NGS utilization for blood group prediction. The discovery of ABO group antigens in 1901 [30] and the creation of Sanger sequencing in 1977 [31] made discovery of the genetic basis ABO possible in 1990 [32]; after this, the completion of the Human Genome Project in 2001 [33,34] and the rise

TABLE 2
Databases of Variant Alleles Coding for Blood Group Antigens

BGMUT [10,11]	(From" Blood Group antigen gene MUTation") Human blood group antigen variant allele database with concurrent serologic phenotypes, created through the Human Genome Variation Society (HGVS). Active from 1999 until transferred under the National Center for Biotechnology Information (NCBI) and National Institute of Health (NIH)'s dbRBC (database Red Blood Cells).
dbRBC [12]	NCBI and NIH's human blood group antigen variant allele database. Included common through extremely rare single-instance variants. BGMUT merged in 1999. Supported through 2017. Foundational to current databases.
RheususBase [13]	At publication (2014), the largest database of variant alleles coding for Rh group antigens.
Blood Group Antigens FactsBook [14]	Published in 1997, updated in 2003 and 2012, this succinct desktop reference outlines 33 blood group systems' antigens, phenotypes and molecular bases.
Erythrogene [13,15]	Database of variant alleles coding for blood group antigens extracted from a diverse cohort of samples (1000 Genomes Project [16], n = 2504 samples from 26 population groups).
bloodantigens.com [5]	Curated database of all known blood group and HPA variants. Publicly available website. Forms the basis for bloodTyper interpretations.

of NGS in the early 21st century led to the first instance of NGS utilization for ABO typing in 2011 [35], followed by the proof of concept work demonstrating NGS exhaustive blood group antigen prediction [8].

Method overview

High-throughput massively parallel sequencing begins with DNA extraction and degradation. Then, library preparation adds oligonucleotide adaptors to dsDNA's 3′ and 5′ fragment ends. Barcoding and/or indexing-specific libraries allow simultaneous sequencing of multiple libraries (multiplexing). After this, the library may be clonally amplified. Sequencing proceeds via the chosen methodology. Then, mapping aligns sequenced reads with concurrent reference genome areas.

Sequence interpretation

History. Many recent approaches to genotyping include SNP-based assays or SNP-focused genomic analysis. Although a leap forward compared with serology, such assays cannot identify novel and rare SNPs not targeted by the assay. *An early algorithm* [36] based on Hidden Markov Modeling (HMM) and the BGMUT database called 94.2% samples (n = 67/71) correctly. Nonetheless, HMM is difficult to iteratively improve, and the allele tables used are not regularly updated. Other algorithms were based on 1000 Genomes [15,37]. Unfortunately, the underlying input coverage included only 15x mean coverage, insufficient to fully resolve heterozygous SNVs and SVs. The bioinformatic basis for NGS RBC genotyping is evolving.

Current algorithms. Specific algorithms facilitate variant calling (Fig. 2 and Table 3). *One algorithm* [5,8] aligned 30x mean coverage whole genome sequencing (WGS) data to the RefSeq transcript database, making variant calls for RBC and platelet antigens where nucleotides differed from the HRG. Aligning HRG and cDNA RefSeq allowed genomic coordinate conversion from variant calling into conventional CDS, allowing comparison with variant allele tables and comprehensive prediction of blood and platelet antigens. Subsequent updates automated and iteratively improved the process via samples' serologic typing and built a collective variant database [5] and permitted whole exome sequencing (WES) [38] input, allowing high-accuracy antigen calling (Table 3).

Interpretation of specific variants

Single nucleotide variants and indels. Simplest among variants to call, exonic SNVs account for the majority of RBC antigen variants. As noted previously, resources list variants in cDNA format, requiring conversion to CDS. Accurate and complete calling of SNVs requires a RefSeq transcript (otherwise variants may be overlooked) and also requires a database containing a thorough compilation of known variants [5,8,15].

Structural variants. Early NGS data analysis for blood group genotyping primarily focused on targeted sequencing able to identify well-defined SNV alterations encoding protein antigens. Now, we and other researchers have used WGS to predict SVs [5,39,40].

Final predicted phenotype depends on accurate SV analysis, but homologous blood group systems with hybrid alleles (eg, Rh and MNS) are seen which are challenging to call with traditional genotyping methods. Much progress, especially in the Rh system, has been made to call these complex SV from NGS data using several different analysis methods including copy number depth analysis (ie, Read Depth Analysis) and split read analysis (SRA) [28,41,42].

An ancestral RHD exon 2 conversion event produced the *RHCE*C* sequence. Thus, this sequence commonly misaligns to *RHD* exon 2 in NGS analysis. Assessment of copy number through sequence depth of coverage can identify this misalignment and correctly call the C/c antigens in both WGS [5,41] and WES [38,43]. Similarly, M antigen sequences align to RefSeq with low efficiency, likely due to RefSeqs encoding only the N, not M, antigen or due to misalignment of M antigen's *GYPA* sequence to a homologous region on *GYPE*. This can be addressed by looking in *GYPE* for misaligned sequence reads with one M-specific and one *GYPA*-specific SNP [38].

Transcription factors. Multiple blood group systems depend on transcription factor function [44]. The *A4GALT*-encoded galactosyl transferase attaches galactose on an RBC glycolipid, producing P1 antigen. A RUNX-1 transcription factor (TF) binding site SNP rs5751348 (NM_017436:c.-188 + 3010G > T) alters the expression of A4GALT, with the G nucleotide associated with P1-positive and T nucleotide with P1-negative phenotypes [45]. Xg^a antigen expression, produced by the X-linked gene *XG*, requires GATA-1 TF binding activity [46]. A GATA-1 TF binding site SNP rs311103 (NC_000023.11:g.2748343 G > C) alters expression of Xg^a, with the G nucleotide producing Xg^a-positive and C producing Xg^a-negative phenotypes. Lane and colleagues screened WGS data to find the same TF changes and integrated them into their *algorithm's variant database* [44]. However, it is only possible to genotype for the Xg^a-associated SNVs in males because the X and Y chromosomes share virtually identical copies of a region called PAR1 that includes the Xg^a TF binding location. Thus, females can have off-target genotyping [44,46].

WGS versus WES versus targeted sequencing. Multiple approaches to sequencing exist (Fig. 3). Whole genome sequencing allows analysis of ~three billion base pairs [34]. Benefits include identification of rare or not previously observed variants and analysis of intronic mutations affecting gene expression. Drawbacks include time and cost of sequencing and analysis and data storage space required (150 GB/genome without backup [47]). Whole exome sequencing generally sequences only exons and immediately adjacent introns, sequencing only ~thirty million base pairs [34], reducing cost, time to sequence, and storage space required, but precluding analysis of some deep intronic variants and requiring pipeline adjustments for accurate calls [38]. Additionally, enrichment may create capture bias, skewing copy number calculations used to call antigens in the Rh and MNS blood group systems. Targeted sequencing, requiring analysis of only 150,000 base pairs (<0.5% of the exome), further compresses time, money, and analytical and storage requirements. Targeted sequencing is least likely of the three methods to sufficiently sequence intronic regions and identify variants therein. An excellent review documents previous studies and approaches undertaken in each [48].

Short read versus long read. Commonly used short-read sequencing produces ~50 to 400 base pair read lengths. Many platforms use short reads for rapid, parallel, accurate sequencing (>99%). Nonetheless, mapping short reads to homologous genes in the HRG is challenging. Similarly, short reads cannot always resolve cis/trans ambiguities. Compared with short-read sequencing, long-read sequencing is generally more expensive, and some methods are less accurate, but long reads allow for essentially unambiguous cis/trans phasing and virtually eliminate ambiguities. Several groups have used long reads in ABO genotyping to phase SNVs [49,50]. Long read have also been used to resolve compound heterozygous SV underlying the U-antigen phenotype [28].

Call out 4: NGS terminology

DNA Microarrays

Introduction

DNA microarrays are a high-throughput and cost-effective tool for ascertaining individual genotypes pertaining to a predetermined set of genetic variants, selected during array design. They were adopted and popularized by early population scale genotyping studies such as The International HapMap project which used several different DNA microarrays to genotype 1397 individuals from several ethnic backgrounds [51]. The aim of the study was to identify loci in the genome for assessing risk of common diseases and variants which control quantitative traits of biomedical interest such as height, weight, and blood cell metrics. In 2006, the Wellcome Trust Case Control Consortium (WTCCC) conducted the first genome-wide association study (GWAS) in which donor samples were used. In this study, DNA samples from 14,000 English National Health Service patients with seven common diseases and 3000 healthy controls (1500 of which were UK blood donors) were genotyped on the Affymetrix GeneChip Mapping Array which contained probes for typing 500,000 DNA variants and captured about 60% of the then known common sequence variation in the genome. The WTCCC study discovered 24 genetically independent loci associated with disease risk, thus validating that DNA microarray-based GWAS could be used as a hypothesis-free method to identify risk loci for human diseases [52].

Today, DNA microarrays are widely used for a wide variety of purposes, and many different array designs exist. The genome-wide typing arrays in recent large-scale studies such as UK BioBank, which used the ThermoFisher Axiom UK BioBank array, now type over 800,000 genetic variants which have been specifically selected to allow for statistical inference of genotypes for untyped variants via imputation and GWAS [53]. There are also large numbers of highly specialized arrays which type a limited number of genetic variants such as the BioArray HEA BeadChip (Immucor, Norcross, GA) for typing select red cell antigens or the CytoScan 750k (Affymetrix, Santa Clara, CA) for genomic copy number characterization of patients with diseases such as hematological cancers [54,55].

How DNA microarrays work

Many different DNA microarray technologies exist, and it would be infeasible to discuss them all within a single book chapter. The authors have therefore selected the ThermoFisher Axiom genotyping platform as an exemplar of how these platforms generally work.

The Thermo Fisher Scientific Axiom ligation-based microarray genotyping platform uses 30-mer DNA oligonucleotide "probe sets", synthesized in situ on "array slides" to genotype-specific genetic variants. Numerous 3-μm squares—"features"—populate glass array slide surfaces. Each feature contains millions of unique 30 base pair oligonucleotide probes complementary to the genomic sequence flanking the variant of interest (forward or reverse). Replicating features numerous times on each array improves specific SNP resolution and protects against failure by adding redundancy. Two fluorescent color channels and each probe's recorded array slide spatial position detect genotypes. A<>T and C<>G variation must also be represented by two spatially separated features as only two dyes are used, one for bases A and T, and another for bases C and G.

In a standard genotyping experiment sample, DNA, amplified by PCR, fragmented, hybridizes to the probe/array complex. A solution of detection probes, many DNA probes representing every possible combination of 9 DNA bases labeled with a base-specific "hapten", wash over the array and covalently bond to the array-probe/genomic-DNA complex. A stringent wash cycle removes unbound solution probes and genomic DNA. After fluorescently labeled antibody staining, laser excitation produces a signal, and fluorescent intensity measurements denote genotype.

An overview of the Axiom genotyping process is given in Fig. 4.

Variant calling

Further statistical analysis of all samples' fluorescence intensity data calculates and extracts genotype information for each typed variant—"genotype clustering" [56]. In simple terms, each probe set on the array consists of two components, an A or B probe. During clustering, the A and B probe fluorescence for each measured variant are used to group samples with similar fluorescence patterns. If all fluorescence is accounted for by probe A, then the individual is of genotype homozygous *AA*, and similarly, if all fluorescence is accounted for by probe B, then the individual is of genotype homozygous *BB*. If fluorescence signal is detected for both probes A and B, then the individual is of genotype AB, or a heterozygote.

Fig. 5 shows a "genotype call plot" and illustrates the separation of samples via A and B probe fluorescence intensity.

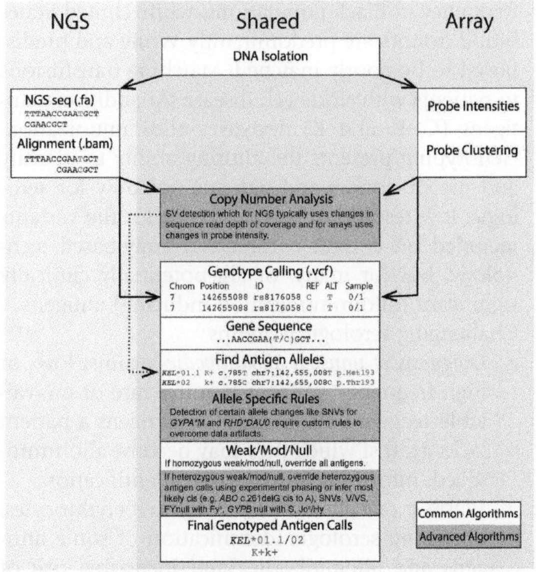

FIG. 2 Flowchart illustrating common and advanced algorithm processes for predicting blood group antigens from NGS sequencing data.

For SNPs and indels where the genetic variation being measured is an A|T <> C|G change for which two different colored fluorescent dyes are used, the intensity of each color for each sample is compared and genotype inferred. In the case if A<>T or C<>G changes, for which the same color dye is used, the probes are physically separated on the surface of the array slide. Importantly, indel identification queries only a particular set of variants consistent with indel presence or absence. No direct, complete indel sequencing occurs.

DNA microarrays may measure larger scale genomic structural variation using "copy number probes." These probes target nonpolymorphic sites spread throughout the genome. The average total fluorescence intensity produced by the copy number probes determines a "baseline" assumed to represent copy number 2. Comparing the average fluorescence intensity of probes in a region of interest to this baseline intensity allows copy number assessment.

DNA microarrays for typing blood group antigens

Owing to being low cost and high throughput, DNA microarrays provide an excellent platform for genotyping large numbers of blood donors for the variants that underpin antigen expression. The main commercial assays on the market today are the HEA BeadChip and the BloodChip assay. The HEA BeadChip is based on a short extension reaction of oligonucleotide probes bound to color-encoded beads using a PCR product as template. The test can type for a few antigens in the RHCE, KEL, FY, DO, LW, CO, SC, LU, DI, JK, and MNS blood group systems but lacks the ability to type for many clinically important antigens [57].

The BloodChip assay is based on allele- and spatial-specific hybridization of PCR products to complementary oligonucleotides affixed to glass arrays and can be used for clinical typing of 13 RBC antigens (JK, FY, KEL, RH, MNS, and DO) [58]. Studies using DNA microarrays in combination with antibody-based typing have shown that the typing data produced can dramatically increase the availability of antigen-negative blood, with *one group reporting* that they were able to provide blood for 99.8% of complex blood requests using just 43,066 donors genotyped for a limited number of antigens [13].

Although the benefits of the previously described assays are clear, they have not been widely applied to all donors by the global blood supply organizations. This is because the currently commercially available RBC antigen genotyping assays can only detect a limited number of antigens, and in comparison to traditional serologic methods, they are expensive for the number of antigens they type. In 2020, an international group of researchers sought to overcome these limitations and redesigned the UK BioBank Axiom genotyping array, a cheap population genetics screening test capable of assaying approximately 800,000 DNA variants, with blood donor genotyping in mind. In the study, 7984 English and Dutch donors were genotyped, and blood types were inferred from the resulting data using the bloodTyper algorithm. In 89,371 comparisons between genotype and serologically determined antigen types, 99.9% concordance was observed, and the total number of antigen typing results was raised from 110,980 to over 1.2 million for the typed donors. The researchers were also able to infer platelet (HPA) and leukocyte (HLA) antigen types from the same data, observing 99.97% and 99.03% concordance in 3016 and 9289 comparisons for HPA and HLA, respectively. Once these tests have achieved regulatory approval and their results can be used for labeling blood products, it is likely that they will be applied to vast numbers of donors worldwide ushering in an era of genomics-based precision transfusion medicine.

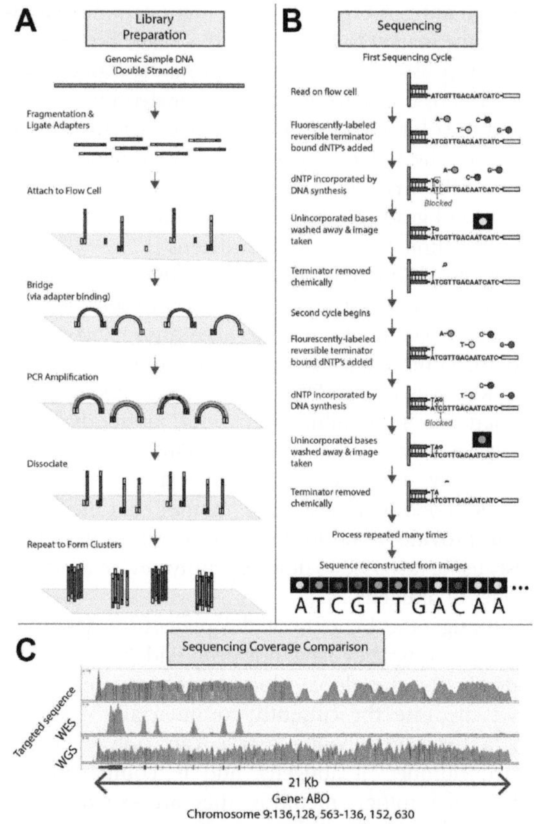

FIG. 3 Description of next-generation sequencing, including library preparation (**A**) and sequencing (**B**). (**C**) Comparison of NGS versus other molecular methods' coverage when sequencing the ABO blood group system's genes.

PRESENT RELEVANCE AND FUTURE AVENUES TO CONSIDER OR TO INVESTIGATE

Clinical Indications for Genotyping

Applications of NGS genotyping for RBC antigen prediction range wide—from selecting healthy donors to provide rare products, diagnosing potentially pathogenic alternate antigens between mother and fetus, and to providing well-matched product for chronically transfused populations (Table 3).

- Patients requiring chronic transfusion: The challenge of providing blood to chronically transfused populations (often patients with sickle cell anemia or thalassemia) is compounded by population-based genetic diversity. Antigen variants (specifically those providing malarial resistance) occur at higher frequency in Black populations, while United States blood donors are predominantly White and predisposed to be poorly matched. Matching transfusions to patients with sickle cell disease for additional antigens (C, E, and K) decreases alloimmunization. Genotyping presents the alluring ability to identify and match donors and patients not only for serologic, low-resolution types, or even for the variants included on current commercial array-based technology, but for many, or all, potentially clinically significant (alloimmunization inducing) antigens.
- Challenging serologic workups
    - *Diagnosis of unusual alloantibodies* against low- or high-frequency antigens requires rare or unavailable reagents. NGS identifies antigens a patient lacks against which they may become alloimmunized, informing alloantibody identification.
    - *Warm or cold autoantibodies* bind self erythrocytes, obscuring serologic identification of some antigens and alloantibodies and increasing risk of further alloimmunization and hemolysis. Serologic techniques remove autoantibodies from plasma but require time and remove other potentially hemolytic alloantibodies. NGS can accurately, exhaustively predict phenotype, expediting compatible product delivery and preventing alloimmunization.
    - *Therapeutic monoclonals* anti-CD38 and anti-CD47 monoclonal antibodies bind patient red cells and populate patient plasma causing false positive serologic phenotyping results and "reverse" ABO typing, respectively. As mentioned previously, NGS can accurately, exhaustively predict phenotype, expediting compatible product delivery and preventing alloimmunization.
- Challenging samples: Recently transfused patients' typing reflects both donor and recipient antigens. NGS typing, collected from recipient nonblood or leukocyte sources, accurately identifies recipient-only type.
- Insufficient sample: HDFN occurs when a pregnant woman forms an alloantibody targeting a fetal RBC antigen. These antibodies may cross into fetal circulation, destroying fetal RBCs (anti-D) or blood-producing cells (anti-K). Neonatal alloimmune thrombocytopenia (NAIT) similarly destroys platelets. Early RBC and platelet typing confirms HDFN and/or NAIT allowing treatment. Fetal blood sampling is impossible early in pregnancy and, later, poses significant fetal risk. Cell-free fetal DNA circulates in maternal plasma. This DNA can predict Rh

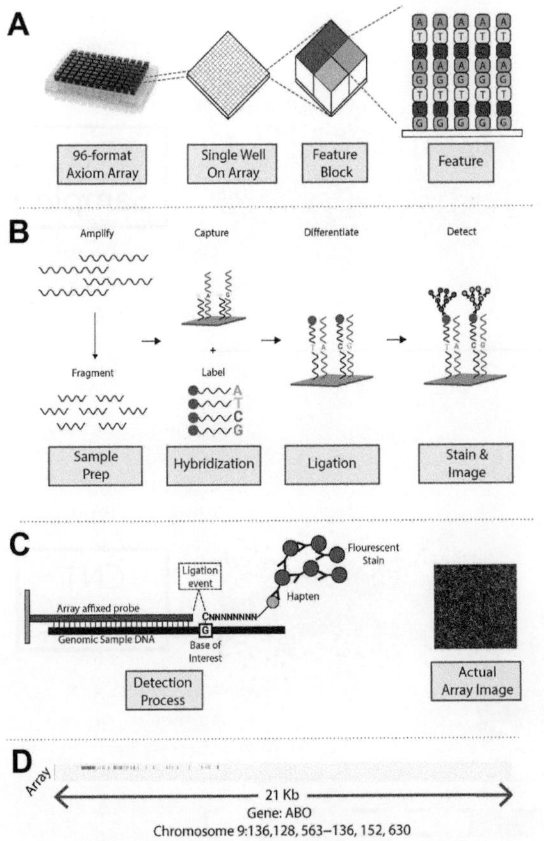

FIG. 4 Overview of Axiom array genotyping. (**A**) A zoomed diagram showing the construction of an Axiom array. (**B**) Axiom genotyping workflow. From left to right, Genomic DNA is amplified then fragmented, fragments are captured and labeled via hybridization to array probes and detection probes, ligation then covalently bonds the genomic DNA to the array/detection probe complex, finally fluorescent staining is performed followed by excitation and imaging. (**C**) Cartoon representation of the genomic DNA and array/detection probe complex. An actual image of array fluorescence during genotyping is included for reference. (**D**) Example array probe coverage for the *ABO* locus, red marks indicate the positions in the locus where probesets for measuring specific DNA changes have been incorporated into the array design.

typing [67], Kell typing [68], and recently Rh, Kell, Duffy, Kidd, MNS, and 5 HPA antigens (implicated in NAIT) [69]. Similarly, sufficient blood for serologic workup can be challenging to obtain from neonates, pediatric patients, and anemic adults. NGS can sequence DNA from nonblood sources, facilitating testing when blood is not available.

- Blood donor screening: Blood donor samples are laboriously serologically typed, antigen by antigen. Additionally, serologic typing cannot reliably recognize variants. NGS typing all donors would undoubtedly reveal numerous rare (or heretofore unrecognized) blood types. Such units could be directed to needy, compatible recipients, and donors' information could be collected and stored for future use.
- Transplant screening: ABO compatibility affects time to engraftment of allogeneic hematopoietic stem cell transplants. Stem cell donor HLAs of recipients are commonly gathered via genotyping pretransplant, and ABO is gathered serologically. Extending genotyping to include *ABO* could allow for screening of stem cell transplant donors from buccal swabs before the collection of a blood sample. Many deceased donors undergo massive transfusion with type O emergency release blood. *ABO* genotyping of deceased donors could help identify deceased donors who have converted their serologic ABO and aid in the resolution of discordant ABO due to these transfusions.

Many challenges to widespread adoption of NGS for blood typing remain [70]:

- Cost and accessibility: Despite decreasing costs, NGS's current cost may still be prohibitive for many. Similarly, storage requirements for the large volumes of information generated by NGS are significant, and ensuring balanced data security and accessibility (ideally for all clinicians caring for a given patient) remain problematic.
- Databases and pipelines: No single, exhaustive source documents all known antigen variants. An exceedingly large number of interacting mutations' effects on antigen expression must be considered. Pipelines continue to reckon with these challenges.
- Clinical significance? NGS frequently identifies novel variations and polymorphisms of unknown significance. Current modeling techniques often cannot accurately predict their effects on antigen structure.
- Alignment: Alignment of sequenced reads—mapping—allows variant calling, but blood group systems coded by multiple homologous chromosomes (Rh, MNS) are particularly challenging, often mapping to either homologue irrespective of origin, preventing variant calls [35,63,71]. Depth of coverage analysis identifies inaccurate mapping. Paired end reads and SRA further inform correct algorithmic placement.

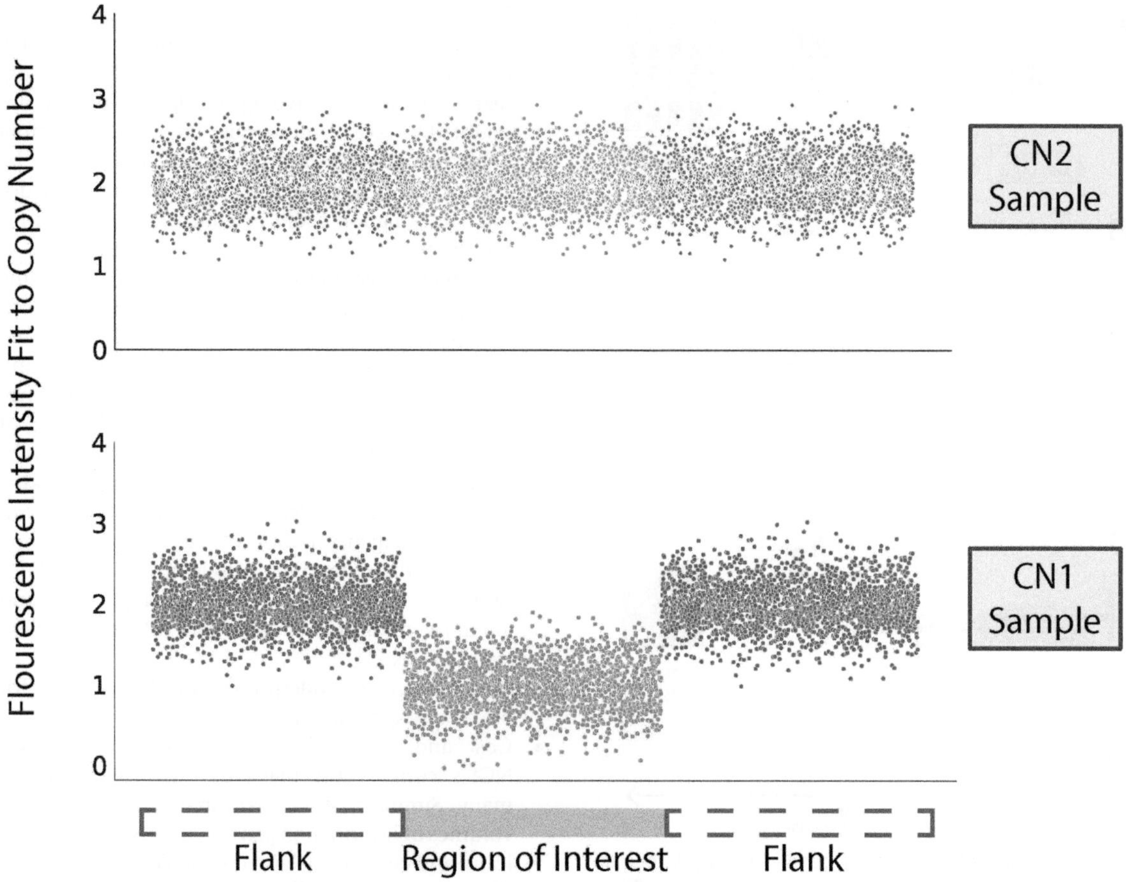

FIG. 5 Fluorescence intensity, fit to copy number, for all copy number probes in an example genomic region. A clear difference in fluorescence intensity over the region of interest can be observed between the copy number one and two samples.

- Rare null alleles: Although NGS can evaluate entire gene regions, it can miss novel null alleles, especially those produced by the introduction of stop codons or exonic indels. It can be especially difficult to predict the effect of novel changes in promoter or intronic regions which can, in theory, affect expression and lead to null states. Miscalling nulls could result in incompatible transfusion, alloimmunization, and hemolysis. Maintaining current, thorough, widely curated variant databases would decrease, but not prevent this, especially in cases of previously undescribed alleles. Encouragingly, recently produced microarrays encompass not only known but also predicted (ie, not yet observed) variants.

Future directions

Historically, serologic antigen or antigen variant discovery precipitated a search for the underlying CDS. As observed in many fields in medicine, NGS analysis commonly inverts this process, identifying variants of unknown clinical significance. As such, by sequencing larger collections of samples and then correlating concurrent serologically typed samples will allow a more complete understanding of the serologic effect of variants. Similarly, historically, blood group discovery proceeded from interesting serologic findings ("Ah! This antibody is confounding my serologic work-up! Huh. It does not target any common known antigens. I should try to identify it!") to erythrocyte surface structure identification and to underlying genetic basis

TABLE 3
Genotyping Software

BOOGIE [36]	First WGS predictive algorithm for a subset of blood group systems. First machine learning-guided software for predicted typing. Called 94.2% samples (n = 67/71) correctly. Difficult to iteratively improve. Not updated with new allele tables.
bloodTyper [5,8,38,44]	Comprehensive genotyping of all known blood group and HPA variants. A curated, regularly updated allele database (bloodantigens.com). Analyzed NGS data producing exhaustive RBC and HPA antigen genotyping from WGS, WES, targeted NGS, and high-density DNA arrays with >99% accuracy. Includes expansive SV support for Rh and MNS hybrids.
RHtyper [42]	Comprehensive, high-throughput RH-typing algorithm utilizing RHD zygosity, allele zygosity and hybrid alleles via coverage profiling, and allele pair prediction via haplotype associations. Open access [59].
Omixon [60]	Monotype ABO amplifies ABO exons 2–7 for NGS sequencing, designed for solid organ transplant compatibility analysis [61].
Erythrogene [15,62]	Imported 1000 Genomes variant data and population information. Compared inputs with a composite antigen table curated from ISBT, Blood Group Antigen Factsbook, and dbRBC. Available as a searchable, online database. 15x input coverage limits SVs identification.
Schoeman et.al. Software [63–66]	Utilizes targeted exome data to interpret 35 blood group systems.
Montemayor-Garcia Software [37]	Evaluated 1000 Genomes data for single SNV and short indels of 42 blood group genes (excluding ABO, Rh and MNS). Extracted coordinates and superpopulation frequencies.

determination. This process undergirds the identification of ABO, Rh, and other blood groups throughout the 20th and early 21st century. Only recently has new blood group identification begun with genetic observations, followed by confirmatory serologic discovery.

Mismatches between blood donor and blood recipient phenotypes theoretically increase the risk for alloimmunization. Such mismatches occur commonly when transfusing patients with sickle cell disease in the United States, where the donor population consists primarily of people who are white. Analysis of other geographic regions of broad-scale blood donor and recipient mismatch would highlight areas where increased alloimmunization surveillance is beneficial. Finally, RBC antigens function in a variety of cellular processes, and varying antigens and/or antigen variants may produce susceptibility or confer resistance to diseases from severe acute respiratory syndrome coronavirus 2 (SARS-CoV-2) [72] to malaria [73]. Gene-wide association studies focused on blood group antigens will likely deepen insight into such connections.

SUMMARY

Historical antibody-based RBC antigen typing accurately calls common antigens but poorly calls many variant antigens. Inaccurately phenotyped blood samples increase the risk of incompatible blood transfusion, potentially resulting in hemolysis and death. SNVs code most blood group antigens, but indels, SVs, and copy number variants or regulatory region variants code others, including variants which are often particularly challenging to phenotype. Enriching standard short-read NGS analysis with copy number, paired end read, and SRA allows accurate prediction of challenging blood group systems such as Rh. Recent advances in array technology provide nearly comparable clinical information. Such NGS and array technology allows challenging serologic case analysis, provides phenotype information when sample blood cannot be obtained, identifies rare blood donors from the donor population, and allows product matching for patients at risk of alloimmunization.

DEFINITIONS

Call Out 1: Blood Group Terms

- Antigen: RBC-surface protein or sugar structure capable of provoking a specific humoral response. Include RBC antigens, human platelet antigens, and "human leukocyte antigens," although RBC antigens are the main focus of the chapter.

- Blood group: Antigen or antigens encoded by a single (or multiple homologous) gene(s).
- Phenotyping: Determining antigen identity, commonly through serologic (antibody) reagents.
- Weak: Lower antigen expression than expected.
- Modified (mod): Significantly lower antigen expression than expected.
- El (from "eluate"): Significantly lower antigen expression than expected, requiring sensitive serologic techniques (absorbtion-elution) to identify.
- Partial: Lack some surface structure portion (some epitope or epitopes) characteristic of the antigen.

Call Out 2: Allele Terminology

- Locus: Gene's fixed chromosomal location.
- Allele: Alternate gene iterations.
- CDS (from "coding sequence"): Sum of an organism's protein-coding sequences.
- Genome Reference Consortium: Multi-institutional collaborative maintaining human reference genomes.
- Contig: Overlain DNA sequences forming a consensus sequence.
- Human reference genome: A representative genome. Not one human's DNA sequence, rather an idealized "normal" human genome composite. Built of contigs.
- hg38 [9]: Human genome reference build, released December 2013, widely used in NGS to make variant calls.
- Genomic coordinates: Denote gene location in relation to the reference genome. Include chromosome number and gene start and end positions.
- Format: File formats relaying NGS data. Include FASTA (reference sequence; eg, RefSeq), FASTQ (unaligned NGS reads with quality scores), SAM (aligned NGS reads), BAM (binary format sequence of SAM files), and VCF (variant call format).
- Single nucleotide variant (SNV): At one genomic position, interchanging one nucleotide with another.
- Single nucleotide polymorphism: SNV occurring in greater than 1% of a population.
- Structural variant: Large changes in chromosome structural (generally >1kb). Include insertions, deletions, translocations, duplications, and *copy number variants*.
- Indels: Nucleotide sequences inserted or deleted, typically less than 100 nucleotides.
- Gene conversion: Interchanging one sequence with a homologue, producing a hybrid gene.
- Hybrid gene: Product of gene conversion.
- Deletion: Nucleotide sequence loss, via removal or nonreplication.
- Insertion: Nucleotide sequence addition.
- Multiallelic site: Genomic position where greater than 2 alternative alleles (or variants) have been detected.

Call Out 3: Blood Group Governance

The ISBT defines blood group antigens under the governance of the Red Cell Immunogenetics and Blood Group Terminology working party, a collaborative of blood group antigen serology and genetics world experts. ISBT recognizes greater than 330 blood group antigen phenotypes across 43 blood group systems, defined by greater than 1700 alleles [74].

Call Out 4: Next Generation Sequencing Terminology

- Read: Nucleotide sequence copied from reference DNA.
- Sequence read: Number of separate sequence reads copying a locus [75].
- Paired read: Two reads separated by a known distance, flanking the sequenced area. Read distance variation from expected implies structural variation. Algorithms use read distance to improve mapping in repetitive portions of the genome.
- Split read: Presumed contiguous read mapping to two separate areas in the reference genome. Indicates structural variation.
- Phased sequencing, "Phasing": Delineating mapped allele maternal versus paternal origin. Allows [76],
  - Compound heterozygote analysis
  - Allele-specific expression measurement
  - Variant linkage identification.

Call Out 5: Array Terminology

- Probe: Oligonucleotide hybridizing with a specific nucleotide target sequence.
- Feature: Geographic array constituent; a "spot" of probes designed to hybridize with one specific target sequence.
- Probeset: Multiple probes targeting one transcript. Separate probes hybridizing with varying transcript sequence lengths.
- Array: Collection of spots identifying selected transcripts.
- Copy number probe: Oligonucleotides hybridizing with transcripts of a specific copy number.
- Probe intensity: Fluorescent antibodies bind probe-transcript hybrids. High fluorescence implies

successful hybridization. Genotype (delineated by known feature position) is inferred by degree of fluorescence.

- Cluster plot: Specific genotypes produce repeatable array fluorescence patterns. Statistical analysis of fluorescence intensity data allows variant calling.
- Contrast: Ratio between fluorescence signal from probe A and probe B in array genotyping determines separability of different genotype clusters. Equals log2 (A signal intensity/B signal intensity).
- Strength: The average strength of the fluorescence signal from probe A and probe B in array genotyping. Usefully highlights signal strength differences between genotype clusters. Equals (log2(A signal) +log2(B signal))/2.

CLINIC CARE POINTS

- Conventional serologic testing and PCR based genotyping cannot be used to routinely identify all known clinically significant blood group antigens, potentially leading to incompatible transfusions.
- Conversely, next generation sequencing (NGS) and high-density DNA array genotyping can identify nearly all known blood group antigens, promoting more compatible transfusions and prevent alloantibody formation.
- Therefore, NGS and high-density DNA array-based genotyping are valuable testing modalities to supplement serologic testing in multiply transfused patients, patients for whom blood samples are not available and patients with complicated serologic workups.

DISCLOSURE

W.J. Lane reports receiving personal consulting fees from CareDx, Inc, and his institution is a founding member of the Blood transfusion Genomics Consortium (BGC) that has received fees from Thermo Fisher Scientific Inc. to help codevelop a high-density DNA genotyping array. J.K. Cone Sullivan has nothing to disclose. N. Gleadall's institution is a founding member of the Blood transfusion Genomics Consortium (BGC) that has received fees from Thermo Fisher Scientific Inc. to help codevelop a high-density DNA genotyping array.

REFERENCES

[1] Table of blood group systems. ISBT. 2021. Available at: https://www.isbtweb.org/fileadmin/user_upload/Table_of_blood_group_systems_v._9.0_03-FEB-2021.pdf. Accessed March 16, 2021.

[2] Hendrickson JE, Tormey CA, Shaz BH. Red blood cell alloimmunization mitigation strategies. Transfus Med Rev 2014;28(3):137–44.

[3] Tormey CA, Stack G. The persistence and evanescence of blood group alloantibodies in men. Transfusion 2009; 49(3):505–12.

[4] Schonewille H, van de Watering LMG, Brand A. Additional red blood cell alloantibodies after blood transfusions in a nonhematologic alloimmunized patient cohort: is it time to take precautionary measures? Transfusion 2006;46(4):630–5.

[5] Lane WJ, Westhoff CM, Gleadall NS, et al. Automated typing of red blood cell and platelet antigens: a whole-genome sequencing study. Lancet Haematol 2018;5(6): e241–51.

[6] Daniels G. Human blood groups. Hoboken, NJ: John Wiley & Sons; 2008.

[7] Westhoff CM. Blood group genotyping. Blood 2019; 133(17):1814–20.

[8] Lane WJ, Westhoff CM, Uy JM, et al. Comprehensive red blood cell and platelet antigen prediction from whole genome sequencing: proof of principle. Transfusion 2016;56(3):743–54.

[9] Genome browser FAQ. Available at: https://genome.ucsc.edu/FAQ/FAQreleases.html#release1. Accessed March 18, 2021.

[10] Patnaik SK, Helmberg W, Blumenfeld OO. BGMUT database of allelic variants of genes encoding human blood group antigens. Transfus Med Hemother 2014;41(5): 346–51.

[11] Patnaik SK, Helmberg W, Blumenfeld OO. BGMUT: NCBI dbRBC database of allelic variations of genes encoding antigens of blood group systems. Nucleic Acids Res 2012;40(Database issue):D1023–9.

[12] Index of/pub/mhc/rbc/Final archive. Available at: https://ftp.ncbi.nlm.nih.gov/pub/mhc/rbc/Final%20Archive/. Accessed March 21, 2021.

[13] Wagner FF, Flegel WA. The rhesus site. Transfus Med Hemother 2014;41(5):357–63.

[14] Reid ME, Lomas-Francis C, Olsson ML. The blood group antigen factsBook. Hoboken, NJ: Academic Press; 2012.

[15] Möller M, Jöud M, Storry JR, et al. Erythrogene: a database for in-depth analysis of the extensive variation in 36 blood group systems in the 1000 Genomes Project. Blood Adv 2016;1(3):240–9.

[16] 1000 Genomes Project Consortium, Auton A, Brooks LD, et al. A global reference for human genetic variation. Nature 2015;526(7571):68–74.

[17] [No title]. Available at: http://www.isbtweb.org/fileadmin/user_upload/Working_parties/WP_on_Red_Cell_Immunogenetics_and/004_RHCE_alleles_v4.0_180208.pdf. Accessed March 18, 2021.

[18] Tournamille C, Colin Y, Cartron JP, et al. Disruption of a GATA motif in the Duffy gene promoter abolishes

erythroid gene expression in Duffy–negative individuals. Nat Genet 1995;10(2):224–8.

[19] Booth PB, Serjeantson S, Woodfield DG, et al. Selective depression of blood group antigens associated with hereditary ovalocytosis among melanesians. Vox Sang 1977;32(2):99–110.

[20] Ogasawara K, Yabe R, Uchikawa M, et al. Molecular genetic analysis of variant phenotypes of the ABO blood group system. Blood 1996;88(7):2732–7.

[21] Olsson ML, Irshaid NM, Hosseini-Maaf B, et al. Genomic analysis of clinical samples with serologic ABO blood grouping discrepancies: identification of 15 novel A and B subgroup alleles. Blood 2001;98(5):1585–93.

[22] Seltsam A, Wagner FF, Grüger D, et al. Weak blood group B phenotypes may be caused by variations in the CCAAT-binding factor/NF-Y enhancer region of the ABO gene. Transfusion 2007;47(12):2330–5.

[23] Yamamoto F-I, McNeill PD, Hakomori S-I. Human histo-blood group A2 transferase coded by A2 allele, one of the A subtypes, is characterized by a single base deletion in the coding sequence, which results in an additional domain at the carboxyl terminal. Biochem Biophys Res Commun 1992;187(1):366–74.

[24] Hosseini-Maaf B, Smart E, Chester MA, et al. The Abantu phenotype in the ABO blood group system is due to a splice-site mutation in a hybrid between a new O1-like allelic lineage and the A2 allele. Vox Sanguinis 2005; 88(4):256–64.

[25] Wagner FF, Frohmajer A, Flegel WA. RHD positive haplotypes in D negative Europeans. BMC Genet 2001;2:10.

[26] Richard M, Perreault J, Constanzo-Yanez J, et al. A newDELvariant caused by exon 8 deletion. Transfusion 2007;47(5):852–7.

[27] Olsson ML, Chester MA. A rapid and simple ABO genotype screening method using a novel B/O2 versus A/O2 discriminating nucleotide substitution at the ABO locus. Vox Sang 1995;69(3):242–7.

[28] Lane WJ, Gleadall NS, Aeschlimann J, et al. Multiple GYPB gene deletions associated with the U- phenotype in those of African ancestry. Transfusion 2020;60(6): 1294–307.

[29] Suzuki K, Iwata M, Tsuji H, et al. A de novo recombination in the ABO blood group gene and evidence for the occurrence of recombination products. Hum Genet 1997;99.

[30] Landsteiner K. On agglutination of normal human blood. Transfusion 1961;1:5–8.

[31] Sanger F, Nicklen S, Coulson AR. DNA sequencing with chain-terminating inhibitors. Proc Natl Acad Sci U S A 1977;74(12):5463–7.

[32] Yamamoto F, Clausen H, White T, et al. Molecular genetic basis of the histo-blood group ABO system. Nature 1990;345(6272):229–33.

[33] Lander ES, Linton LM, Birren B, et al. Initial sequencing and analysis of the human genome. Nature 2001; 409(6822):860–921.

[34] Venter JC, Adams MD, Myers EW, et al. The sequence of the human genome. Science 2001;291(5507):1304–51.

[35] Stabentheiner S, Danzer M, Niklas N, et al. Overcoming methodical limits of standard RHD genotyping by next-generation sequencing. Vox Sang 2011;100(4):381–8.

[36] Giollo M, Minervini G, Scalzotto M, et al. BOOGIE: predicting blood groups from high throughput sequencing data. PLoS One 2015;10(4):e0124579.

[37] Montemayor-Garcia C, Karagianni P, Stiles DA, et al. Genomic coordinates and continental distribution of 120 blood group variants reported by the 1000 Genomes Project. Transfusion 2018;58(11):2693–704.

[38] Lane WJ, Vege S, Mah HH, et al. Automated typing of red blood cell and platelet antigens from whole exome sequences. Transfusion 2019. https://doi.org/10.1111/trf.15473.

[39] Pirooznia M, Goes FS, Zandi PP. Whole-genome CNV analysis: advances in computational approaches. Front Genet 2015;6:138.

[40] Baronas J, Westhoff CM, Vege S, et al. RHD zygosity determination from whole genome sequencing data. J Blood Disord Transfus 2016;7(5). https://doi.org/10.4172/2155-9864.1000365.

[41] Wheeler MM, Lannert KW, Huston H, et al. Genomic characterization of the RH locus detects complex and novel structural variation in multi-ethnic cohorts. Genet Med 2019;21(2):477–86.

[42] Chang T-C, Haupfear KM, Yu J, et al. A novel algorithm comprehensively characterizes human RH genes using whole-genome sequencing data. Blood Adv 2020; 4(18):4347–57.

[43] Chou ST, Flanagan JM, Vege S, et al. Whole-exome sequencing for RH genotyping and alloimmunization risk in children with sickle cell anemia. Blood Adv 2017;1(18):1414–22.

[44] Lane WJ, Aguad M, Smeland-Wagman R, et al. A whole genome approach for discovering the genetic basis of blood group antigens: independent confirmation for P1 and Xga. Transfusion 2019;59(3):908–15.

[45] Westman JS, Stenfelt L, Vidovic K, et al. Allele-selective RUNX1 binding regulates P1 blood group status by transcriptional control of A4GALT. Blood 2018;131(14): 1611–6.

[46] Möller M, Lee YQ, Vidovic K, et al. Disruption of a GATA1-binding motif upstream of XG/PBDX abolishes Xga expression and resolves the Xg blood group system. Blood 2018;132(3):334–8.

[47] Storage and computation requirements. Available at: https://www.strand-ngs.com/support/ngs-data-storage-requirements. Accessed March 29, 2021.

[48] Orzinska A, Guz K, Brojer E. Potential of next-generation sequencing to match blood group antigens for transfusion. IJCTM 2019;7:11–22.

[49] Lang K, Wagner I, Schöne B, et al. ABO allele-level frequency estimation based on population-scale genotyping by next generation sequencing. BMC Genomics 2016;17:374.

[50] Wu PC, Lin Y-H, Tsai LF, et al. ABO genotyping with next-generation sequencing to resolve heterogeneity in donors with serology discrepancies. Transfusion 2018; 58(9):2232–42.

[51] International HapMap Consortium. The international HapMap project. Nature 2003;426(6968):789–96.

[52] Wellcome Trust Case Control Consortium. Genome-wide association study of 14,000 cases of seven common diseases and 3,000 shared controls. Nature 2007; 447(7145):661–78.

[53] Bycroft C, Freeman C, Petkova D, et al. The UK Biobank resource with deep phenotyping and genomic data. Nature 2018;562(7726):203–9.

[54] Veldhuisen B, van der Schoot CE, de Haas M. Blood group genotyping: from patient to high-throughput donor screening. Vox Sang 2009;97(3):198–206.

[55] Berry NK, Scott RJ, Rowlings P, et al. Clinical use of SNP-microarrays for the detection of genome-wide changes in haematological malignancies. Crit Rev Oncol Hematol 2019;142:58–67.

[56] Rabbee N, Speed TP. A genotype calling algorithm for affymetrix SNP arrays. Bioinformatics 2006;22(1):7–12.

[57] Hashmi G, Shariff T, Seul M, et al. A flexible array format for large-scale, rapid blood group DNA typing. Transfusion 2005;45(5):680–8.

[58] Beiboer SHW, Wieringa-Jelsma T, Maaskant-Van Wijk PA, et al. Rapid genotyping of blood group antigens by multiplex polymerase chain reaction and DNA microarray hybridization. Transfusion 2005;45(5):667–79.

[59] Company Profiles: DNAnexus Inc. Available at: https://platform.dnanexus.com/app/RHtyper. Accessed August 13, 2021.

[60] HLA Typing. Available at: https://www.omixon.com/. Accessed March 17, 2021.

[61] Monotype ABOTM. Available at: https://www.omixon.com/products/monotype-abo/. Accessed March 17, 2021.

[62] Möller M, Hellberg Å, Olsson ML. Thorough analysis of unorthodox ABO deletions called by the 1000 Genomes project. Vox Sang 2018;113(2):185–97.

[63] Schoeman EM, Roulis EV, Liew Y-W, et al. Targeted exome sequencing defines novel and rare variants in complex blood group serology cases for a red blood cell reference laboratory setting. Transfusion 2018; 58(2):284–93.

[64] Sano R, Nakajima T, Takahashi K, et al. Expression of ABO blood-group genes is dependent upon an erythroid cell-specific regulatory element that is deleted in persons with the B(m) phenotype. Blood 2012;119(22): 5301–10.

[65] Schoeman EM, Lopez GH, McGowan EC, et al. Evaluation of targeted exome sequencing for 28 protein-based blood group systems, including the homologous gene systems, for blood group genotyping: SEQUENCING FOR BLOOD GROUP GENOTYPING. Transfusion 2017;57(4):1078–88.

[66] RBC-FluoGeneNX ABO plus Published May 12, 2020.Available at: https://www.inno-train.de/en/news/produkte/details/detail/rbc-fluogenenx-abo-plus/. Accessed March 17, 2021.

[67] Lo YM, Hjelm NM, Fidler C, et al. Prenatal diagnosis of fetal RhD status by molecular analysis of maternal plasma. N Engl J Med 1998;339(24):1734–8.

[68] Rieneck K, Bak M, Jønson L, et al. Next-generation sequencing: proof of concept for antenatal prediction of the fetal Kell blood group phenotype from cell-free fetal DNA in maternal plasma. Transfusion 2013. https://doi.org/10.1111/trf.12172.

[69] Orzińska A, Guz K, Mikula M, et al. Prediction of fetal blood group and platelet antigens from maternal plasma using next-generation sequencing. Transfusion 2019; 59(3):1102–7.

[70] Montemayor-Garcia C, Westhoff CM. The "next generation" reference laboratory? Transfusion 2018;58(2): 277–9.

[71] Fichou Y, Le Maréchal C, Bryckaert L, et al. Variant screening of the RHD gene in a large cohort of subjects with D phenotype ambiguity: report of 17 novel rare alleles. Transfusion 2012;52(4):759–64.

[72] Wu S-C, Arthur CM, Wang J, et al. The SARS-CoV-2 receptor-binding domain preferentially recognizes blood group A. Blood Adv 2021;5(5):1305–9.

[73] Rowe JA, Opi DH, Williams TN. Blood groups and malaria: fresh insights into pathogenesis and identification of targets for intervention. Curr Opin Hematol 2009; 16(6):480–7.

[74] E T. Red Cell Immunogenetics and Blood Group Terminology. Available at: https://www.isbtweb.org/working-parties/red-cell-immunogenetics-and-blood-group-terminology. Accessed March 18, 2021.

[75] Sims D, Sudbery I, Ilott NE, et al. Sequencing depth and coverage: key considerations in genomic analyses. Nat Rev Genet 2014;15(2):121–32.

[76] Phased sequencing. Available at: https://www.illumina.com/techniques/sequencing/dna-sequencing/whole-genome-sequencing/phased-sequencing.html. Accessed March 21, 2021.

Advances in Molecular Pathology 4 (2021) 145–171
ADVANCES IN MOLECULAR PATHOLOGY

Artificial Intelligence in Anatomic Pathology

Joshua J. Levy, PhD[a,b,c,*], Louis J. Vaickus, MD, PhD[c]
[a]Program in Quantitative Biomedical Sciences, Geisel School of Medicine at Dartmouth, Hanover, NH 03755, USA; [b]Department of Epidemiology, Geisel School of Medicine at Dartmouth, Hanover, NH 03755, USA; [c]Emerging Diagnostic and Investigative Technologies, Department of Pathology, Dartmouth Hitchcock Medical Center, 1 Medical Center Drive, Borwell Building Floor 4th, Lebanon, NH 03756-1000, USA

KEYWORDS
• Machine learning • Deep learning • Whole slide images • Histopathology • Virtual staining • Classification • Regression • Artificial intelligence

KEY POINTS

- Whole slide images (WSIs) are large digitized representations of tissue/cytology specimen and are of prohibitive dimensionality, costly to store and integrate with the clinical workflow in high throughput.
- Machine learning approaches, particularly deep learning, can mine complex microarchitectural and macroarchitectural patterns across the tissue to form nuanced disease associations.
- Supervised learning algorithms learn associations (classification and regression) when the data have been labeled a priori. Unsupervised learning algorithms learn from data to group patients when it is unlabeled. Models are trained and evaluated after partitioning collected data into training, validation, and test cohorts.
- Statistics across sub-images/patches/cells are tabulated to form final predictions. Segmentation and cell detection neural networks may be used to decompose a slide into its constituent cells.
- Weakly supervised, graph-based approaches, virtual staining, spatial omics, multi-modal, and hierarchical Bayesian modeling approaches are emerging technologies for digital pathology that warrant additional investigation.

INTRODUCTION

Board-certified anatomic pathologists spend years developing domain-specific visual skills and heuristics, which allow them to efficiently (both temporally and mentally) detect and classify thousands of perturbations of normal architecture and cytology. Over the past few decades, there has been an explosive increase in methods designed to encapsulate this expert knowledge into computer programs which can emulate their thought processes. However, clinical decision-making is highly nuanced and thus automated computer analyses that rely on hard-coded rulesets can easily be fooled by deviations from these assumptions (eg, the shape of a nucleus is always round, and hematoxylin stain intensity is invariant to fixation, lighting, etc.). Like all physicians, pathologists desire tools which can resolve ambiguity and bias while providing efficient, simple outputs. In designing these tools, there is therefore a precarious cost-benefit balance of providing enough new information to negate any increases in processing time. Ideally, any such tool will be faster and better than the current standard of care, but in the real world, this is seldom possible. Artificial intelligence (AI) techniques (machine learning, deep learning, etc.) that effectively "learn" their own set of heuristics from experience/instruction by human experts are

*Corresponding author, *E-mail address:* joshua.j.levy.gr@dartmouth.edu

https://doi.org/10.1016/j.yamp.2021.07.005
2589-4080/21/

ideally poised to provide these ideal tools given their flexibility, relative insensitivity to high-dimensional data, and ability to detect correlations that are beyond the ability of human practitioners [1]. The creative, intuitive, socially adept pathologist can thus be partnered with an indefatigable, quantitative algorithm with limitless attention to detail.

In this review article, we provide a brief introduction of AI, machine learning and deep learning techniques and technologies. Then we discuss emerging methodologies and their applications in pathology. Finally, we contemplate some of the logistical, legal, and ethical concerns surrounding the safe and pragmatic implementation of AI anatomic pathology technologies.

SLIDES AT SCALE

Pathologists generally diagnose patients by examining a tissue under a microscope after it has been biopsied, fixed with formalin, embedded in paraffin, sectioned into 5uM slices, and stained with chemicals optimized to highlight particular cellular features (the most common being hematoxylin and eosin, H&E) [2]. Digitized representations of the tissue—whole slide images (WSIs)—are large multidimensional ($N \times M \times 3$) arrays/matrices (Fig. 1A). The digital format has many advantages over glass slides, the most trivial of which is portability. However, this digital format also comes with significant disadvantages when treated analogously to a glass slide, chief among them being that it is much less efficient to screen a WSI in the same manner as one might screen a glass slide. While other data modalities are available to the anatomic pathologist (clinical chemistry, NGS, other imaging modalities, etc.), none is as vital to the future practice of pathology and as familiar to the pathologist as the WSI and we will spend the bulk of the article discussing them.

WSI may span hundreds of thousands of pixels in any given spatial dimension and typically require 5 to 25 GB of storage space per slide. As individual pathology laboratories may process tens of thousands to hundreds of thousands of slides per year, data storage costs can become intractable for most academic medical centers [3]. Other common issues include memory usage and a surfeit of image features (eg, a WSI can contain millions of cells, not all of which are relevant). Analyses operating on an entire WSI at once thus face a 2-fold challenge: (1) graphics processing units (GPUs; the most common computational device used for machine learning) have limited RAM, which must house all data under consideration as well as the model and (2) irrelevant features can represent a majority of the data gleaned from an image (eg, white space in a large histologic slide and other irrelevant features). Thus, WSIs are typically assessed using small image patches or other functional subunits (eg, cells) and results are then aggregated to make predictions on the slide level (Fig. 1A–C) [4]. These concerns are in addition to the stress placed on a file storage system

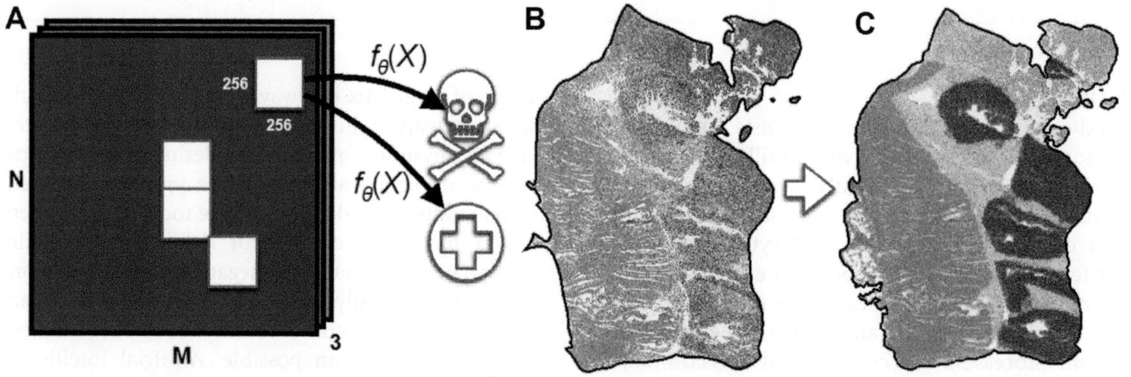

FIG. 1 Overview of Patch-Based Analysis of WSI. (**A**) WSI is an NxMx3 array and, because of the high dimensionality of the data, WSIs are typically broken into patches/subimages, which are analyzed separately using a machine learning model. Visualized here are predictions being made over 256 × 256 pixel image patches (eg, benign/malignant) and these statistics from these patches may be tabulated across the slide. (**B**) Example of WSI from Colon which has been stained with a Hematoxylin (*purple*) and Eosin (*pink*) stain. (**C**) Machine learning algorithms are trained to predict on a patch-by-patch basis different Colon subcompartments, from epithelium to fat/serosa and tumor as common examples; information from these subcompartments may be aggregated/tabulated to form inferences across the WSI.

when millions of input/output (I/O) requests are generated on a daily basis.

INTRODUCTION TO MACHINE LEARNING

When the number of predictors (eg, image tiles in a WSI) greatly surpasses the number of observations/patients, it becomes incredibly difficult to develop efficient heuristics and rules which capture the necessary information from a WSI. For instance, prior expert-driven rule-based systems relied on the development of human-specified shapes and patterns to look for in images [5]. However, the number of rules from which to enumerate is now much greater than can be enumerated and registered, which has spurred the development of AI technologies which can flexibly devise their own rules to make inferences on well-defined tasks. Machine learning algorithms can capture unintuitive relationships (eg, predictors that are nonlinear with respect to the outcome and interact with one another or some pattern or shape that is spatially defined/relevant at many levels of analysis) in big data by developing new rules and patterns that capture the relationship between the input and target which have not been previously specified; in essence, they "teach" themselves through trial and error. When the target is known, we refer to this as supervised learning which encompasses classification and regression tasks (eg, automated assignment of tumor stage based on image) (Fig. 2A). When the target is unknown, we refer to this as unsupervised learning, where similarities and differences between the observations capture groups in the data which may be more prognostically relevant (eg, delineating ambiguous cellular morphology into further subgroupings) (Fig. 2B) [6].

Supervised learning tasks predict either continuous (regression) or binary/multi-class targets (classification). Examples of supervised learning techniques include:

1. Tree-based approaches: Also known as classification and regression tree methodologies, these methods can render decisions on data given a set of input predictors by asking a series of questions about

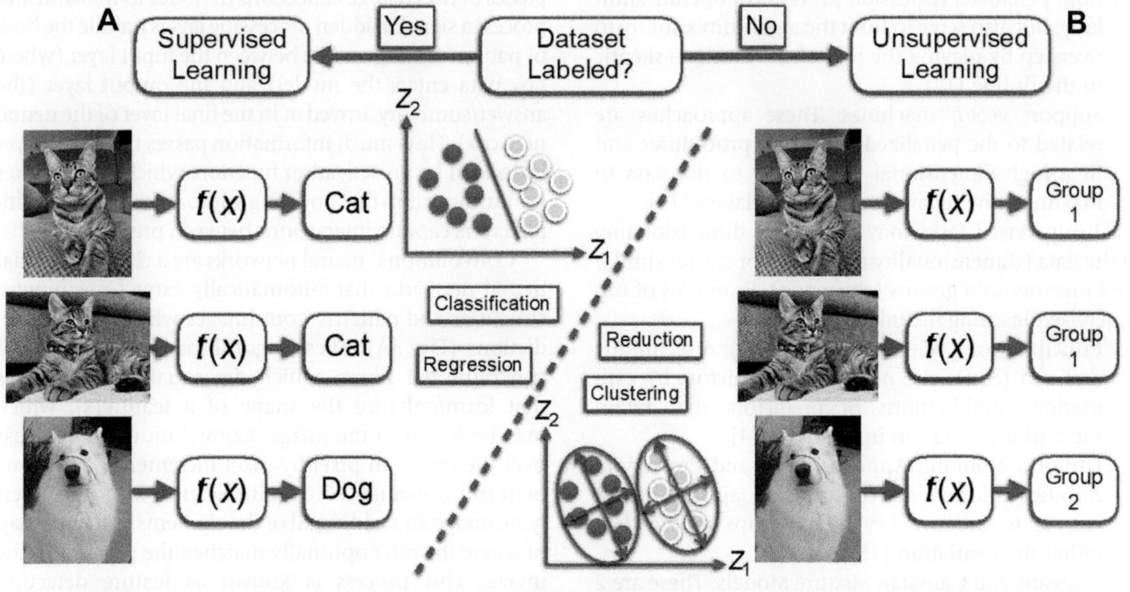

FIG. 2 Quick Description of Types of Machine Learning Tasks. If data are labeled, opt for (**A**) the supervised learning task, while if data are not labeled, opt for (**B**) unsupervised learning tasks. For (**A**) supervised learning tasks, it is known whether images are of cats or dogs, and common subtasks include classification (categorical outcome) and regression (continuous outcome) tasks; scatterplot demonstrates how data of 2 different classes (*gray* and *green*) are separated using machine learning algorithm (*line*). For (**B**) unsupervised learning tasks, it is not known whether images are of cats or dogs, and common subtasks include dimensionality reduction (visualize high dimensional data and capture meaningful components) and clustering (group similar objects) tasks; scatterplot demonstrates how data of 2 different clusters (*gray* and *green*) are separated using machine learning algorithm (ellipses summarize distribution of cluster which has been estimated).

specific predictors. Predictors or features are selected based on their ability to partition the data more purely into specific classes/disease states. A set of these decision splits form a decision tree, and results aggregated over many such trees form the basis of Random Forest (RF) and XGBoost models, which more completely explore the space of all of the high dimensional predictors [7–9].
2. Nearest neighbor approaches: Nearest neighbor approaches use labeled outcomes to establish points of reference for assessing new input data. A new datapoint is compared to its neighbors from the reference set, where the decision rendered by most of the reference neighbors is the decision adopted by the new input data point [10].
3. Discriminant analyses: These approaches learn the optimal combinations of predictors, which when added, are able to maximize the distance between data belonging to one class versus another [11].
4. Penalized regression: Although traditional regression procedures may fit a line to the data or use a line to separate benign versus malignant information, penalized regression procedures operate similarly, but also serve to limit the algorithm's ability to overstep by playing the role of the cautious skeptic to the fit line [12].
5. Support vector machines: These approaches are related to the penalized regression procedures and fit a high-dimensional hyperplane to the data to maximize the separation between classes [13].

Unsupervised tasks may reduce the dimensionality of the data (dimensionality reduction) or cluster similar data together into groups (clustering). Examples of unsupervised learning include:

1. Principal Component Analysis (PCA): A technique that can reduce the number of predictors by estimating combinations of predictors that retain most of the variation in the data [14].
2. Uniform Manifold Approximation and Projection: Another information compression approach that is able to preserve key relationships in the data rather than variation [15,16].
3. K-Means and Gaussian Mixture Models: These are 2 related approaches that are able to iteratively assign points to a cluster based on some measure of distance to the center of the cluster, then reassigns clusters [17,18].
4. Spectral Clustering: A clustering approach that models relationships in the data using graphs and cuts regions of weak connectivity in the graph to establish the clusters [19].
5. Density-Based Clustering (eg, HDBSCAN): Uses density estimation algorithms to find characteristic highly dense pockets of points [20].

Selection of the appropriate machine learning approach depends on the task at hand (type of data, question, complexity, etc.). We have included an abridged decision guide for the reader (see Fig. 2) as to which algorithms should be used depending on the time of study.

DEEP LEARNING

Artificial neural networks, a part of the deep learning methodologies (a distinct branch of machine learning that does not require structured or manually curated input data for analysis), are algorithms that are organized into multiple processing layers to represent objects at multiple levels of analysis [21–23]. These algorithms are inspired by but not analogous to processes of the central nervous system (eg, they are far simpler than biological neural networks). The basic unit of analysis is a node, where a signal passes between large collections of nodes to transmit and process a signal. Hidden processing layers handle the bulk of pattern mining and lie between the input layer (where raw data enters the model) and the output layer (the answer/summary arrived at in the final layer of the neural network). How much information passes through a layer is decided by an activation function, which incorporates nonlinearity into the modeling approach while the multiple layers capture interactions between predictors [24].

Convolutional neural networks are a class of artificial neural networks that automatically extract meaningful structures and patterns from images when making predictions (Fig. 3A). These algorithms are composed of convolutional filters, which are square-grid matrices that form/enhance the shape of a feature(s), which may be found in the image. Convolutional filters pass over the image in pixel-by-pixel increments, each time performing elementwise multiplication with the underlying image and adding all of the elements to form a map of where the filter optimally matched the patterns in the image. This process is known as feature detection (Fig. 3B–C). A familiar example is the Sobel edge detection filter, found in many image manipulation software platforms (eg, PhotoShop). Multiple features may be detected through the application of multiple filters. Detected features are then grouped using pooling operations, which slide windows of fixed width and height across the image and summarize the most dominant features in a given region through a process that is akin to compression (Fig. 3B,D) [23,25]. Instead of performing

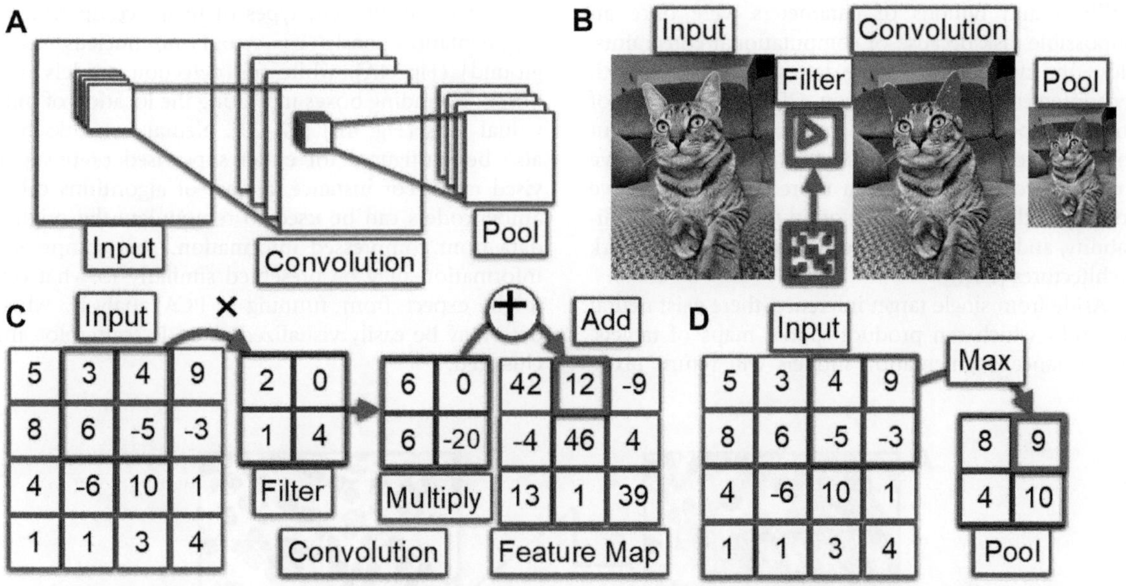

FIG. 3 Demonstration of Deep Learning Components. (**A**) Convolutional neural networks are primarily composed of convolutional layers, which detect features from input image, and pooling layers, which summarize the relationships between the lower-level features by shrinking the spatial dimensions of the image. (**B**) Example of convolution and pooling mechanism applied to cat. Deep learning algorithm starts with filter that is random noise and overtime learns filter in shape of an ear; this ear filter is convolved with the original input to highlight in red where filter matched image. Pooling mechanism has collapsed information in image of cat, reducing spatial dimensions. (**C**) Mathematical representation of convolution operation, where filter is multiplied elementwise with input values in red square, then these elements after multiplication are added together to collapse values in 2 × 2 square into a single value in the feature map. (**D**) Mathematical representation of pooling operation, where red 2 × 2 square in input has been collapsed into a single value by taking the maximum of the 4 values.

element-wise multiplication and addition like the convolution, pooling operations collapse the information in these windows by averaging the values, which decreases the spatial resolution of the image when performed across the image. Then, new filters are passed over the resultant compressed image to capture more complex spatial relationships between features to further abstract the object. For a human-relevant example, consider looking at a person's face and realizing "I know them," the raw image arriving at the retina was reduced to a single thought/feeling after processing. The application of convolution and pooling operations are iterated until the higher-order complexities of the image are encapsulated into a small set of predictors which may be directly converted into a vector of probabilities, the elements of which are correspondent to the selection of specific outcomes or classes (eg, [0.4,0.3,0.3], [Cat, Mouse, Dog]). These types of neural networks may be used for disease classification tasks, among other tasks that require the output of a single target.

When training a model from scratch, the ideal filter values in the various convolutional layers are unknown (and hence are instantiated randomly) and the prediction offered by the nascent neural network is very likely to be erroneous/random (see Fig. 3B). The deviation of the model's predictions from reality is measured through a *loss* function (eg, "how wrong am I?"). Based on this *loss*, errors are propagated backward to alter filters (eg, up-weighting successful filters, down-weighting unsuccessful filters and changing filter values) to ensure that the next time the data passes through, the prediction is correct. Optimization algorithms, such as gradient descent, search for the filters that best delineate the targets of interest given the input image through iterative applications of backpropagation (essentially searching for loss minimums on a surface that cannot be fully visualized without trying every possible combination of filter values and weights) until the *loss* converges (decreases and plateaus). Backpropagation processes over large neural network architectures with millions and billions of parameters were once an impossible task because of computational constraints. Now, the availability of large data sets combined with technological advancements in GPUs (composed of small independent processing cores that can carry out thousands of simple operations simultaneously) have made inferences on big data more feasible and have consequently led to a revolution in the accuracy, applicability, and development speed of new neural network architectures [26].

Aside from single target inference, there exist neural networks which can produce spatial maps of targets. For instance, segmentation models will return pixel-wise maps of different types of image compartments (segmentation masks eg, cytoplasm, nucleus, background) (Fig. 4A), while cell detection models may output bounding boxes indicating the location of individual cells (Fig. 4B) [27–29]. Neural networks may also be configured for either supervised or unsupervised tasks. For instance, a class of algorithms called autoencoders can be used to recapitulate the original data from compressed information. This compressed information may be presented similarly to what one might expect from running a PCA analysis, where data may be easily visualized in a 2D scatterplot and clustered.

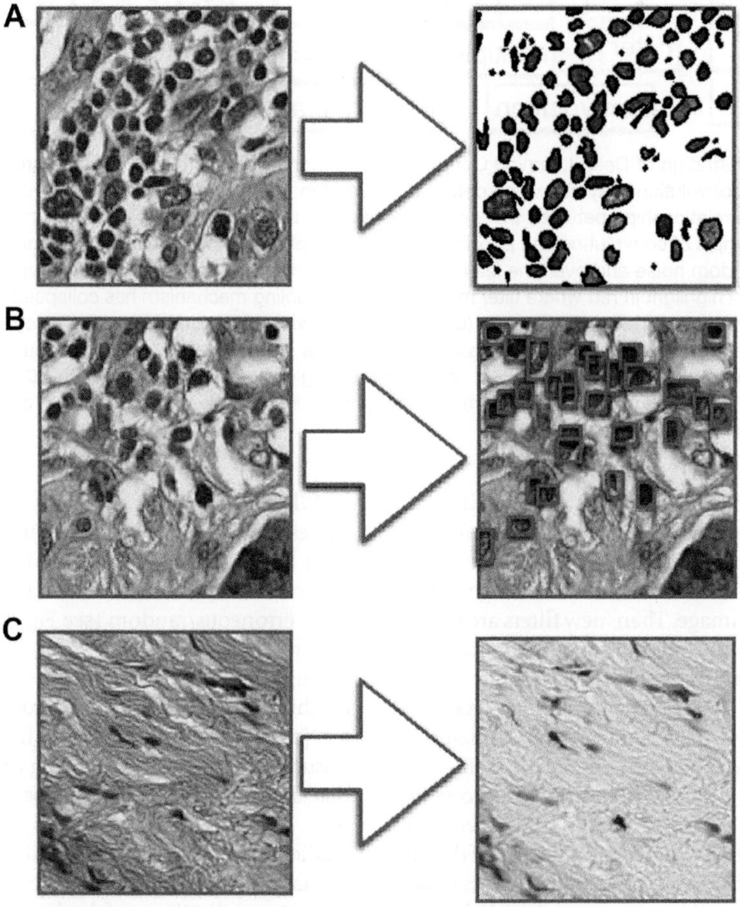

FIG. 4 Examples of Common Cell-Based Tasks and Explainable AI. (**A**) Common output from coarse nuclei segmentation, where a pixel-wise map has been generated that details locations of nuclei. (**B**) Common output from nuclei detection model, where bounding boxes are drawn over nuclei. (**C**) Common output from gradient-based model explanation approach for a classification task, where highlighted in green are image features which contribute positively toward the class in question, while image features in red were negatively associated with the outcome.

TRAINING AND VALIDATING MODEL

To train a machine learning algorithm, large amounts of image data must be collected (Fig. 5A). The data are then annotated by a domain expert (eg, practicing pathologist) through annotation programs such as QuPath/ASAP or by manually dragging and dropping images into labeled folders [30]. Unfortunately, most annotation software is either not user-friendly for nontechnical pathologists or cannot handle gigapixel images. Most, however, do offer the functionality to outline both macroarchitectural and microarchitectural features of tissues/cells using polygons, boxes, dots, and splines. Alternatively, labeling information is unnecessary if opting for the unsupervised approaches; however, much more data are typically needed. Once the data have been collected and labeled, the data are then partitioned into 3 separate cohorts: the training, validation, and test cohorts. Machine learning models learn directly from the training cohorts, where errors in prediction of the target may be used to improve the model parameters (Fig. 5B). However, *overfitting* or memorization of the input data can occur, which results in a model that may poorly generalize to new data. The validation cohort is used to prevent/detect overfitting. By assessing

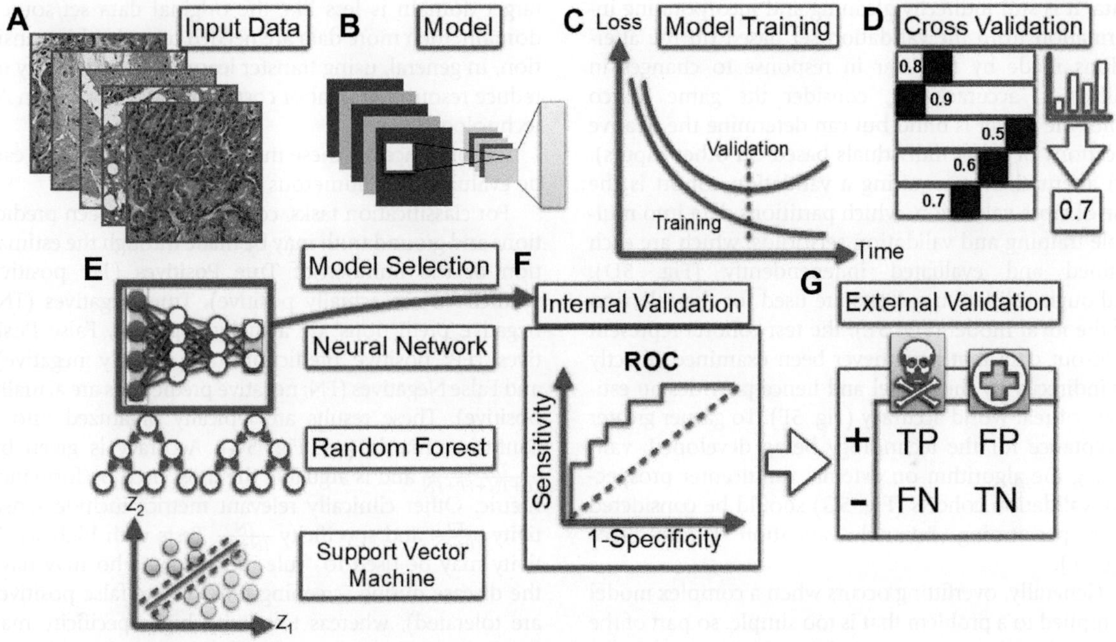

FIG. 5 Common Workflow for Training and Validating Machine Learning Model for Clinical Deployment. (**A**) Histopathological images are collected and labeled. (**B**) Images pass through machine learning model (in this case a convolutional neural network) to make predictions as well as update the model parameters. (**C**) To identify when to stop training the model or to select parameters, the training loss is compared to the validation loss over time, when the validation loss is at its lowest point, a snapshot/record model is saved and this model is used. As training loss continues to decrease, validation loss increases, which means that the model is memorizing/overfitting the data. (**D**) Cross-validation is applied to evaluate the performance of the model across parts of the data which it has not seen, averaging performance on these validation sets across all cross-validation folds gives an overall metric of model performance given the model selection/configuration. (**E**) Final model is selected based on its cross-validation performance and then the model is trained across training/validation data. Here, neural network has outperformed random forest and support vector machine. (**F**) Model performance is assessed across a held-out test set within the institution which was not used to inform model selection. receiver operating characteristic curve (ROC)/area under the receiver operating characteristic curve (AUC) is reported as final performance for model for internal validation test. (**G**) Then, perhaps with some additional training data, model is then trained and validated across multiple institutions for external validity. Here, the model's positive and negative predictions are compared against actual assignment of benign versus malignancy to form confusion matrix.

model accuracy using both the training set (which the model directly interrogates) and a separate validation set (which the model never directly examines), the user can spot deviation in training and validation accuracy. When overfitting begins to occur, the training and validation accuracies, which typically progress in parallel will begin to deviate (eg, the training accuracy will continue to increase while the validation accuracy plateaus or decreases; alternatively, training loss accuracy decreases while validation loss increases) (Fig. 5C). Typically, the validation accuracy/loss is used to determine the overall fitness of the model and inform changes to the model hyperparameters. Thus, even though the model never directly "sees" the validation data, it is still indirectly gleaning and incorporating information from the validation set based on the alterations made by the user in response to changes in validation accuracy (eg, consider the game Marco Polo, the seeker is blind but can determine the relative locations of other individuals based on other inputs). An alternative to acquiring a validation cohort is the use of cross-validation, which partitions data into multiple training and validation sets/folds, which are each trained and evaluated independently (Fig. 5D). Although validation cohorts are used for the selection of the ideal model (Fig. 5E), the test cohorts represent held-out data that have never been examined directly or indirectly by the model and hence provides an estimate of real-world accuracy (Fig. 5F). To garner greater acceptance for the technology being developed, validating the algorithm on external multicenter prospective validation cohorts (Fig. 5G) should be considered after performing internal validation studies (see Fig. 5F).

Generally, overfitting occurs when a complex model is applied to a problem that is too simple, so part of the art of choosing a proper architecture is scoping the complexity of the problem and experimenting with multiple architectures of varying complexity. The general goal is to use the simplest model that achieves superior accuracy (eg, if linear regression can solve your problem, deep learning is unlikely to prove superior and may have inferior real-world performance). In addition to selection of model architectures and hyperparameters, overfitting can also be reduced by augmenting the data. That is, applying random transformations to the data during training such as vertical and horizontal flips, rotations, crops, and perturbations to the color space, among many others, can help increase the effective sample size of the data set and reduce overfitting by exposing the algorithm to more scenarios which it may have never considered and thus making the algorithm more flexible [31,32]. Ensuring the staining qualities of the tissue are consistent/standardized within the dataset using what are called stain normalization techniques can improve performance [33].

Transfer learning approaches are also incredibly helpful for improving model performance while minimizing the amount of new data which should be acquired. These procedures adapt knowledge learned from similar histology to reduce the data burden. For instance, a model that has been trained to detect malignancy in skin histology could be fine-tuned for malignancy detection in the colon, allowing for fewer colon cases than would normally be required when training from scratch. As a rule of thumb, if the new data set/target domain is less like the original data set/source domain, then more data are needed to make this transition. In general, using transfer learning is a great way to reduce resource and labor costs when developing an AI technology [34].

Performance for these machine learning models can be evaluated via numerous techniques.

For classification tasks, comparisons between predictions and ground truth may be made through the estimation of the number of True Positives (TP; positive predictions are actually positive), True Negatives (TN; negative predictions are actually negative), False Positives (FP; positive predictions are actually negative), and False Negatives (FN; negative predictions are actually positive). These results are typically organized into a confusion matrix (see Fig. 5G). Accuracy is given by $\frac{TP+TN}{TP+TN+FP+FN}$ and is arguably the most used performance metric. Other clinically relevant metrics include sensitivity $\frac{TP}{TP+FN}$ and specificity $\frac{TN}{TN+FP}$. Tests with high sensitivity may be used to "rule-in" anyone who may have the disease during screening tests (where false positives are tolerated), whereas tests with high specificity may be used to "rule-out" anyone who does not have the disease during diagnostic tests (where a false negative would be intolerable). Before establishing which patients are positive and negative for a condition, machine learning models will generate probabilities between 0 and 1, which indicates some measure of confidence in a given diagnosis. These probabilities are cut at values between 0 and 1 to yield the positive (probability greater than threshold) and negative (probability less than threshold) predictions, where each threshold corresponds to different sensitivities and specificities. A receiver operating characteristic curve plots the complete range of sensitivities and specificities which are obtainable when considering all different probability cutoffs and can be used to establish a clinically actionable probability cutoff depending on the use case ("rule-in"/"rule-out") (see

Fig. 5F). The F1-Score balances the sensitivity and specificity in its assessment, and overall performance of the algorithm across all sensitivities and specificities may be obtained using the area under the receiver operating characteristic curve.

Performance metrics for regression tasks include the R^2 coefficient of determination, which is the proportion of total variation which is explained by the model. The mean squared error and median absolute error are also metrics which look at the overall differences between the predicted continuous value and observed values.

EMERGING TECHNOLOGIES, APPLICATIONS, AND CHALLENGES

Over the past decade, the sheer quantity of machine learning methods that have been developed for anatomic pathology is staggering. In this section, we discuss the development and application of deep learning methods to various aspects of tissue analysis.

Patch-Based Approaches

The predominant approach for making predictions on WSI are patch-based approaches, which break up large WSI into smaller image patches, each of which may be operated on by neural networks to predict a patch-level label. This technique is very common for large images which would not be able to fit into the memory of the GPU. These patch labels may be tabulated to form inferences on the slide level based on, for instance, the percentage breakdown of specific histologic features or a weighted average of features. Training patch-based models requires highly detailed image annotations, and mistakes and omissions in annotation can degrade the quality of predictions and their subsequent validation. Normally, this requires using a group of expert pathologists to perform tens of thousands of annotations across hundreds of slides to yield an accurate prediction model. However, several expert-in-the-loop (EITL) *semi-supervised* annotation systems have been developed, which use prior annotations to suggest new annotations to the pathologist to incorporate into the new training set. This EITL approach can range in sophistication from using an intermediate model to classify unsorted data which the pathologist approves of or corrects in an iterative fashion to fully automated dynamic training environments [35].

Popular examples of patch-based approaches include segmentation of different colon polyp morphologies, recapitulating patterns of lung adenocarcinoma, segmenting portal and parenchymal regions of the colon, or segmenting patterns of colon into their constituent subcompartments. Other popular applications include work in NASH, or Non-Alcoholic Steatohepatitis, where a common computational task for evaluating NASH biopsies is the prediction of fatty vacuoles, done using segmentation networks [36–38].

Cell-Based Approaches

Another common task in anatomic pathology is counting the number and type of cells and other small micro-architectural features which comprise the specimen which are often important for disease grading and offer a more natural way of subdividing an image. For instance, the NAS score for the grading of Non-Alcoholic Steatohepatitis requires a percentage breakdown on the number of hepatocytes undergoing ballooning degeneration, necrosis, and subsequent inflammation, which is subjectively estimated by the pathologist. This requires the identification of individual cells or small clusters, typically by identifying nuclei. Two types of neural networks that are well equipped toward studying cellular morphology in tissue include segmentation and detection networks (previously covered; see Fig. 4A–B). Other popular examples include Signet ring cell detection, tumor invading lymphocyte detection, and melanocyte detection, among numerous others [39–42].

Other popular cell-based approaches are used on cytology specimen, which are acquired after placement of cytology specimen on a slide, but that may be difficult to assess because of their hypervariable cellularity and since cytology slides are less structured than tissue slides. Deep learning and morphometric approaches are particularly well suited for the assessment of cytology specimen because the practicing cytologist may have tens of thousands of cells per slide and take on many cases per day, which can be an absolutely exhausting process. A particularly successful application of these technologies was for the automated assessment of urine cytology specimen for high-grade urothelial carcinoma. Before the incorporation of these automated analyses, the Paris system was a semisubjective assessment guideline, which is heavily used by cytologists to render a diagnosis of negative, atypical, suspicious, or positive high-grade urothelial carcinoma. The system is currently subject to high inter-rater variability in some places which can impact diagnosis. The Auto Paris system, a deep learning workflow system used to automate tasks under the Paris system, can automatically generate findings one would obtain through manual inspection of tens of thousands of cells per slide. Deep learning approaches can be used here to retain cells in the analysis which are urothelial, estimate for each of these cells a subjective score of cellular atypia as based on pathologist interpretation, and estimate the nuclear to cytoplasm ratio as a more objective measure of atypia by decomposing the cell image into its nucleus and cytoplasm components (Fig. 6) [43].

In contrast to the heavy reliance on cellular morphology within cytology specimen, it should be noted that cells are not necessarily the defining aspects of the tissue histology, and current limitations in algorithms for cell detection (which can be quite unintuitive) may not be accurate enough to make the cell the standard, basic unit of analysis.

Unsupervised and Self-Supervised Approaches

Both the cell and patch-based approaches require an ample number of high-quality annotations from which to train these models. Such annotations may be costly to procure and are heavily subject to the interpretation of the rater, which may vary depending on the complexity of the case, the scoring criteria, or their background and training, among other factors. Thus, finding ways to reduce the burden of the amount of data collection and annotation is often advantageous. In addition, *unsupervised/self-supervised* learning techniques may increase the number of training instances by generating labels based on natural variation (Fig. 7). Here, autoencoders, which compress the data while revealing nuances, have been heavily used to cluster data and estimate novel prognostic histologic subtypes [44–47]. Meanwhile, self-supervised algorithms operate by learning to predict tasks that are tangential (eg, detect some perturbation to the image or compare images to others in the cohort) related to the main image prediction task (eg, classification). Learning this unrelated task can help these neural networks capture meaningful morphologic and architectural patterns in the data. A promising application of self-supervised techniques in histopathology is the application of contrastive predictive coding techniques, which operate by predicting surrounding image patches from the current ones. This method can capture some of the surrounding tissue architecture, which can be particularly advantageous to contextualizing cells. Many unsupervised approaches

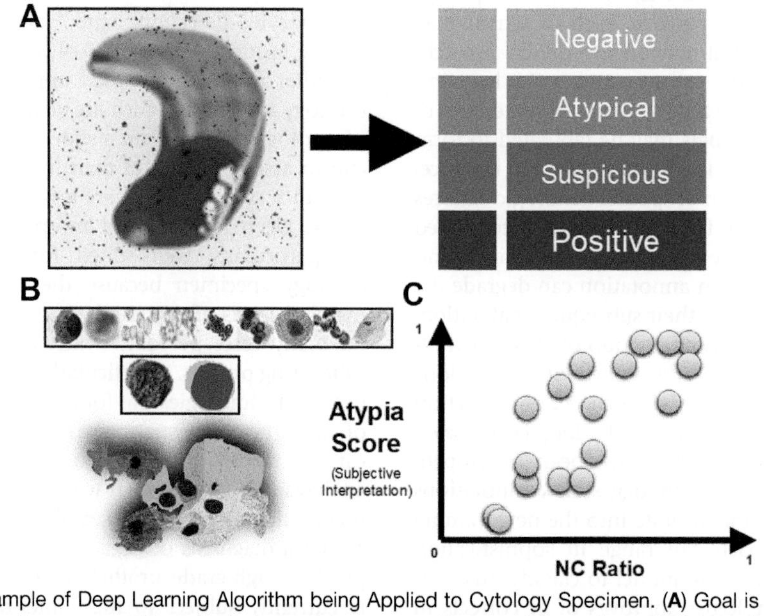

FIG. 6 Example of Deep Learning Algorithm being Applied to Cytology Specimen. (**A**) Goal is to label cytology specimen as negative, atypical, suspicious, or positive for high-grade urothelial carcinoma. (**B**) Morphometric techniques break up cytology specimen into constituent cells, which are further binned based on cell-type by deep learning algorithm. A separate segmentation deep learning model breaks up urothelial cells into nucleus and cytoplasm. Additional morphometric and/or deep learning techniques use segment clusters of cells to assign NC ratios to specific urothelial cells. (**C**) Another deep learning model predicts the degree of cellular atypia based on subjective interpretation of cytologist, while Nuclear to Cytoplasm ratio is calculated as a more objective measure of atypia. Integrating all malignancy information from all urothelial cells assists with diagnosis for specimen.

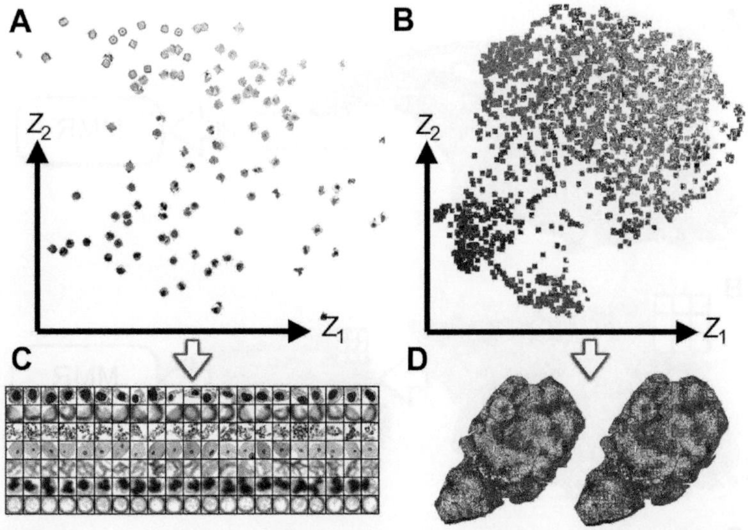

FIG. 7 Examples of Unsupervised Learning Approaches, for example, Variational Autoencoder, Applied to Cytology Specimen and Assessment of Liver Fibrosis. (**A, B**) 2D scatterplot of neural network features learned via autoencoder, where each point represents: (**A**) a cell and original image of cell has been laid over deep learning features, and (**B**) subimages of liver biopsy stained for trichrome stain, where images of tissue patches overlay 2D scatter points, revealing clustering by liver function. (**C**) Deep learning clustering approaches sort cells into 6 distinct classes/clusters (rows) without *a priori* knowledge of the classes. (**D**) Regions of trichrome slide highlighted by formed clusters from (**A**), where here clusters highlight meaningful information in biopsy, segmenting steatosis tissue from hepatic and fibrotic tissue without ground truth.

focus on the cellular morphology [48], whereas contrastive self-supervised approaches consider the surrounding tissue context to learn more about cellular interaction [49,50].

Weakly Supervised Approaches

Labeling data is often the most time-consuming portion of developing a machine learning algorithm because of the (1) the difficulty in securing expert time for labeling, (2) the difficulty or tedium of creating the labels, and (3) the lack of human experts in the domain being studied (eg, morphologic to molecular correlations). Fortunately, many weakly supervised approaches have been developed to make predictions across a WSI after being trained on examples that are assigned one label per slide [51]. As compared to the patch-based approaches, which make changes to the neural network based on local information in the slide, here we are presented with single data object that is often composed mostly of irrelevant tissue (hence there is less informative data per slide to train the model). As such, these models require significantly more data (thousands to hundreds of thousands of additional slides) as compared to patch and cell-based approaches, most of which may be unavailable outside of international data consortiums and collaborations [52]. This is because the information on patches and cells are far more specific and small-scale versus these weakly supervised approaches (more labels and examples for patches and cells). Meanwhile, weakly supervised approaches have a far greater potential to overfit because they are considering far more features at once and thus need more data or constraints placed to ensure successful modeling.

Weakly supervised approaches consider the WSI as a bag of patches or cells. The most successful WSI representation techniques use a mechanism called attention, where each element of the bag is assigned some importance weight for how much to incorporate the patch/cell's information. The final representation of the WSI is a weighted average of its constituent parts and the neural network learns over time how to establish the weights/importance scores (Fig. 8A) [53,54]. Other attention mechanisms use square-grid convolutions, which sample a lot of irrelevant tissue (Fig. 8B) [55]. More recent attention mechanisms are able to consider the spatial context/adjacency of the patches/cells using graphs, to be covered in the next section (Fig. 8C) [56].

Many attention-based weakly supervised approaches are being used to predict the presence of some molecular alteration across the tissue, and several large

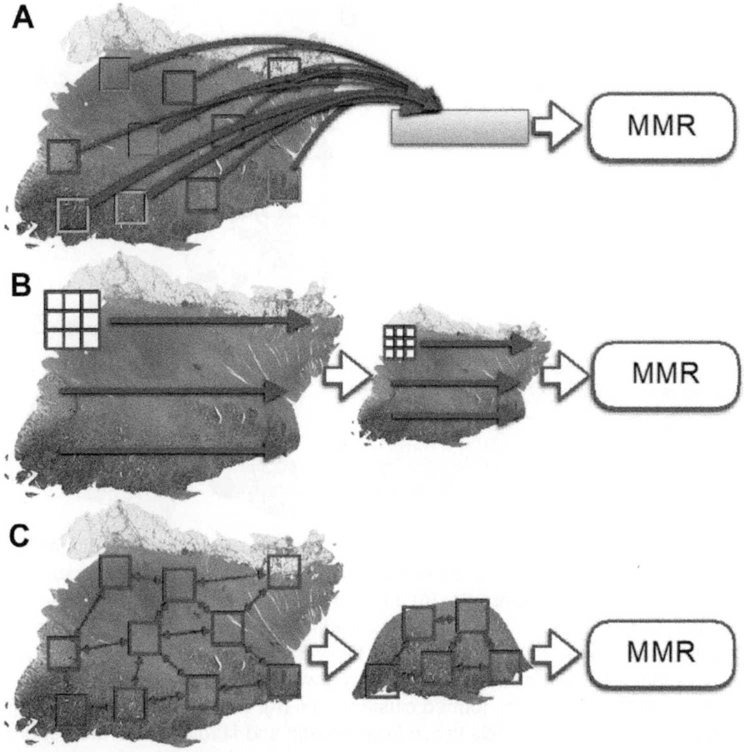

FIG. 8 Example of Whole Slide Aggregation Approaches to Predict MMR Status for Bulk Specimen. (**A**) Attention-based approaches weight contributions from individual image patches but may not relate adjacent patches to one another. Here, attention score demonstrates how much to weigh (importance of) each patch and is visualized by the lightness of the squares and thickness of the connection arrow to the vector (*gray*) which summarizes the slide. (**B**) Classical convolutional neural network slides large square-grid convolutions across the entire image and attempts to do away with patch-based approaches, but this approach may be hard to fit into memory and can capture irrelevant information (orientation, positioning, whitespace). (**C**) Graph-based approaches learn to upweight subgraphs/subarchitectures in the slide which are the most relevant for prediction, capture the topology and shape of the tissue, incorporate spatially adjacent tissue macroarchitecture, and may be combined the attention approaches from A).

international consortia have pooled together tens of thousands of slides to train such models. For instance, recently multiple large-scale efforts have been undertaken to predict MMR status from slides [57] and modeling frameworks have been developed to use these approaches to infer tumor site of origin or delineate different tumor subtypes.

Graph-Based Learning

Most forms of machine learning-based histologic analysis make predictions based on some aggregation of statistics generated from subunits of the WSI (ie, patches and cells). However, many of the commonly used techniques for WSI feature aggregation neglect one crucial component: they assume that these subunits of the slide are entirely independent of one another. This assumption dismisses spatial colocalization and corresponding statistical dependencies between the subunits, which in turn ignores vital contributing information from the surrounding tissue microarchitecture (eg, if tile 1 contains lamina propria, adjacent tiles are much more likely to also contain lamina propria as opposed to serosa). Treating patches as independent of one another leads to noisy predictions because there is over-reliance on the morphologic presentations encoded in the local image tiles. Graph neural networks (GNN) offer a potential solution in that they consider features in an inherently spatial manner. Graphs are essentially networks of "nodes" connected to each other by "edges". If we were to break a WSI down into tiles (nodes), the edges for any node would connect it most closely to its 8 nearest neighbors (if the image is broken down into a grid). GNNs thus capture spatially dependent information such that architectural information is allowed to "flow" across the slide to inform the predictions for adjacent regions (social media sites use similar technology to infer people you are likely to know and suggest that you connect with them) (Fig. 9D) [56]. GNNs operate by updating the morphologic information from an individual tile (node) via messages that are passed from its neighbors (see Fig. 9E–G). This, in turn, can increase the confidence in assigning if a region is epithelium by noticing surrounding images are epithelial. Unlike traditional neural networks, which operate in square-grid geometry, for GNNs, the number of neighbors is not fixed and does not depend on patch ordering. This makes predictions invariant to the rotation and orientation of the tissue. Various pooling mechanisms have been developed to locally aggregate information within a slide to capture the key relationships. For instance, topological techniques collapse irrelevant structures in data to reveal key interactions between adjacent tissue subcompartments and graph-pooling mechanisms use attention-based techniques to assign which subgraphs/subregions are most important for predicting some outcome of interest (see Fig. 8C; Fig. 10). In contrast, other *weakly supervised* attention-based approaches may obtain suboptimal or less predictable results because they either ignoring contributions from the surrounding architecture or may obtain different results if the tissue was displaced or rotated because they do not naturally consider the structure, shape, or boundaries of the tissue (see Fig. 8A, B, Fig. 9A–C) [58]. Popular graph-based approaches consider cells as the basic unit of analysis, but as aforementioned are bottlenecked by accurate detection of cells and place the assumption that they contribute most vitally to the tissue architecture.

Multimodal Approaches

While the practicing pathologist may observe cellular phenomena and microarchitectural/cytologic

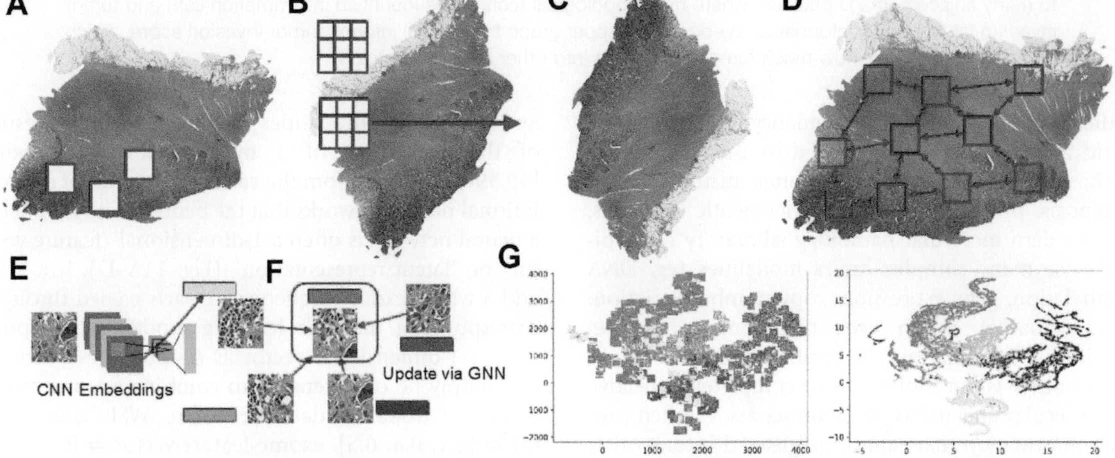

FIG. 9 Description of Graph-Based Techniques. (**A–C**) Previous modeling approaches, which (**A**) model image patches as independent entities, which is too noisy for clinical implementation; (**B**) treat a WSI as an image, where the square-grid convolutions pick up irrelevant whitespace; and (**C**) fail to respect the orientation and positioning of the tissue. (**D**) Graphs over slides place subimages into context of the surrounding tissue macroarchitecture by modeling the spatial dependencies between the constituent parts of the image. Information in graphs is invariant to the orientation and rotation of the tissue, which captures the shape and topology of the tissue. (**E**) GNN first use convolutional neural networks to extract morphologic information from independent tissue patches, then (**F**) update the information in the patch by the surrounding image patches through a message passing/weighted average like operation, where subsequent applications of graph convolutions increase the neighborhood from which information travels around the WSI. (**G**) Information encoded using GNN encapsulates both spatial relationships and morphologic presentations, where here features from one slide have been plotted in 2D scatter plot with clear class/subcomponent separation and overlaid with actual images of patches.

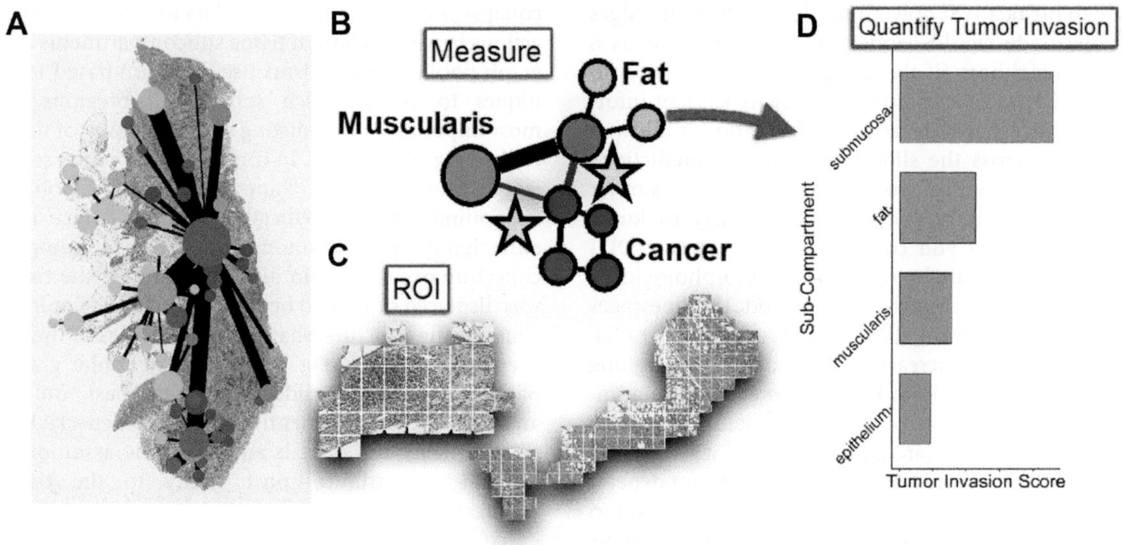

FIG. 10 Topological Techniques Summarize Information Across a WSI. (**A**) Mapper generates a graph which simplifies relationships across tissue macroarchitecture and slide subcomponents, visualization of Mapper graph for one slide. (**B**) Graphical demonstration of Mapper graph, where muscularis, fat, and tumor information are related to one another. The thickness of the edge/line between cancer and other regions details how much cancer is invading other tissue subcompartments. (**C**) Each region of interest corresponds to many adjacent image patches, where here, topological techniques identified inflammation (*left*) and tumor invading fat (*right*). (**D**) Information in edges of Mapper graph from (**A, B**) informs tumor invasion score, which depicts quantitatively how much tumor is invading into other regions of Colon.

indications of atypia and malignancy, ultimately, genetic, and epigenetic alterations drive oncogenesis. As such, the morphology alone is often insufficient for diagnosis, prognostication, and therapeutic decisions. The modern molecular pathology laboratory can typically use many complex omics modalities (eg, DNA methylation, gene expression, copy number variation, DNA variants), which each offer unique disease-specific information. Furthermore, because morphology is not thought to be completely reflective of molecular alterations, these omics assays often provide information that cannot be gleaned in any other way. As such, combining all available information could potentially improve diagnostic and prognostic performance. However, the data at hand often exist in formats that render them noninteroperable. For example, how does one concatenate the morphologic findings from a WSI with a whole exome in a way that synergistically increases prognostic power? To do so, it would be necessary to transform both input data types to a higher-level abstraction where they were readily comparable.

As such, multimodal learning methods take as input the compact representations of information from WSI and other omics modalities that are created as a result of the operations of a machine learning model [50,59–63]. Recall from the earlier discussion of convolutional neural networks that the penultimate output of a neural network is often a 1-dimensional "feature vector" or "latent representation" (Fig. 11A–D). If a WSI and a whole exome sequence are each passed through corresponding machine learning models which produce a 1-dimensional vector as output, these vectors can simply be concatenated to combine features from 2 wholly disparate data types (eg, WSI-feature-vector = [0.1, 0.4, 0.5], exome-feature-vector = [0.2, 0.7, 0.9], combined-feature-vector = [0.1, 0.4, 0.5, 0.2, 0.7, 0.9]). For WSI, these could be low dimensional vectors that encapsulate information from the graph or attention-based approaches. Information from omics modalities and clinical/demographic variables can be similarly vectorized (where neural networks are used to project the data to a lower-dimensional manifold) (Fig. 11E) to form a look-up service or complementary and slightly disjoint information may also prove beneficial for prediction (Fig. 11F).

For these methods to succeed, the predictive performance offered by each modality must be reasonably

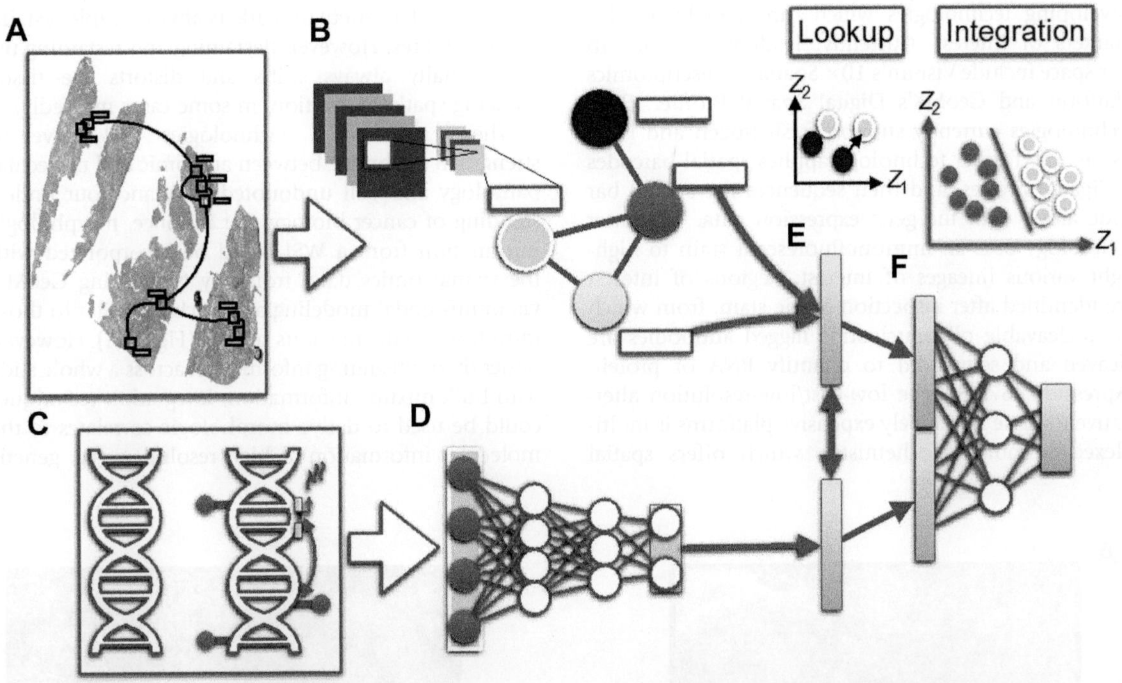

FIG. 11 Visual Description of Multi-Modal Modeling Approaches. (**A**) WSI serves as one data input into multimodal modeling. (**B**) WSI is processed using convolutional neural network (CNN) and GNN to create vector that summarizes slide, though other approaches may be used. (**C**) Genetic/Epigenetic/Omics/Clinical information is extracted and transformed using (**D**) neural network, which summarizes other modalities. (**E**) After WSI and omics information are extracted, they may be compared to one another to establish correspondence (ie, WSI and omics profile from same patient should be maximally aligned). This creates a "look-up" retrieval service which matches omics to WSI, shared information from the other modality can be inferred by input of other. (**F**) WSI and omics data also contain complementary information, which is not shared between both data types, the information from both modalities may be combined through concatenation-like operations from their vector representations to form a more powerful, robust, and informative prediction.

high to warrant incorporation, or else noise may be added which could reduce the model's predictive performance rather than enhance it (eg, if one model was 90% accurate and the other was 50% accurate, combing the 2 data types would be unlikely to lead to superior performance). Currently, paired imaging and genomic features are available via large harmonized public data repositories such as The Cancer Genome Atlas. These data sets have been leveraged to establish correspondence between two or more unrelated modalities (see Fig. 11E) as well as integrate these data sources together for pan-cancer prognostic prediction [64] models (see Fig. 11F).

Spatial Omics Information

Most omics modalities process bulk mixtures of tissue that contain varying percentages of diagnostically interesting tissue (tumor) and surrounding tissue (stroma, leukocytes, etc.). In other words, bulk mixtures are also composed of many different types of cells, and while algorithms have been developed which can approximate the relative contribution of cell types to the mixture, where the cells exist (i.e., positional information within the biopsy relative to other important cell populations) is difficult to ascertain beyond morphologic presentation. In addition, bulk mixtures do not capture the spatial heterogeneity in signal across a slide, which may inform, for instance, cellular communication, activation, and response to tissue damage. The spatial distribution of certain biomarkers may inform diagnosis and prognostication (eg, the location of cells expression various immune regulatory markers may be vital to the development of metastases) [65,66]. These challenges provide ample motivation for developing technologies which can spatially resolve markers of interest. Currently, leading solutions in this space include Visium's 10× Spatial Transcriptomics platform and GeoMX's Digital Spatial Profiler. Both technologies currently support fresh frozen and FFPE tissue. The former technology applies spatial barcodes to ligated probes, and then sequences the spatial bar code along with the gene expression data. The latter technology uses an immunofluorescent stain to highlight various lineages of interest. Regions of interest are identified after inspection of the stain, from which photocleavable oligonucleotide tagged antibodies are cleaved and sequenced to quantify RNA or protein expression [67,68]. The low-cost/low-resolution alternative to these 2 relatively expensive platforms is multiplexed immunohistochemistry, which offers spatial resolution of a variety of markers after multiple restaining procedures. However, destaining and restaining tissue virtually always shifts and distorts the tissue reducing spatial resolution, in some cases markedly.

These multimodal technologies will serve to strengthen the bridge between anatomic and molecular pathology and will undoubtedly enhance our understanding of cancer biology. For instance, morphologic information from a WSI could be incorporated with the spatial omics data, from say Nanostring GeoMx, via multi-modal modeling approaches similar to those introduced in the previous section (Fig. 12A). However, rather than integrating information across a whole slide with bulk mixture information, integration techniques could be used to derive morphologic correlates to the molecular information at high resolution (eg, genetic

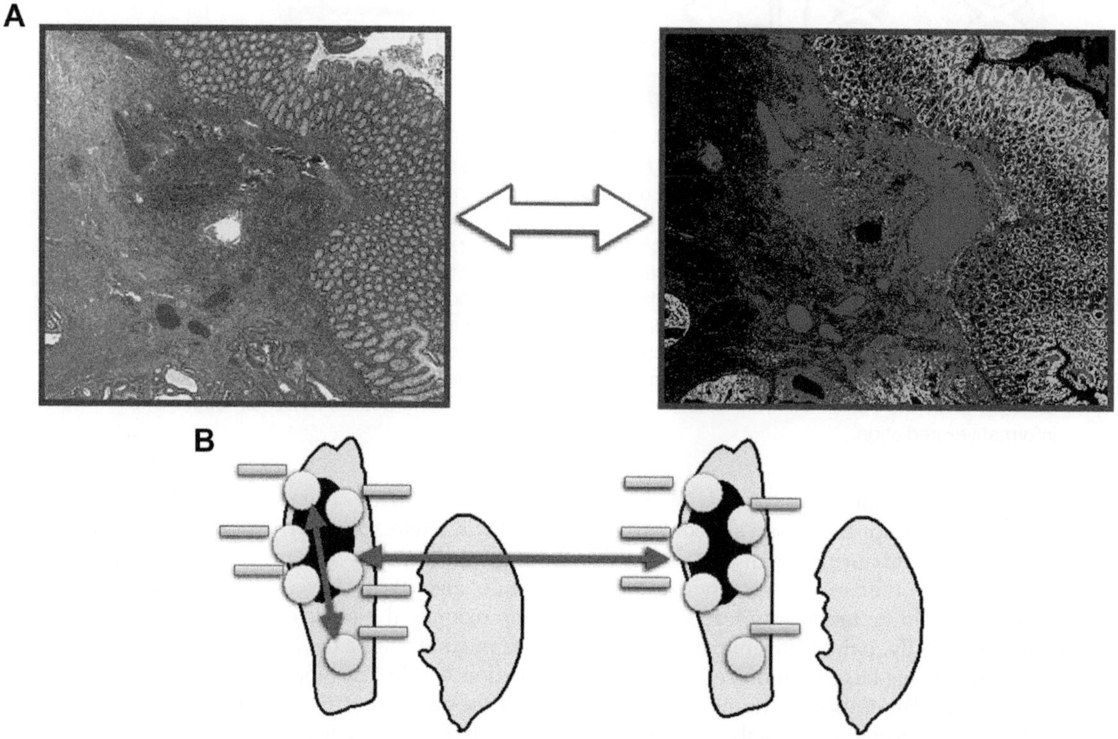

FIG. 12 Opportunity Space for Spatial Omics Approaches. (**A**) Morphologic information contained within H&E WSI may exhibit correspondence to spatial molecular information on right. Visualized on right are three fluorescent antibody stains, a nuclear (hidden) stain, an epithelial/tumor stain, and a lymphocyte stain. When these regions are further profiled using GeoMX and Visium platforms, they reveal highly nuanced and multiplexed molecular information, which offer greater spatial resolution than markers profiled in bulk specimen. (**B**) Representation of spatial molecular information profiled from adjacent/different tissue sections, where black oval represents tumor, green circles are profiled regions of interest and gray rectangles represent signal readout. Common analyses compare across sections/biopsies and spatially within them, as demonstrated by the green lines.

profiles could be matched to individual cells) [69,70]. In addition, when morphological-genomic correspondence is not attainable, the model could "fall back" to contextualizing disease features based on the surrounding macroarchitecture. Many machine learning approaches have also been recently developed to increase the resolution of the spatial omics information while revealing spatially variable molecular patterns within and between tissue specimens (Fig. 12B).

Image Registration, Generative Adversarial Networks (GANs), and Virtual Staining

To facilitate correspondence between molecular and morphologic information (Fig. 13A), information from both modalities must be in optimal spatial alignment. The process of aligning images is commonly referred to as registration. These techniques work by aligning 2 or more images to a reference coordinate system where the images may be compared (Fig. 14A), where the degree of correspondence is an optimization problem summarized by a cost function. Unfortunately, optimization problems are often incredibly computationally intensive and the only way to verify that the optimum solution has been discovered is to try every combination of parameters [71,72]. As such, current image alignment algorithms define a set of simplified transformations to the image, such as rotations, scaling, and affine transforms which work fine for macroscale

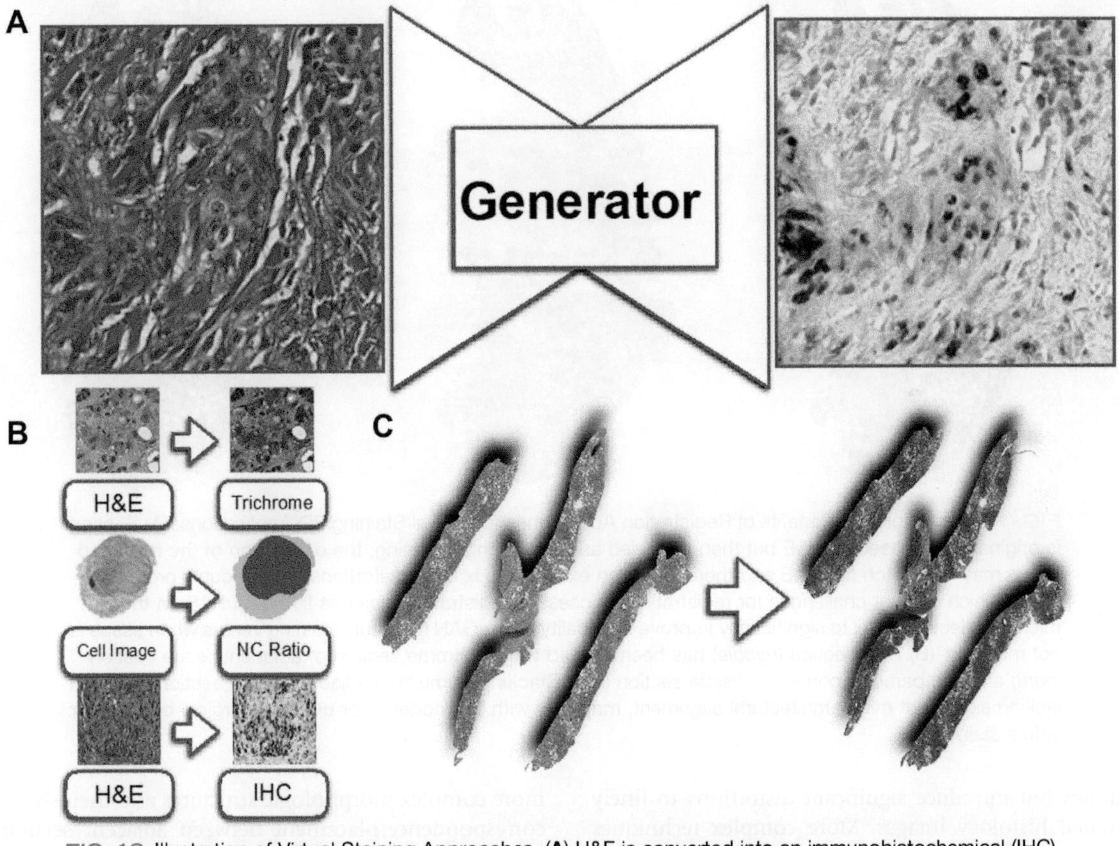

FIG. 13 Illustration of Virtual Staining Approaches. (**A**) H&E is converted into an immunohistochemical (IHC) stain using a GAN to reveal the presence of important biomarkers, where the morphology allows. (**B**) Common tasks with GANs include converting H&E stains into trichrome stains, calculating the nuclear to cytoplasm ratio across cytology specimen, and the H&E to IHC conversion, all of which may provide immediate benefits to Pathology departments aiming to cut down on costs associated with tissue processing, reagents, labor costs, and time. (**C**) The virtual staining techniques are scaled to convert the entire WSI at a time into the specialized stain, here the H&E stain is being converted to the trichrome stain and then is staged to assess the clinical efficacy of the technology.

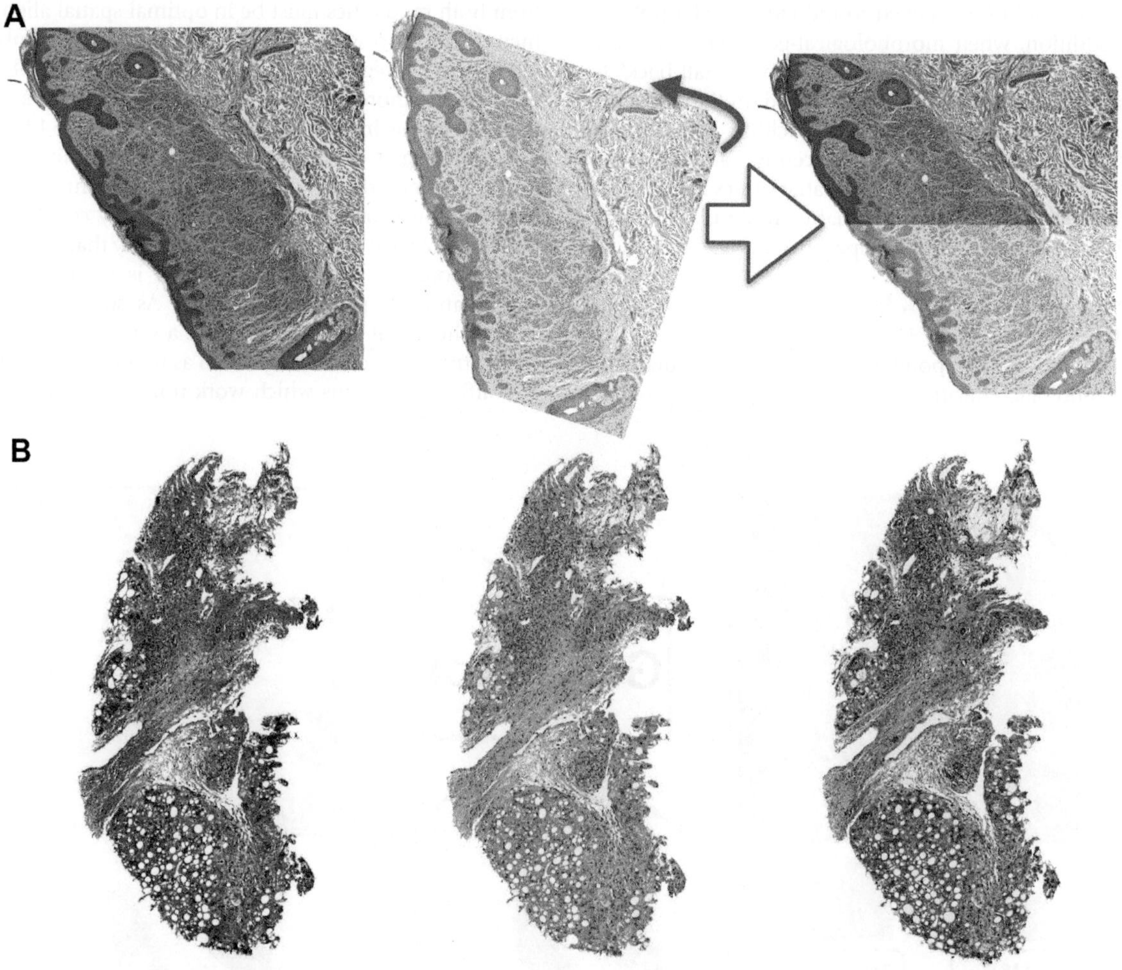

FIG. 14 Illustration and Benefits of Registration Approaches for Virtual Staining/3D Applications. (**A**) Section is originally processed as H&E but then restained as IHC. During scanning, the orientation of the restained tissue may not match the H&E and there may also exist unpredictable distortions in the doubly processed tissue which present challenges for registration. Successful registration matches IHC with H&E on the microarchitectural level to significantly improve the quality of the GAN for virtual staining versus when tissue is not matched. (**B**) H&E section (*middle*) has been aligned with trichrome section of adjacent tissue section (*right*) and compared to converted tissue section (*left*). Stacking of multiple adjacent tissue sections, though lacking significant microarchitectural alignment, may help with 3D modeling or provide marginal benefits for virtual staining.

features but introduce significant distortions to finely detailed histology images. More complex techniques often use too many parameters to be tractable for use on a gigapixel image (for instance, defining alignment on a pixel-by-pixel basis). Deep learning technologies have shown promise in solving complex optimization problems through a learned process akin to intuition (eg, AlphaFold [73]) and may be able to improve alignment procedures through their ability to understand more complex morphologic structures and their shared correspondence/placement between adjacent sections [74]. Once tissue has been registered, information can be integrated across serial layers of tissue, where there exist several deep learning algorithms that operate on 3D patterns and volumes [75].

GANs are neural networks that can create new augmented data in the absence of sufficient input and can be used to convert between 2 different types/sources of data (see Fig. 13A). These algorithms are particularly applicable when studying the morphologic and molecular correspondence after a successful registration though can also be used when images are unpaired. GANs are composed of two types of neural networks: a generator, which generates realistic looking images from input signal/noise, and a discriminator, which decides whether an input image is real or synthetic. The generator uses information from the discriminator to update its parameters and generate images that are better able to fool the discriminator, while the discriminator modifies its parameters to better discern the real from synthetic images. This adversarial game played between the generator and discriminator, in turn, improves the quality of the synthetic images and the effectiveness of the discriminator. A successfully trained GAN can generate hyper-realistic images that often are indistinguishable from real images (deep fakes). GANs have recently been used in the histopathology space to augment data sets for deep learning models to artificially increase the sample size by creating synthetic data and to remove technical artifacts by inferring realistic "filler" pixels to replace the artifact (similar to PhotoShop Context Aware Fill) [76,77].

GANs can also be configured to convert images from a source domain *A* to assume the qualities of images from a target domain *B* (Fig. 13) [41,74,78,79]. Examples include the creation of cell compartment masks (eg, nucleus, cytoplasm, background) from cell images and the inference of immunohistochemistry from H&E images (see Fig. 13). In the former case, GAN-based cell segmentation models were shown to be more accurate than other segmentation techniques. In the latter case, GANs have been used to infer specialized stains from the H&E where the morphology allows (eg, there must be a morphologically visible cue to inform the model, such as subtle copper granules in liver that are difficult to appreciate without a specialized stain). Successful examples include inferring Masson's trichrome stain from liver H&E and predicting SOX10 nuclear staining from skin H&E. Here, using paired imaging data for the GAN can provide better conversion results than when images are unpaired, but care must be taken to ensure optimal alignment (Fig. 14B).

GANs can also be used to normalize histologic stains across institutions are over time to for instance convert outside slides to internal standards or generate a multi-institutional ideal H&E. Stain normalization is also an essential task to standardize images before training a machine learning model (eg, consider the situation where two institutions contribute slides to a study and the bulk of slides showing a particular diagnosis come from a single institution, where the model may learn to focus on an erroneous feature, such as the intensity of hematoxylin) [79].

Text/EHR-Based Analyses

Hospitals use armies of coders to pour through medical documentation and assign standardized billing codes. Simultaneously, insurance companies task their own coders with finding every mistake that hospital coders may have made to deny claims. The process is fraught with human error, bias, and fatigue. To address these issues, algorithmic approaches to billing, including tree-based and deep learning natural language processing pipelines, have been used to mine for patterns and important words which are indicative of the assignment of the diagnostic and procedural code (Fig. 15). Such textual information may also provide rich supplemental information to train deep learning models on WSI, more effectively than dichotomized outcomes of features which may be found through the pathology reports. Interpretation techniques such as the gradient-based backpropagation techniques [80], SHAP (a technique that uses permutation to measure the importance of words input to a tree) [81], and attention-based approaches all serve to weigh the importance of words in each document subsection [82] (covered in greater detail in the Explainable AI section [83]).

Explainable Artificial Intelligence

Currently, machine learning algorithms are perceived to be "black boxes." Signal enters the box, the machinery within the box works its magic, and an outcome is registered. In many cases, understanding what a model finds interesting is truly beyond human comprehension (eg, a model that makes predictions based on analysis of a 1000-dimensional genomic problem space), but in most cases, summaries can be created to aid human understanding. To build trust and adoption for these machine learning technologies, the models must be able to communicate to the user which features in the original input data were indicative of the diagnosis. This may include the construction of saliency maps, which are heatmaps placed over the image to denote the important regions. For matched omics data, model interpretability techniques return the strength and directionality of associations for individual input predictors. There is intensive ongoing research into model interpretability techniques, and it is very much a developing field. Here, we will briefly focus on gradient backpropagation techniques since those have the greatest application for deep learning methods. Gradient-based methods propagate information backward from the outcome to infer

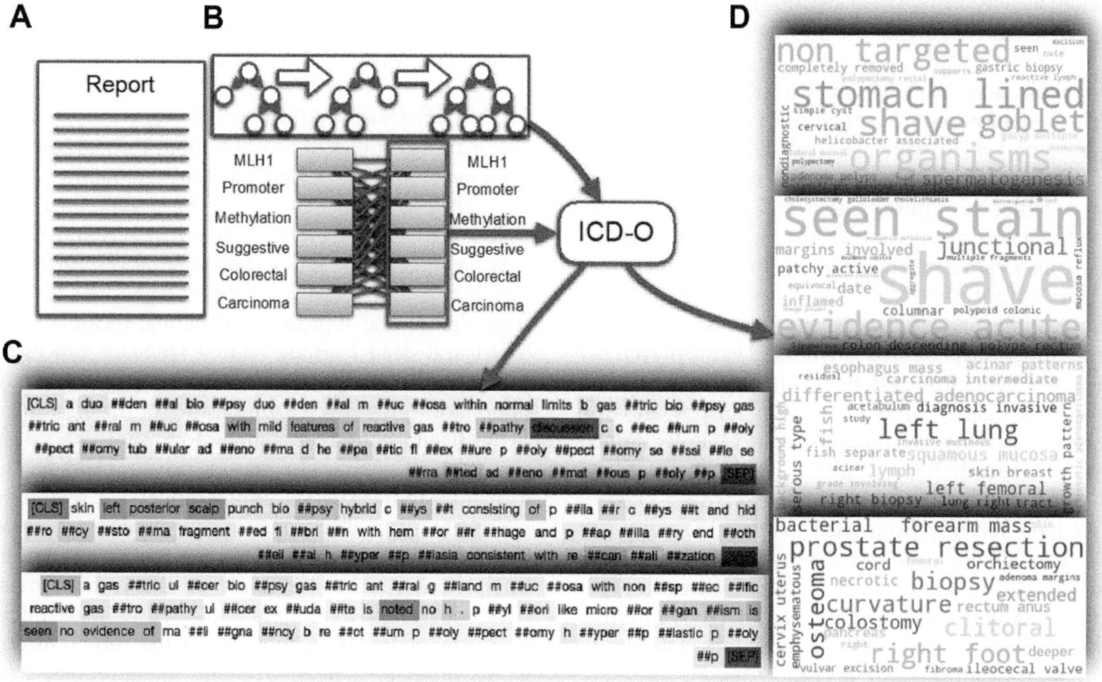

FIG. 15 Natural Language Processing Modeling and Interpretation. (**A**) Pathologist inputs report into machine learning algorithm. (**B**) Random Forest/CART model or BERT attention-based deep learning models can assign a collection of diagnostic and procedural codes to the document. A deep learning approach that models dependencies in sentence and encodes information in a way which can be combined with other data modalities via multimodal modeling approaches. (**C**) Deep learning model passes through gradient-based explainable AI algorithm to highlight words which were pertinent (*green*) and irrelevant (*red*) for prediction of diagnostic/procedure code. (**D**) Similarly, random forest model reveals the most important words for prediction using the SHAP algorithm, where important words are revealed using word cloud where larger words are more important.

which predictors in the image are important. Gradients specify the degree to which the outcome would change based on changes to the input. When the input is an image, these changes correspond to small alterations to the original image. The value of the gradient in these regions is where the local perturbations in the image result in the greatest changes in the outcome [80]. Although the gradient is a coarse approximation of how the output changes with the input, more complex gradient-based methods exist which are beyond the scope of this review, but are incredibly powerful tools for gaining a deeper understanding of the outputs of machine learning models and invaluable for identifying systematic sources of bias in machine learning models. These gradients can be visualized in the slide to highlight cells indicative of the diagnosis (Fig. 4C). Popular alternative modeling techniques include SHAP, which is a model explanation technique that is agnostic to any machine learning model which has been selected. Recently, attention-based transformer deep learning architectures have demonstrated relevance for modeling both text and imaging data and have built in interpretability, as their attention importance scores that are estimated during inference highlight important data attributes [84].

Hierarchical Bayesian Methods

Two problems that have not been well explored in the biomedical machine learning space are as follows: (1) repeated observations and (2) what to do when there is ambiguity in disease grading and staging.

Repeated measurements represent a phenomenon where multiple measurements are made on observations (eg, patients, slides, or biopsies) at a certain experimental unit of analysis. For instance, multiple biopsies may be extracted and analyzed per patient, perhaps tracking a treatment over time. Multiple slides may use the same slide scanner at a particular institution.

Many pathologists may grade or stage the same biopsy. These observations are statistically related to one another and as such present some form of redundant yet variable data which should be accounted for rather than averaged out, removed, or ignored. When repeated measurements are not accounted for in an experimental design, bias or some overstatement of the effectiveness of the machine learning technology may occur (Fig. 16A). As an example, if measurements made from the same patient are placed in both the training and test set, the test set performance may appear erroneously high. This is because having data from the same patient in the training and test set presents a form of data leakage (Fig. 16B) whereby the model is tested on data it has been indirectly exposed to during training (caveat: the extent to which individuals may or may not have characteristic histology is not known). When testing such a model against extra-institutional data, the results may be inferior with no clear indication as to why. As another example, if all the slides pertaining

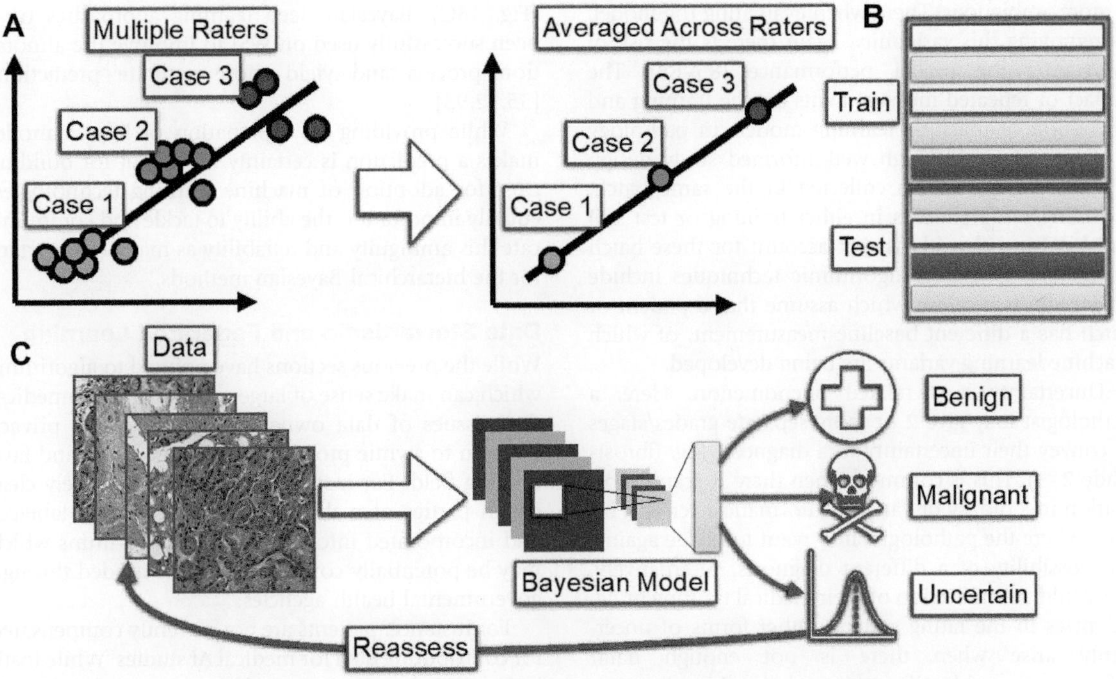

FIG. 16 Illustrating Some of the Issues Associated with Repeated Measurements and Measurement Uncertainty. **(A)** Illustration of how machine learning studies can be biased when using multiple raters to assess the same case. Here, 3 cases are being rated by multiple raters on the continuous scale, where multiple points were color indicate variation in ratings between the multiple raters. We can see there is some variability in the ratings. When properly considering this variability, fitting the model on all the data, the performance captures this ambiguity. However, on the right, ratings have been averaged across raters, revealing a line which is better fit than before. Because the variation was reduced, the model performance is significantly overstated. **(B)** Data comes from 3 different institutions, represented by white, green, and gray rectangles; however, data from the 3 institutions are present in both the training and test sets. Because, for instance, all the green observations may be statistically related between the training and test set, this presents as a form of data leakage and may lead to an overstatement of performance in the test set, which may not generalize to new data and should be communicated as such before conducting such a trial. **(C)** Data are inputted into a Bayesian Deep Learning model, which not only suggests whether case is benign or malignant, but also provides a degree of uncertainty/reliability in the estimate. This information may be incorporated into the clinical triage or used to either relabel or collect more data to build a better model. However, in some medical problems, uncertainty may persist regardless of the degree of model refinement and should be communicated as such to assess the potential for clinical utilization.

to cases were imaged at one institution and the controls scanned at another institution, the machine learning algorithm may pick up on technical artifacts pertaining to the differences in staining and imaging procedures rather than features pertaining to the disease (eg, one institution has Leica scanners with a bluer backlight tint). Finally, it is common to average ratings across multiple pathologists to give a final stage measurement or use a consensus diagnostic rating. However, when relying on a consensus rating where, say 3 of 5, pathologists agree on the same rating, this may skew the training of a machine learning model to confidently assign the majority class where in reality the diagnosis is more ambiguous. Then, when evaluating the model, by removing this variability, again there is the risk of overstating the model performance [85–88]. The impact of repeated measurements on the training and evaluation of machine learning models in pathology may be reduced through well-informed study design (eg, cases and controls collected in the same batch, including same patients in either training or test set) and by using algorithms that account for these batch differences. Common algorithmic techniques include mixed effects models, which assume that a patient or batch has a different baseline measurement, of which machine learning variants are being developed.

Uncertainty is a related phenomenon. Here, a pathologist may give 2 or more separate grades/stages to convey their uncertainty in a diagnosis (eg, fibrosis grade 2–3). This is common when there is scant information in a biopsy or variable information across a biopsy where the pathologist may want to hedge against the possibility of a different diagnosis. Alternatively, this could be a reflection of their medical training or deficiencies in the rating system. Other forms of uncertainty arise when there is not enough data/information to identify strong relationships between the input and outcome. In the former case, *ad hoc* procedures are often applied to select one of the two or more stages as the ground truth. Potentially, this can remove additional variability in the data, which may make the model look better than it really is. In the latter case, the lack of data will lead to a model that is less generalizable as the model is biased to the qualities of the training data, which may not encompass the test data. Under extreme scenarios, this may heavily impact clinical decision-making. When the amount of training data is small, every time the model is trained, it may converge on different sets of parameters, which when making predictions, may result in different predicted disease probabilities [89–91]. The differences in these probabilities may lead to different clinical decisions, so estimating the reliability of the machine learning model becomes crucial. Common solutions to these problems include adopting Bayesian techniques which are able to consider multiple "hypotheses" simultaneously. By taking into account uncertainty, Bayesian methods are able to weigh how much to consider one measurement versus another or one deep learning model versus another, which serves to reduce bias and communicate better the uncertainty or reliability of the prediction. This adds a third dimension to clinical decision-making in addition to the probability that a case is positive or negative, the uncertainty, which can be used to inform new clinical triage practices (Fig. 16C). Bayesian deep learning approaches have been successfully used on WSI to improve the annotation process and yield more accurate predictions [35,92,93].

While providing an explanation of how a model makes a prediction is certainly important for building trust for adoption of machine learning technologies, equally important is the ability to tackle and communicate this ambiguity and reliability as may be important for the hierarchical Bayesian methods.

Data Stewardship and Federated Learning

While the previous sections have pointed to algorithms which can make sense of large quantities of biomedical data, issues of data ownership, security, and privacy threaten to stymie progress in this innovative and fast-moving field. For instance, it is still not entirely clear which parties own the data being produced, labeled, and incorporated into the design of algorithms which may be potentially commercialized or funded through governmental health agencies.

For instance, patients are not currently compensated for contributing data for medical AI studies. While Institutional Review Boards are designed to ensure HIPAA (Health Insurance Portability and Accountability) compliance/data privacy (does not disclose identifiable information pertaining to the individuals) [94], under this system, data are freely available for research and commercial enterprises.

Another party often overlooked in the data creation process are the pathologists, who often spend countless hours and resources acquiring and annotating data, yet their perspectives are not often incorporated into the design process of the downstream applications. An example of this is augmented reality microscopes [95], which can produce creative digital displays for pathologists who are looking at tissue in real time, but it remains to be seen whether pathologists are interested in using this technology and if such technologies can actually result in better patient outcomes/less physician burn-out. In addition to discussing with pathologists AI technologies which are in optimal alignment with clinical utility through user-centered design processes, a system of incentives and rewards are required for engagement in the design process. For instance, clinicians and AI researchers may benefit from serving as co-investigators on research grants, where this experience may provide a career advancement opportunity for the practicing pathologist and a chance for equal influence in the design process [96–99].

Issues of data ownership naturally lend themselves to security (data used as outlined by the authorizing agency) issues, which can often muddy intrainstitutional and interinstitutional collaborations. In a system devoid of adversarial actors (where such actors may unintentionally or purposefully compromise the integrity, quality, or security of the data), data may be pooled across large consortium to serve a greater good (eg, The Cancer Genome Atlas). However, as data becomes more readily identifiable, it becomes less tractable to share information on a digital data commons out of privacy concerns. In addition, such data sharing does not benefit smaller institutions, from which larger institutions may leverage resources unavailable to the smaller institution (eg, compute resources, workforce, in-house validation data) to translate such data into funded grant proposals. In addition, malicious actors and multi-institutional politicking may dissolve trust in collaborative efforts. Thus, there remain numerous incentives to silo data, from which they may not be of benefit to the greater scientific community.

To promote collaboration among multi-institutional actors, there now exists a plethora of algorithms and accompanying software ecosystems which can enable training on multi-institutional data while attending to security and privacy concerns. For instance, federated learning and cryptographic technologies such as secure multiparty compute and homomorphic encryption offer potential solutions toward democratization of data access and scientific advancement. Federated learning environments are systems from which data are stored across multiple host institutions, where machine learning models are trained locally at each center, and then models are sent to a central collaborator, which combines information from these models such that the "averaged" model performs better than any of the models from any of the host institutions. Then, the model is sent back to each of the institutions in the collaborative for further fine-tuning and iteration of the federated averaging process. Recent iterations of this software have demonstrated successful integration of digital pathology data [100] and envisioned how such systems can be designed to scale [101]. However, the process of setting up federated collaborations has not been well documented.

SUMMARY

In summary, digital histology WSIs are incredibly rich, complex, and high dimensional sources of information on patient diagnosis and prognosis but require algorithms which can make sense of these complexities. Machine learning technologies, particularly deep learning, are able to capture many of these complexities and will become increasingly integrated into the clinical workflow to make timely and reliable decisions. While it remains to be seen which technologies can adequately capture information on WSI (in all likelihood many approaches will find niche applications), perhaps more meaningful is that such technologies are in optimal alignment with the needs and practices of the pathologist, pathology assistant, cytotechnologist, resident, and so forth. The machine learning technologies of the future in anatomic pathology should be informed by user-centered design processes and mindful of the role that content creators play in the process of developing new technologies. These fundamental values should not be sidelined by excitement over the potential of these technologies. The progression of technology has time and time again invented new roles for professionals even as it invalidates older practices. Fear of replacement always follows automation. As medical professionals we should not fear that machine learning will "take our jobs" but instead begin to consider a future where algorithms "take the worst parts of our jobs" and free us to explore more interesting and important topics.

ACKNOWLEDGEMENTS

We would like to acknowledge Harshavardhan Harish and Christian Haudenschild for contributions to Figure 7. We also acknowledge support of the Laboratory for Clinical Genomics and Advanced Technology in the Department of Pathology and Laboratory Medicine of Dartmouth Hitchcock Health System and Pathology Shared Resource, at the Norris Cotton Cancer Center at Dartmouth with NCI Cancer Center Support Grant 5P30 CA023108-37. Additional funding support from Burroughs Wellcome Fund Big Data in the Life Sciences training grant, and Dartmouth College Neukom Institute for Computational Science CompX award.

CLINICS CARE POINTS

- When training a machine learning model, monitor the performance of the validation set over time and across model configurations to select the best model. Select a model where the accuracy on the validation set is maximized, else the model may become overfit to the training data and will not perform well on external cohorts.
- Use explainable AI techniques to observe the model's decision-making with saliency heatmaps overlaid on the images. This can help assess systematic points of bias which can be remedied in the design/annotation stage of the study.
- When designing a clinical study, be weary of the potential for confounded disease associations. For instance, the presence of a mutation to be predicted may differ by age, sex, or body mass index, make sure to adjust for these factors directly in the modeling approach by incorporation into the machine learning model or by making sure cases and controls are matched by these and other relevant (eg, disease stage) clinical covariates.
- Batch effects may also confound prediction models and artificially inflate model performance. For instance, if cases are primarily from one institution and controls from another, the model may pick up on technical artifacts (eg, differences in staining, tissue preparation, lighting, etc.). Avoid batch effects by separating data from different batches into the training and test sets and by applying hierarchical modeling procedures in the development and validation of the model. The reliability of the model can be supplied using Bayesian methods.
- If number of slides numbers in the hundreds, consider using a patch-based annotation approach to train the deep learning model, where applicable. When the number of WSIs are in the thousands, consider using weakly supervised learning methods. To boost the amount of training data, data can be augmented using a generative adversarial network (GAN) and unsupervised/semisupervised approaches can be used. Transfer learning approaches reduce the amount of training data required by first learning a model from a similar domain.
- Pathologists have the unique perspective of having seen and understood the advantages and drawbacks of medical interventions that quantitative biomedical researchers aim to benefit. Thus, the design and implementation of digital pathology technologies should be informed through user-centered design processes, where iterative design and stakeholder interviews/feedback are commonplace.

REFERENCES

[1] Serag A, Ion-Margineanu A, Qureshi H, et al. Translational AI and deep learning in diagnostic pathology. Front Med 2019;6:185.

[2] Fischer AH, Jacobson KA, Rose J, et al. Hematoxylin and eosin staining of tissue and cell sections. Cold Spring Harb Protoc 2008 pdb.prot4986 (2008).

[3] Levy JJ, Salas LA, Christensen BC, et al. PathFlowAI: a high-throughput workflow for preprocessing, deep learning and interpretation in digital pathology. Pac Symp Biocomput 2019;25:403–14.

[4] Wei JW, Tafe LJ, Linnik YA, et al. Pathologist-level classification of histologic patterns on resected lung adenocarcinoma slides with deep neural networks. Sci Rep 2019;9:3358.

[5] Jordan MI, Mitchell TM. Machine learning: trends, perspectives, and prospects. Science 2015;349:255–60.

[6] Chan S, Reddy V, Myers B, et al. Machine learning in dermatology: current applications, opportunities, and limitations. Dermatol ther (Heidelb) 2020;10:365–86.

[7] Quinlan JR. Induction of decision trees. Mach Learn 1986;1:81–106.

[8] Breiman L. Random forests. Mach Learn 2021;45:5–32.

[9] Chen T, Guestrin C. XGBoost: a scalable tree boosting system. In: Proceedings of the 22Nd ACM SIGKDD international conference on knowledge discovery and data mining. San Francisco: Association for Computing Machinery; 2016. p. 785–94. https://doi.org/10.1145/2939672.2939785.

[10] Cover T, Hart P. Nearest neighbor pattern classification. IEEE Trans Inf Theor 1967;13:21–7.

[11] Lachenbruch PA, Sneeringer C, Revo LT. Robustness of the linear and quadratic discriminant function to certain types of non-normality. Comm Stat 1973;1:39.

[12] Hesterberg T, Choi NH, Meier L, et al. Least angle and angle and nd certain types of non. Stat Surv 2008;2:61–93.

[13] Hearst M, Dumais ST, Osman E, et al. Support vector machines. IEEE Intell Syst App 1998;13:18–28.

[14] Wold S, Esbensen K, Geladi P. Principal component analysis. Chemometr Intell Lab Syst 1987;2:37–52.

[15] Becht E, McInnes L, Healy J, et al. Dimensionality reduction for visualizing single-cell data using UMAP. Nat Biotechnol 2018;37:38.

[16] McInnes L, Healy J, Saul N, et al. Uniform manifold approximation and projection. J Open Source Softw 2018;3:861.

[17] Likas A, Vlassis N, Verbeek J, et al. The global k-means clustering algorithm. Pattern Recognition 2003;36:451–61.

[18] Reynolds D. Gaussian mixture models. In: Li SZ, Jain A, editors. Encyclopedia of biometrics. New York: Springer; 2009. p. 659–63.

[19] von Luxburg U. A tutorial on spectral clustering. Stat Comput 2007;17:395–416.

[20] McInnes L, Healy J, Astels S. hdbscan: hierarchical density based clustering. J Open Source Softw 2017;2:205.

[21] LeCun Y, Bengio Y, Hinton G. Deep learning. Nature 2015;521:436–44.

[22] Esteva A, Chou K, Yeung S, et al. Deep learning-enabled medical computer vision. NPJ Digital Med 2021;4:1–9.

[23] Krizhevsky A, Sutskever I, Hinton GE. ImageNet classification with deep convolutional neural networks. In: Pereira F, Burges CJC, Bottou L, et al, editors. Advances in neural information processing systems. Twenty-sixth Conference on Neural Information Processing Systems, Lake Tahoe, Nevada, vol. 25 2012;. 2012. p. 1097–105.

[24] Ching T, Chou K, Yeung S, et al. Opportunities and obstacles for deep learning in biology and medicine. J R Soc Interf 2018;15:20170387.

[25] Lo S-CB, Chan HP, Lin JS, et al. Artificial convolution neural network for medical image pattern recognition. Neural Networks 1995;8:1201–14.

[26] Zhang A, Lipton ZC, Li M, et al. Dive into deep learning 2020. Available at: https://d2l.ai.

[27] Ronneberger O, Fischer P, Brox T. U-Net: convolutional networks for biomedical image segmentation. In: Navab N, Hornegger J, Wells WM, et al, editors. Medical image computing and computer-assisted intervention al Networks. New York: Springer Science+Business Media; 2015. p. 234–41. https://doi.org/10.1007/978-3-319-24574-4_28.

[28] Vuola AO, Akram SU, Kannala J. Mask-RCNN and U-Net ensembled for nuclei segmentation. In: 2019 IEEE 16th international Symposium on biomedical imaging (ISBI 2019). Venice, Italy: International Symposium on Biomedical Imaging; 2019. p. 208–19. https://doi.org/10.1109/ISBI.2019.8759574.

[29] Redmon J, Farhadi A. YOLOv3: an incremental improvement 2018 arXiv:1804.02767 [cs].

[30] Bankhead P, Loughrey MB, Fernández JA, et al. QuPath: open source software for digital pathology image analysis. Sci Rep 2017;7:1–7.

[31] Perez L, Wang J. The effectiveness of data augmentation in image classification using deep learning 2017 arXiv: 1712.04621 [cs].

[32] Wei J, Suriawinata A, Vaickus L, et al. Generative image translation for data augmentation in colorectal histopathology images. Vancouver, Canada: ML4H@NeurIPS MLR Press; 2019.

[33] Macenko M. et al. A method for normalizing histology slides for quantitative analysis. In 2009 IEEE international symposium on biomedical imaging: from nano to macro 1107-1110. Boston, Massachusetts, 28 June-1 July, 2009. https://doi.org/10.1109/ISBI.2009.5193250.

[34] Shallu, Mehra R. Breast cancer histology images classification: training from scratch or transfer learning? ICT Express 2018;4:247–54.

[35] Zkowski RR, Moowski M, Zambonelli J, et al. Accurate, reliable and active histopathological image classification framework with Bayesian deep learning. Sci Rep 2019;9:14347.

[36] Heinemann F, Birk G, Stierstorfer B. Deep learning enables pathologist-like scoring of NASH models. Sci Rep 2019;9:18454.

[37] Ramot Y, Zandani G, Madar Z, et al. Utilization of a deep learning algorithm for microscope-based fatty vacuole quantification in a fatty liver model in mice. Toxicol Pathol 2002;48:702–7.

[38] Davison BA, Harrison SA, Cotter G, et al. Suboptimal reliability of liver biopsy evaluation has implications for randomized clinical trials. J Hepatol 2020;73:1322–32.

[39] Stringer C, Wang T, Michaelos M, et al. Cellpose: a generalist algorithm for cellular segmentation. Nat Methods 2021;18:100–6.

[40] Ziemys A, Kim M, Menzies AM, et al. Integration of digital pathologic and transcriptomic analyses connects tumor-infiltrating lymphocyte spatial density with clinical response to BRAF inhibitors. Front Oncol 2020;10: 757.

[41] Jackson CR, Sriharan A, Vaickus LJ. A machine learning algorithm for simulating immunohistochemistry: development of SOX10 virtual IHC and evaluation on primarily melanocytic neoplasms. Modern Pathol 2020;33(9):1638–48.

[42] Hou L, Gupta R, Van Arnam JS, et al. Dataset of segmented nuclei in hematoxylin and eosin stained histopathology images of ten cancer types. Sci Data 2020; 7:185.

[43] Vaickus LJ, Suriawinata AA, Wei JW, et al. Automating the paris system for urine cytopathologytopathologyancer types. C and evaluation on primar. Cancer Cytopathol 2019;127:98–115.

[44] Karim MR, Beyan O, Zappa A, et al. Deep learning-based clustering approaches for bioinformatics. Brief Bioinform 2021;22:393–415.

[45] Kingma DP, Welling M. Auto-encoding variational bayes 2014 arXiv:1312.6114 [cs, stat].

[46] Yamamoto Y, Tsuzuki T, Akatsuka J, et al. Automated acquisition of explainable knowledge from unannotated histopathology images. Nat Commun 2019;10:5642.

[47] Feng Y, Zhang L, Mo J. Deep manifold preserving autoencoder for classifying breast cancer histopathological images. IEEE/ACM Trans Comput Biol Bioinform 2020; 17:91–101.

[48] Hu B, et al. Unsupervised learning for cell-level visual representation in histopathology images with generative adversarial networks. IEEE J Biomed Health Inform 2018;23:1316–28.

[49] Lu MY, Chen RJ, Mahmood F. Semi-supervised breast cancer histology classification using deep multiple instance learning and contrast predictive coding (Conference Presentation). In: Tomaszewski J, Ward A, editors. Medical imaging 2020: digital pathology, vol. 11320. Houston, TX: International Society for Optics and Photonics; 2020. p. 113200J.

[50] Chen RJ, et al. Pathomic fusion: an integrated framework for fusing histopathology and genomic features for cancer diagnosis and prognosis 2019.

[51] Ianni JD, Soans RE, Sankarapandian S, et al. Tailored for real-world: a whole slide image classification system validated on uncurated multi-site data emulating the prospective pathology workload. Sci Rep 2020;10:3217.

[52] Campanella G, Hanna MG, Geneslaw L, et al. Clinical-grade computational pathology using weakly supervised deep learning on whole slide images. Nat Med 2019;25:1301–9.

[53] Lu MY, Williamson DFK, Chen TY, et al. Data-efficient and weakly supervised computational pathology on whole-slide images. Nat Biomed Eng 2021;5(6):555–70.

[54] Lu MY, Chen TY, Williamson DFK, et al. AI-based pathology predicts origins for cancers of unknown primary. Nature 2021;594:106–10.

[55] Tomita N, Abdollahi B, Wei J, et al. Attention-based deep neural networks for detection of cancerous and precancerous esophagus tissue on histopathological slides. JAMA Netw Open 2019;2:e1914645.

[56] Levy J, Haudenschild C, Barwick C, et al. Topological feature extraction and visualization of whole slide images using graph neural networks. Pac Symp Biocomput 2020;285–96.

[57] Yamashita R, Levy J, Haudenschild C, Barwick C, et al. Deep learning model for the prediction of microsatellite instability in colorectal cancer: a diagnostic study. Lancet Oncol 2021;22:132–41.

[58] Adnan M, Kalra S, Tizhoosh HR. Representation learning of histopathology images using graph neural networks. Proceedings of the IEEE/CVF Conference on Computer Vision and Pattern Recognition (CVPR) Workshops. 2020. p. 988–9.

[59] Ash JT, Darnell G, Munro D, et al. Joint analysis of expression levels and histological images identifies genes associated with tissue morphology. Nat Commun 2021;12:1609.

[60] Carmichael I, et al. Joint and individual analysis of breast cancer histologic images and genomic covariates 2019 arXiv:1912.00434 [eess, q-bio, stat].

[61] Zheng H, Momeni A, Cedoz P-L, et al. Whole slide images reflect DNA methylation patterns of human tumors. NPJ Genomic Med 2020;5:11.

[62] Hao J, Kosaraju S, Tsaku N, et al. Interpretable and integrative deep learning for survival analysis using histopathological images and genomic data. Pac Symp Biocomputing 2020;25:355–66.

[63] Zhan Z, Jing Z, He B, et al. Two-stage Cox-nnet: biologically interpretable neural-network model for prognosis prediction and its application in liver cancer survival using histopathology and transcriptomic data. NAR Genom Bioinform 2021;3:lqab015.

[64] Cheerla A, Gevaert O. Deep learning with multimodal representation for pancancer prognosis prediction. Bioinformatics 2019;35:i446–54.

[65] de Vries NL, Mahfouz A, Koning F, et al. Unraveling the complexity of the cancer microenvironment with multidimensional genomic and cytometric technologies. Front Oncol 2020;10:1254.

[66] Zhang M, Sheffield T, Zhan X, et al. Spatial molecular profiling: platforms, applications and analysis tools. Brief Bioinform 2021;22(3):bbaa145.

[67] Van TM, Blank CU. A user's perspective on GeoMxTM digital spatial profiling. Immuno-Oncology Technol 2019;1:11-8.

[68] Goytain A, Ng T. NanoString nCounter technology: high-throughput RNA validation. In: Li H, Elfman J, editors. Chimeric RNA: methods and protocols. New York: Springer Nature; 2020. p. 125–39.

[69] Tan X, Su A, Tran M, et al. SpaCell: integrating tissue morphology and spatial gene expression to predict disease cells. Bioinformatics 2020;36:2293–4.

[70] He B, Bergenstråhle L, Stenbeck L, et al. Integrating spatial gene expression and breast tumour morphology via deep learning. Nat Biomed Eng 2020;4:827–34.

[71] Levy JJ, Jackson CR, Haudenschild CC, et al. PathFlow-mixmatch for whole slide image registration: an investigation of a segment-based scalable image registration method. bioRxiv 2020. https://doi.org/10.1101/2020.03.22.002402.

[72] Paknezhad M, et al. Regional registration of whole slide image stacks containing highly deformed artefacts 2020 arXiv:2002.12588 [cs, eess].

[73] Senior AW, Evans R, Jumper J, et al. Improved protein structure prediction using potentials from deep learning. Nature 2020;577:706–10.

[74] Levy J, Jackson C, Sriharan A, et al. Preliminary evaluation of the utility of deep generative histopathology image translation at a Mid-sized NCI Cancer Center. In: Proceedings of the 13th International Joint Conference on Biomedical Engineering Systems and Technologies (BIOSTEC 2020), vol. 3. Valletta, Malta: Bioinformatics SCITEPRESS; 2021. p. 30.

[75] Pichat J, Iglesias JE, Yousry T, et al. A survey of methods for 3D histology reconstruction. Med Image Anal 2018; 46:73–105.

[76] Goodfellow I, Pouget-Abadie J, Mirza M, et al. Generative adversarial networks. *Advances in Neural Information Processing Systems* 2014;3.

[77] Zhu JY, Park T, Isola P, et al. Unpaired image-to-image translation using cycle-consistent adversarial networks. in Proceedings of the IEEE international conference on computer vision. Venice, Italy: IEEE; 2017;2223–2232.

[78] Levy JJ, Azizgolshani N, Andersen MJ, et al. A large-scale internal validation study of unsupervised virtual trichrome staining technologies on nonalcoholic steatohepatitis liver biopsies. Mod Pathol 2021;34:808–22.

[79] Ghazvinian Zanjani F, Zinger S, Ehteshami Bejnordi B, et al. Stain normalization of histopathology images using generative adversarial networks. In 2018 IEEE 15th International Symposium on Biomedical Imaging (ISBI 2018), Washington DC. https://doi.org/10.1109/ISBI.2018.8363641.

[80] Sundararajan M, Taly A, Yan Q. Axiomatic attribution for deep networks. in *Proceedings of the 34th International*

Conference on Machine Learning. Sydney, Australia: Association for Computing Machinery; 017;70: 3319–28

[81] Lundberg SM, Erion G, Chen H, et al. From local explanations to global understanding with explainable AI for trees. Nat Machine Intell 2020;2:56–67.

[82] Devlin J, Chang M-W, Lee K, et al. BERT: pre-training of deep bidirectional transformers for language understanding. In: Proceedings of the 2019 conference of the North American chapter of the association for computational linguistics: human language technologies, vol. 1. Minneapolis, Minnesota: Association for Computational Linguistics; 2019. p. 4171. https://doi.org/10.18653/v1/N19-1423, Long and short papers.

[83] Levy J, Vattikonda N, Haudenschild C, et al. Comparison of machine learning algorithms for the prediction of current procedural terminology (CPT) codes from pathology reports. medRxiv 2021. https://doi.org/10.1101/2021.03.13.21253502.

[84] Tosun AB, Pullara F, Becich MJ, et al. Explainable AI (xAI) for anatomic pathology. Adv Anat Pathol 2020; 27:241–50.

[85] Bürkner PC. Advanced Bayesian Multilevel Modeling with the R Package brms. R J 2018;10:395.

[86] Bürkner PC. brms: an R package for bayesian multilevel models using Stan. J Stat Softw 2017;80:1–28.

[87] McElreath R. Statistical rethinking: a Bayesian course with examples in R and Stan. Boca Raton, Florida: CRC Press; 2020.

[88] Young AT, Fernandez K, Pfau J, et al. Stress testing reveals gaps in clinic readiness of image-based diagnostic artificial intelligence models. NPJ Digit Med 2021;4:10.

[89] Kompa B, Snoek J, Beam AL. Second opinion needed: communicating uncertainty in medical machine learning. NPJ Digital Med 2021;4:4.

[90] Cabitza F, Ciucci D, Rasoini R. A giant with feet of clay: on the validity of the data that feed machine learning in medicine. In: Cabitza F, Batini C, Magni M, editors. Organizing for the digital world. New York: Springer International Publishing; 2019. p. 121–36. https://doi.org/10.1007/978-3-319-90503-7_10.

[91] Djulbegovic B, Paul A. From efficacy to effectiveness in the face of uncertainty: indication creep and prevention creep. JAMA 2011;305:2005–9.

[92] Begoli E, Bhattacharya T, Kusnezov D. The need for uncertainty quantification in machine-assisted medical decision making. Nat Mach Intell 2019;1:20–3.

[93] Pasetto S, Gatenby RA, Enderling H. Bayesian framework to augment tumor board decision making. JCO Clin Cancer Inform 2021;5:508–17.

[94] Gerke S, Minssen T, Cohen G. Ethical and legal challenges of artificial intelligence-driven healthcare. Artif Intell Healthc 2020;295–336.

[95] Razavian N. Augmented reality microscopes for cancer histopathology. Nat Med 2019;25:1334–6.

[96] Grote T, Berens P. On the ethics of algorithmic decision-making in healthcare. J Med Ethics 2020;46: 205–11.

[97] Rigby MJ. Ethical dimensions of using artificial intelligence in health care. AMA J Ethics 2019;21:121–4.

[98] Jackson BR, Ye Y, Crawford JM, et al. The Ethics of Artificial Intelligence in Pathology and Laboratory Medicine: Principles and Practice. *Acad Pathol* 2021;8.

[99] Abras C, Maloney-krichmar D, Preece J. User-centered design. In: Bainbridge W, editor. Encyclopedia of human-computer interaction. Thousand Oaks: *Sage Publications* (Publications); 2004.

[100] Lu MY, et al. Federated learning for computational pathology on gigapixel whole slide images 2020 arXiv: 2009.10190 [cs, eess, q-bio].

[101] Warnat-Herresthal S, Schultze H, Shastry KL, et al. Swarm learning for decentralized and confidential clinical machine learning. Nature 2021;594:265–70.

Solid Tumors

Advances in Molecular Pathology 4 (2021) 173–185

ADVANCES IN MOLECULAR PATHOLOGY

Operationalizing Genomic Medicine

Laboratory Practice Considerations Beyond the Assay

Nikoletta Sidiropoulos, MD[a,b,*]

[a]The Robert Larner, M.D. College of Medicine at The University of Vermont, Burlington, VT, USA; [b]Genomic Medicine, Department of Pathology and Laboratory Medicine, University of Vermont Medical Center, Burlington, VT 05401, USA

KEYWORDS

• Genomic • Precision • Preanalytic • Service • Stewardship • Pathologist • Value • Champion

KEY POINTS

- Clinical value of genomic testing is realized via investment in a laboratory professional that champions efforts comprising a genomic medicine service that supports the assay.
- Components of a genomic medicine service include tissue, workflow, and educational stewardship.
- Key expertise for operationalizing a genomic medicine service includes broad training in pathology and laboratory medicine inclusive of next-generation sequencing coupled with clinical training.
- Medical interpretation of genomic results is a professional service requiring mastery of medical communication and underpins effective translation of complex testing for clinical action.
- Recognition for information systems supportive of genomic medicine is underestimated yet it is a necessity for delivering on any investment otherwise in precision medicine.

INTRODUCTION

The Human Genome Project along with the development of next-generation sequencing technology were two foundational factors that ignited the ongoing endeavor to realize the clinical practice of "precision medicine". Another term for this practice is "genomic medicine", partly defined by the National Human Genome Research Institute as "an emerging medical discipline that involves using genomic information about an individual as part of their clinical care (eg, for diagnostic or therapeutic decision-making)" [1]. Generally speaking, the clinical practice of genomic medicine is achieved by an arduous process whereby genomic-based research findings pertinent to human health are published, validated, evaluated for safety and clinical efficacy via clinical trials, and then finally incorporated into clinical care via professional guidelines, and ideally into insurance coverage policies as well.

Increasingly, the medical field is experiencing approval of molecular biomarkers into many different facets of clinical care [2]. And while regulatory approval and incorporation of this information into professional guidelines are gatekeeping aspects to the clinical practice of genomic medicine, the realization of this practice requires optimization of the so-called "precision medicine ecosystem" [3] (Fig. 1). The ecosystem is complex and often conceptually oversimplifies the nature of the "Laboratory". Addressed here forth, will be the clinical laboratory, specifically the molecular diagnostic laboratory as defined by the ownership and expertise to develop, deploy, maintain, and scale genomic testing using next-generation sequencing. It is important to consider the optimization of this sector of the ecosystem as it is responsible for generating precise,

*Corresponding author, *E-mail address:* Nikoletta.sidiropoulos@uvmhealth.org

https://doi.org/10.1016/j.yamp.2021.07.006
2589-4080/21/

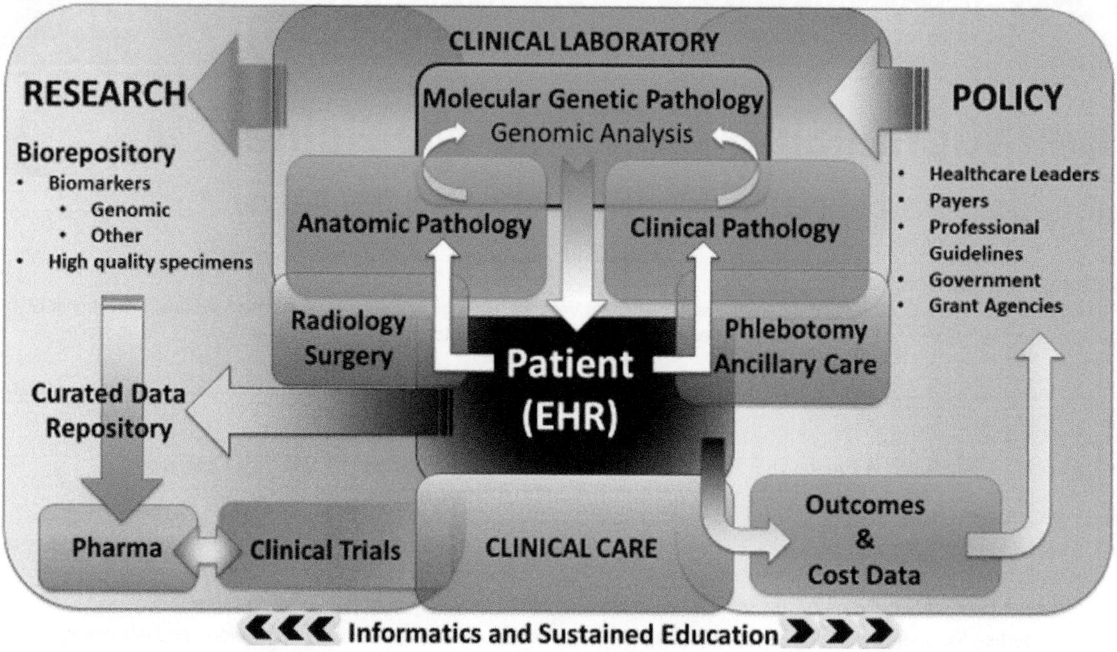

FIG. 1 The "precision medicine ecosystem". The successful practice of precision medicine occurs in a complex ecosystem within the overarching health care system. Although the ecosystem can be visualized from different perspectives, it is generally accepted that the center of the system is the patient. The patient is often defined by personal health information that is documented in the electronic health record (EHR) which *ideally*, in an equitable system, is the basis for the clinical care a patient receives. A growing component of precision medicine is genomic information. This information is derived from specimens that are the direct extension of the corporeal patient and should be treated as such via thoughtful and informed stewardship. The laboratory is ideally suited for this role because proper specimen management underpins successful laboratory testing that thereby is a significant factor driving clinical care. All too commonly, however, the "clinical laboratory" is conceptually oversimplified in the precision medicine ecosystem. Successful incorporation of genomic information in the effort to achieve a precision medicine care model ultimately relies on linkage of clinical, genomic, and laboratory data not only for clinical care but also to prime related research through to clinical trials. Although many regulators define clinical trials as "research," patients often times consider the care they receive via clinical trials as "clinical care". Ultimately, the clinical-research spectrum generates outcomes and cost data that drive policy at many different levels. It is policy and guidelines that then have a feedback impact on the ecosystem. Just recognizing the different components of the ecosystem is not enough for *adoption* of precision medicine. This complex system requires heavy investment in informatics and sustained education. *Adapted from* Ginsburg GS, & Phillips KA. Precision medicine: from science to value. Health Aff (Millwood). 2018 May; 37(5): 694–701. doi: 10.1377/hlthaff.2017.1624

accurate, and clinically relevant molecular results, which some would argue is the basis for the clinical practice of genomic medicine.

The implementation of next-generation sequencing is resource intensive as evidenced by countless instructional resources and "how to" guides. Yet increasingly, laboratories are choosing to insource the technology assuming "it" will meet the clinical demand for and enable the growing clinical practice of precision medicine. This assumption often does not take into account that to achieve these goals, the technology must be deployed in parallel with the consideration of preanalytic and postanalytic variables within the local "ecosystem" that transcend practice in the molecular diagnostics laboratory.

Significance

First and foremost, it is important to review some key housekeeping considerations. Most molecular laboratories considering insourcing next-generation sequencing in an effort to meet the ever-expanding clinical demands for genomic medicine have a general awareness that this is a relatively expensive endeavor. Medical systems as a whole have many competing priorities and limited resources. Therefore, it behooves the laboratory to proactively assess the vision of the health system at large, identify and engage key stakeholders that constitute the precision medicine ecosystem, and foster leadership engagement (Fig. 2). These are key components for establishing an ecosystem that can move from a concept of implementing "just genomic testing" to embracing adoption of a genomic medicine "service". Early identification and ongoing engagement with key stakeholders is useful in (1) defining test performance expectations and (2) building processes that support and enhance clinical workflow. These are two components that when considered together, foster efficient use of resources and adoption of genomics into clinical care, which is the ultimate return on investment.

It is the *simultaneous* consideration of (1) processes that support and enhance clinical workflow, along with (2) intralaboratory considerations of test design and validation that is important. It is useful to define what the former concept entails. Although it can technically be defined by the consideration of preanalytical and postanalytical factors surrounding the test itself, there is risk in this definition to not think more broadly beyond factors about which the laboratory is aware. Herein arises the concept of the "care pathway", where genomically informed clinical care involves strategic integration of the best genomic technology with people and processes beyond the laboratory to realize the promise of precision medicine for each unique patient (Fig. 3). From the molecular laboratory perspective, simultaneous effort to design a care pathway alongside the development and validation of a test is the logistical exercise for developing a genomic medicine service. It is the "care pathway" that significantly informs the components of the "service" that is supportive beyond the test.

A final housekeeping item is the recognition that "sequence data does not equal a clinical report". Within the laboratory, there are many steps composing tests that are performed using next-generation sequencing. At a very high level, the next-generation sequencing workflow can be divided conceptually into the "wet bench" and the "dry bench". The "wet bench" includes all processes that involve working with a physical sample, from receipt of the accessioned sample to the generation of sequence. The "dry bench" includes all processes that involve working with the sequence data all the way through to medical interpretation culminating in report generation (Fig. 4). Establishing high-quality processes for both the wet and dry benches that have consistent performance parameters is of foundational importance for the molecular diagnostics laboratory yet is outside the scope of this article. That said, while establishing solid "testing fundamentals", awareness of and commitment to care pathway development, inclusive of preanalytical and postanalytical variables in the laboratory at large and beyond, will guide simultaneous development of a nuanced genomic medicine service.

It was about a decade ago when molecular testing was effectively stripped of a professional interpretation component [4,5]. The G code (G0452), designating physician interpretive work for molecular interpretation, does not adequately reflect the medical interpretive component required for clinically relevant genomic reports derived via next-generation sequencing. This negatively impacted the molecular diagnostic field with ripple effect into the clinical sphere as the practice of precision medicine/genomic medicine evolved to be intimately associated with genomic testing that relies on next-generation sequencing. The economic impact of the coding change disrupted the investment in medical staffing of clinical molecular diagnostic laboratories, thereby decoupling molecular biology expertise from clinical expertise. It takes careful coordination to create clinical-grade assays that adequately interrogate the genome and thereby deliver meaningful clinical results. Even with an assay that is designed to effectively interrogate the genome, the interpretation of the results for clinical care is a highly specialized practice that requires a mastery of medical communication which underpins the effective translation of complex testing for clinical action. This is optimally accomplished in laboratories and health centers that value the coupling of molecular biology and clinical expertise. Clinically relevant genomic interpretation for precision medicine requires medical judgment and professional time commitment beyond that which is reflected in the G code (Fig. 5). Therefore, a baseline consideration for building a genomic medicine service is investment in medical interpretation, which is a necessity for delivering on any investment otherwise in the practice of precision oncology.

To further illustrate the importance of some aforementioned considerations, it is worthwhile to consider the example of *MET* exon 14 skipping mutations. These mutations constitute a category of oncogenic abnormalities in non-small cell lung cancer (NSCLC) that are

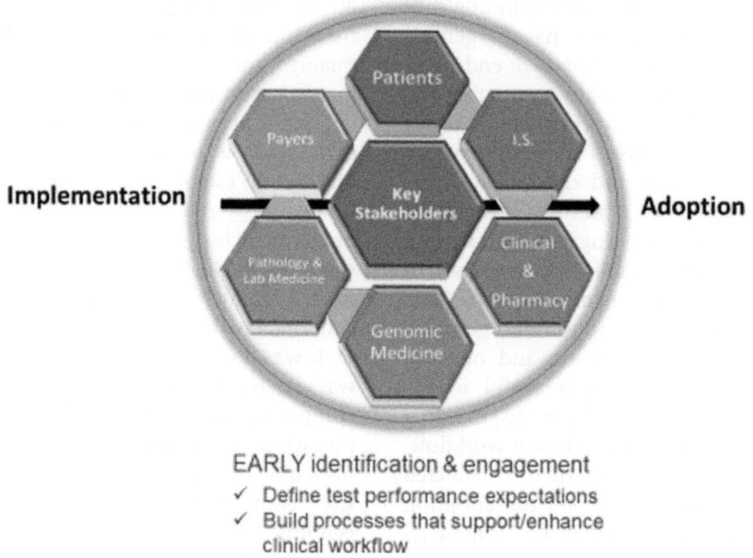

FIG. 2 Key stakeholders in the precision medicine ecosystem. It is advised that the laboratory proactively assess the vision of its health care system at large, engage key stakeholders that constitute the precision medicine ecosystem, and foster leadership engagement. This is foundational in the establishment of an ecosystem that can move from a concept of implementing "just genomic testing" to embracing adoption of a genomic medicine "service". Early identification and ongoing engagement with key stakeholders is useful in (1) defining test performance expectations and (2) building processes that support and enhance clinical workflow. These are two components that when considered together, foster efficient use of resources and adoption of genomics into clinical care, which is the ultimate return on investment.

predictive of response to targeted cancer therapy [6,7]. Consequently, awareness of *MET* exon 14 skipping mutations and an understanding of molecular diagnostic approaches that detect these variants is necessary in modern multifaceted clinical and laboratory care of NSCLC.

Molecular detection of *MET* exon 14 skipping events can be achieved via DNA or RNA-based next-generation sequencing. That being said, most molecular diagnostic laboratories are not yet using RNA-based sequencing regularly. This is mentioned because it has implications for the delivery of clinically relevant testing in NSCLC since a large degree of genomic variation underlies resultant *MET* exon 14 skipping. The diversity spans many mutations that either do not involve canonical splice site sequences or lie outside regions captured and interpreted for *MET* analysis via DNA-based next-generation sequencing [8–10]. Therefore, these mutations can go undetected with DNA-based next-generation sequencing alone. However, if RNA is being sequenced, the direct result of altered splicing (as the direct fusion of exons 13 and 15) must be detected and it is the latter, the abnormal fusion product, that is ultimately the outcome regardless of the underlying DNA mutation [10,11].

MET exon 14 skipping mutations illustrate why understanding the complexity of the molecular biology, the strengths and limitations of next-generation sequencing, *and* up-to-date clinical implications are all important facets that should not be "decoupled" in molecular diagnostic laboratories that are considering or are actively involved in genomic testing (Fig. 6). The aforementioned expertise domains are necessary for meaningful, professional report interpretation and they also are important a priori for efficient and relevant assay design and development.

Anyone with experience in the laboratory practice of genomic medicine will attest to the fact that next-generation sequencing-based assay implementation in the clinical laboratory takes longer and requires more resources than is anticipated, even with the most insightful a priori plans. Owing to the time that elapses from assay design to launch, and given the relatively rapid evolution of the biomarker space in oncology, before comprehensive genomic profiling availability, there needed to be carefully informed planning at the

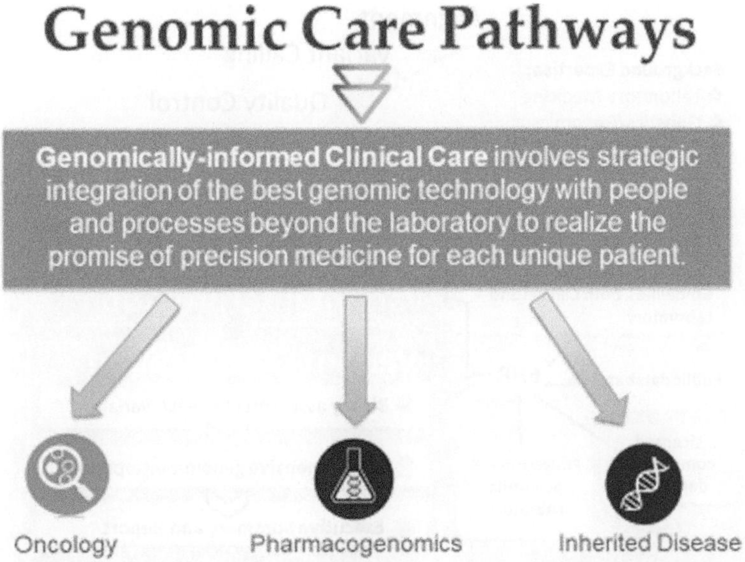

FIG. 3 The Genomic Care Pathway. When considering how to design a care pathway, it is useful to consider the test in terms of the patient population and health care category it will inform. It is then important to consider processes that support and enhance clinical workflow in the defined health care setting in parallel with intralaboratory test design and validation. From the molecular laboratory perspective, *simultaneous* effort to design a care pathway alongside the development and validation of a test is the logistical exercise for developing a genomic medicine service. It is the "care pathway" that significantly informs the components of the "service" that is supportive beyond the test.

early assay design phase to future proof the assay in anticipation for biomarker needs at the point of launch and beyond (Fig. 7). This is a challenging activity and if inaccurate predictions are made, then often times a laboratory is behind the times at the time of assay launch thereby having to invest more resources and time into iterative assay upgrades. At this point, comprehensive genomic profiling options inherently future proof assay development in this regard and in the end, are currently hypothesized to be an economically sound option for clinical laboratories with the mission to provide clinically relevant biomarker testing [12–14].

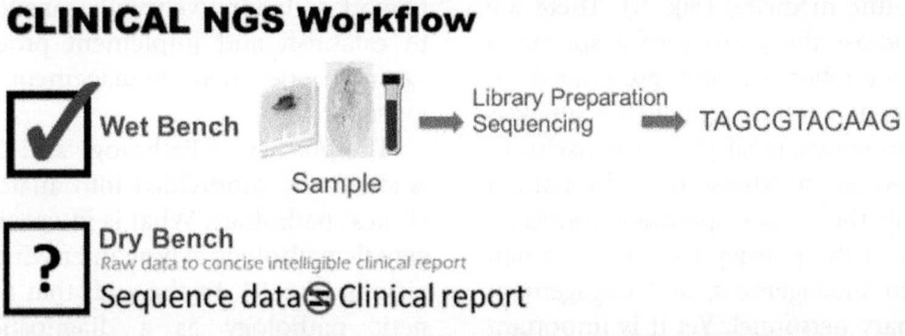

FIG. 4 Sequence data do not equal a clinical report. An assay that uses next-generation sequencing is composed of many workflow steps divided conceptually into the "wet bench" and the "dry bench". The "wet bench" includes all processes that involve working with a physical sample, from receipt of the accessioned sample to the generation of sequence. The "dry bench" includes all processes that involve working with the sequence data all the way through to medical interpretation culminating in report generation. Establishing processes for both benches that have consistent performance parameters is of foundational importance for the molecular diagnostics laboratory. The ultimate value of a genomic assay however is intimately related to the genomic service of *how* the assay information is "delivered" for use in the precision medicine ecosystem.

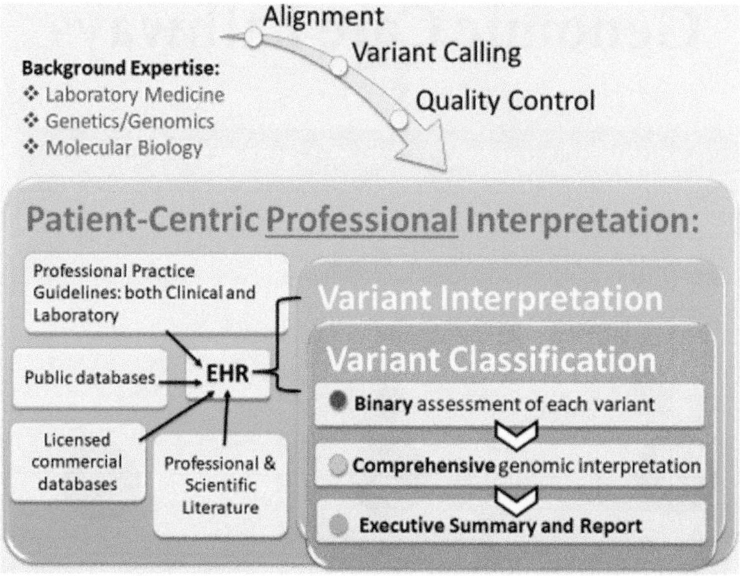

FIG. 5 Clinically relevant genomic testing requires professional interpretation. Genomic results are not binary. Each genomic assay generates results on more than one gene. It is not enough to report on each gene variant without considering and addressing the implications of co-occurring variants. Annotation requires laborious data mining for each variant and then for concomitant variant profiles. Pertinent information from the data sources must be extracted then interpreted based on the clinical profile of the patient. This process of ensuring pertinent data is reviewed, then how it is interpreted and whittled down to executive reporting statements is a professional activity. Clinically relevant genomic interpretation for precision medicine requires medical judgment and professional time commitment beyond that which is reflected in the G code.

Yet even when a laboratory can offer genomic testing that comprehensively interrogates clinically relevant biomarkers, assay performance is ultimately dependent on the specimen that is submitted for testing. This is why the concept of "tissue (or specimen) stewardship" is a key factor underlying successful genomic testing and practice of genomic medicine (Fig. 8). There are plenty of variables across the journey of a specimen from the patient to the laboratory that are critical for the reliability of next-generation sequencing analysis where standardization is beneficial [15]. It is useful to consider the specimen as an extension of the patient when conceptualizing the "tissue/specimen journey". In general, key steps of the journey include specimen acquisition, specimen management, and engagement of key multidisciplinary personnel. Yet it is important to have awareness that specimen journeys invariably differ according to local practices.

Of central importance for successful genomic analysis is the alignment of next-generation sequencing assay requirements with clinical and non-molecular pathology practice considerations. The transdisciplinary alignment is best served when there is investment in a champion of this effort. It is the role of the champion to identify, engage, and educate key personnel in the tissue/specimen journey about pertinent information related to specimen requirements for genomic testing and how successful testing underpins the delivery of genomic medicine. It is also the role of the champion to work collaboratively with transdisciplinary personnel to establish and implement procedures that ensure optimal specimen management across the tissue journey.

The practice of Pathology and Laboratory Medicine is classically subdivided into anatomic pathology and clinical pathology. What is interesting about molecular genetic pathology is how intertwined it is with both divisions (Fig. 9). In the end, that means molecular genetic pathology as a diagnostic practice is best delivered when the service being offered is informed by leadership that understands the lifecycle of specimens derived from both divisions. The concept of more information from less or the same amount of specimen is very well understood and generally a universal challenge regardless of practice type. Therefore, a molecular diagnostic professional with broad training

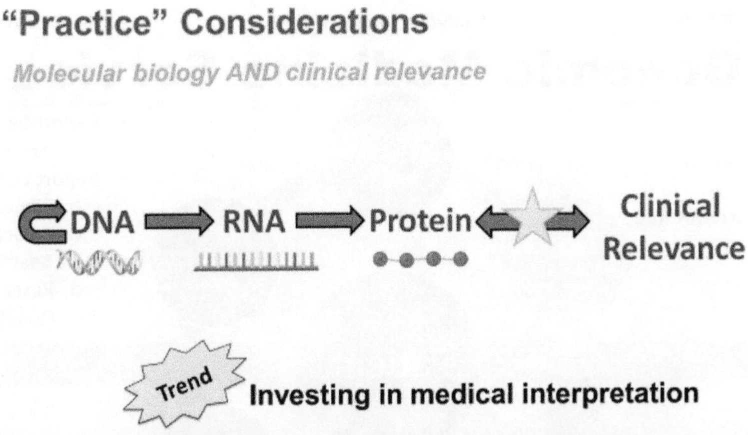

FIG. 6 Recoupling molecular biology and clinical expertise. A clinical assay that effectively interrogates the genome generates results that require medical interpretation for translation to clinical care. There is a high-stakes translation from assay output to report signout that requires a mastery of medical communication which underpins the effective translation of complex testing for clinical action. Understanding the complexity of the molecular biology, the strengths and limitations of next-generation sequencing, *and* up-to-date clinical implications of genomic results should not be "decoupled".

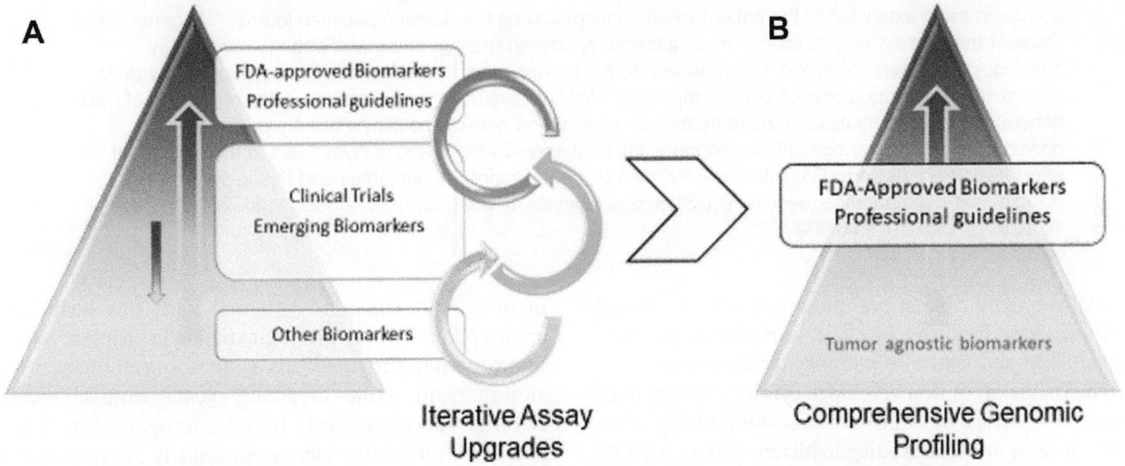

FIG. 7 The shift to comprehensive genomic profiling. Implementation of next-generation sequencing-based assays in the clinical laboratory typically takes longer and requires more resources than is anticipated. (***A***) Owing to time that elapses from assay design to launch, and given the relatively rapid evolution of the biomarker space in oncology, before comprehensive genomic profiling availability, there needed to be carefully informed planning at the early assay design phase to future proof the assay in anticipation for biomarker needs at the point of launch and beyond. This is a challenging activity and if inaccurate predictions are made, then oftentimes a laboratory is behind the times at the time of assay launch thereby having to invest more resources and time into iterative assay upgrades. (***B***) Comprehensive genomic profiling options inherently future proof assay development and are currently hypothesized to be an economically sound option for clinical laboratories with the mission to provide clinically relevant biomarker testing.

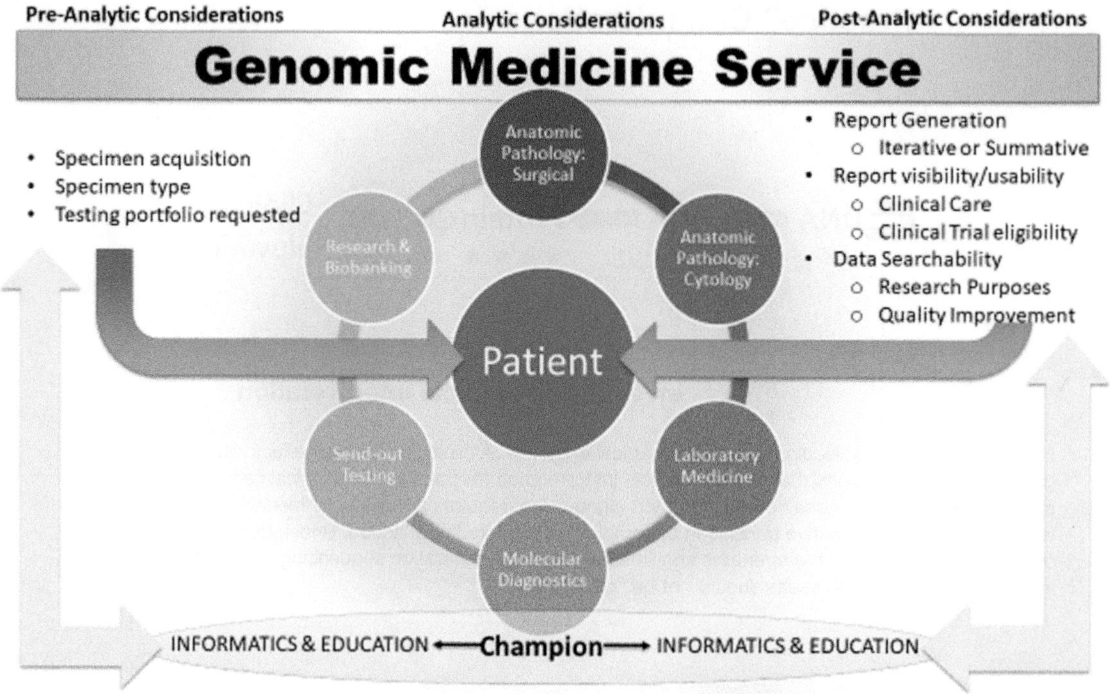

FIG. 8 The Tissue/Specimen Journey. Assay performance is ultimately dependent on the specimen that is submitted for testing. There are plenty of variables across the journey of a specimen from the patient to the laboratory that are critical for the reliability of next-generation sequencing analysis. It is useful to consider the specimen as an extension of the patient when conceptualizing the "tissue/specimen journey". In general, key steps of the journey include specimen acquisition, specimen management, and engagement of key multidisciplinary personnel. Yet it is important to have awareness that specimen journeys invariably differ according to local practices. Of central importance for successful genomic analysis is the alignment of next-generation sequencing assay requirements with clinical and non-molecular pathology practice considerations. The transdisciplinary alignment is best served when there is investment in a champion of this effort. *Data from* Ascierto PA, Bifulco C, Palmieri G, et al. Preanalytic variables and tissue stewardship for reliable next-generation sequencing (NGS) clinical analysis. *J Mol Diagn*. 2019 Sep; 21(5): 756-767. doi: 10.1016/j.jmoldx.2019.05.004

in anatomic *and* clinical pathology (as well as clinical training) is well-poised to champion tissue/specimen stewardship and lead care pathway development.

The inclusion of non-cell block cytology material for genomic analysis of solid tumors wonderfully illustrates how a molecular diagnostician, when broadly trained in anatomic pathology, can bring value to a genomic medicine service. Cytopathology is a subdivision of anatomic pathology and while it can be practiced with subspecialty fellowship training and board certification via the American Board of Pathology, it can also be incorporated into practice following anatomic pathology residency with subsequent board certification. Fine needle aspiration is a commonly used cytologic technique to obtain diagnostic material in oncology. The cells obtained with this technique are prepared for morphologic diagnosis using a variety of cytopreparatory methods aside from cell block preparation. And while for many years, non-cell block cytology specimens were broadly recognized as a rich source of tumor, the relative complexity of cytopreparation was a barrier to specimen acceptability for molecular diagnostics [16].

As there is increasingly more information required from small biopsy specimens for the practice of genomically-informed oncologic care of solid tumors, it is important to validate genomic testing for all relevant sources of tumor material. It behooves molecular professionals to have a keen awareness of cytopathology and anatomic pathology practices to thereby

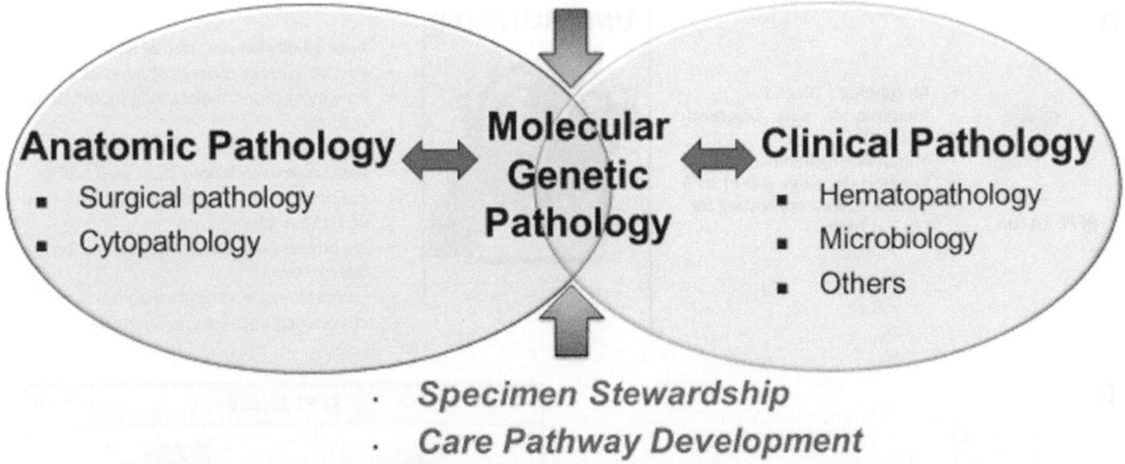

FIG. 9 Organizational structure considerations for the practice of Pathology and Laboratory Medicine. The practice of pathology and laboratory medicine many times is divided into anatomic pathology and clinical pathology each of which has subdivisions. The practice of molecular genetic pathology, when considered broadly, is intimately intertwined with both divisions. The organizational structure of molecular genetic pathology within the overall organizational chart can have significant implications for practice performance.

establish carefully coordinated validation studies that can unlock access to cytology material prepared in ways other than cell blocks (Fig. 10). These specimens have been shown to have superior nucleic acid quality when compared with that derived from formalin-fixed paraffin-embedded tissue and when incorporated into genomic analysis, result in lower quantity not sufficient rates [16].

Many of the concepts considered thus far illustrate the complexity of the "laboratory" and the laboratory's intricate interactions with stakeholders beyond the laboratory. To build a successful genomic medicine program, there must be investment in a champion of the program. This calls for an awareness of and commitment to the significant time and effort that is required to operationalize a program, much if not all of which is not reimbursable in the current health care delivery system. Yet it is imperative to recognize that even with all the aforementioned support and resources, even the best implementation team will fall short if there is not a significant investment in relevant clinical informatics. This is not the same as the dry-bench and bioinformatics in the laboratory. As defined by the American Medical Informatics Association (AMIA), "Clinical Informatics is the application of informatics and information technology to deliver healthcare services. It is also referred to as applied clinical informatics and operational informatics" [17].

The champion has a duty to educate leadership about the foundational need to support clinical informatics underpinning a genomic medicine program. Ideally, it is advised that all business plans for precision or genomic medicine programs include significant resources for information services, inclusive of supportive personnel. In addition, it is imperative that the champion engages with information services leadership to understand local processes and thereby inform business and implementation planning for genomic medicine.

Informatics and the associated information systems are foundational for complex laboratory testing and transdisciplinary communication throughout the tissue/specimen journey [3,18]. Efforts to establish a genomic medicine service, which underpins the effective delivery of precision medicine, will be stunted and delayed without parallel approval of necessary information services. Delays equate to inefficient use of limited resources and ultimately risk eroding institutional morale.

Informed implementation of information systems to support the clinical informatics of precision medicine not only support the laboratory practice of the genomic testing. These systems are the necessary infrastructure that support highly complex clinical communication and also serve quality control, quality assurance, and ongoing quality improvement endeavors [19]. This concept may seem distant and relatively simple,

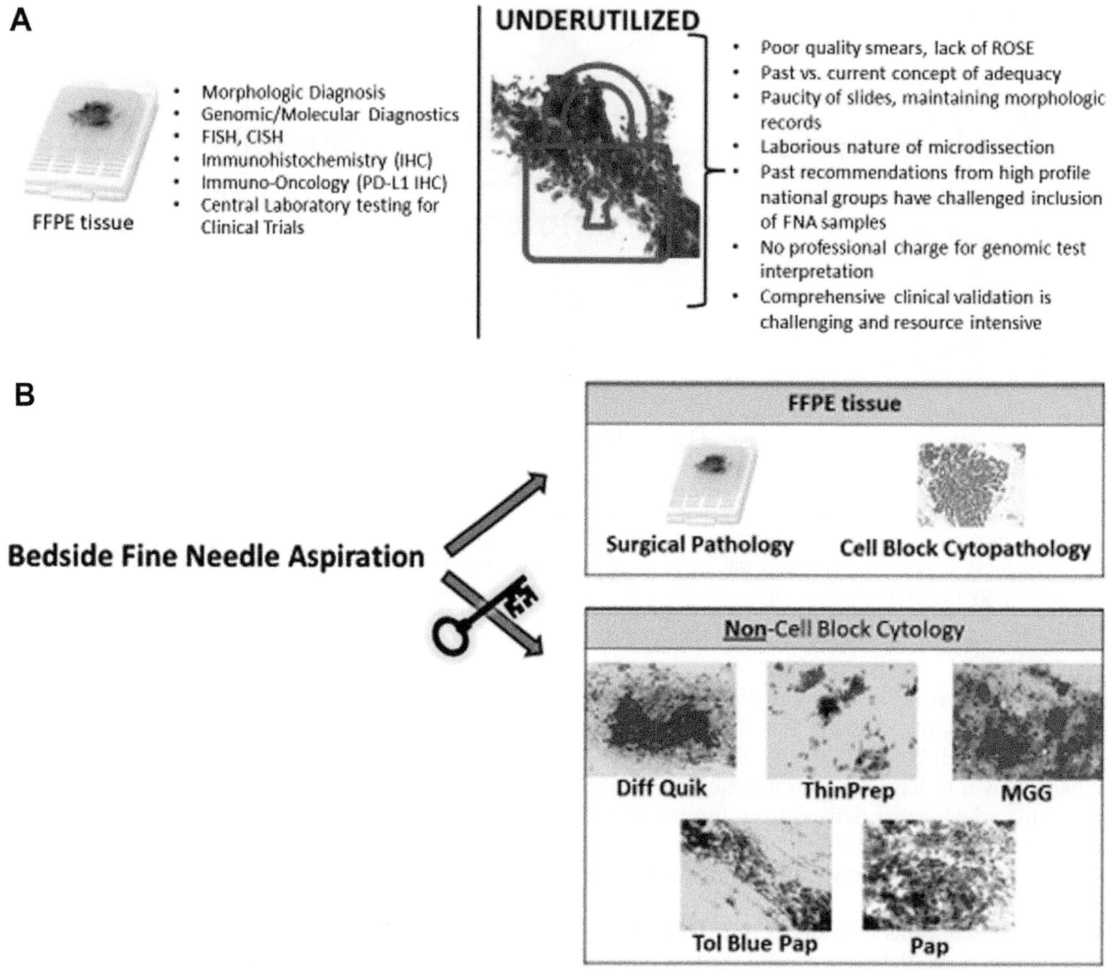

FIG. 10 Tissue/Specimen stewardship—An example of optimization. Non-cell block cytology specimens are broadly recognized as a rich source of tumor. (***A***) Commonly perceived barriers to utilization of non-cell block cytology specimens for molecular diagnostic testing. (***B***) When properly validated for specimen acceptability in genomic analysis, a previously underutilized category of specimens mitigates "quantity not sufficient" rates for genomic analysis and alleviates uncertainty and consternation during bedside FNA procedures regarding specimen collection and triage. Original magnification: Cell block ×40; Non-cell block cytology ×100. FFPE, formalin-fixed paraffin-embedded; ROSE, rapid on-site evaluation; FISH, fluorescent in-situ hybridization; CISH, chromogenic in-situ hybridization; Diff Quik, Differential Quik; MGG, May Grünwald Giemsa; Tol Blue Pap, Toluidine Blue, subsequent Progressive Gill's-modified Papanicolaou stain; Pap, Papanicolaou stain.

especially when getting into the business of bringing on clinical next-generation sequencing and building a service to deliver genomics for bedside care. Although there have been many key considerations beyond the test addressed herein, it is probably fair to assume the most underestimated facet of this topic at large is the effort, energy, and expertise necessary to implement information systems to support a genomic medicine program. As the background expertise necessary to inform this aspect of implementing genomic medicine is difficult to obtain without dedicated informatics practice or a fellowship in clinical informatics, one consideration for laboratories is the investment in a laboratory systems architect. This expertise, so long as it bridges similar expertise outside of the laboratory, has the potential to serve the laboratory both for and

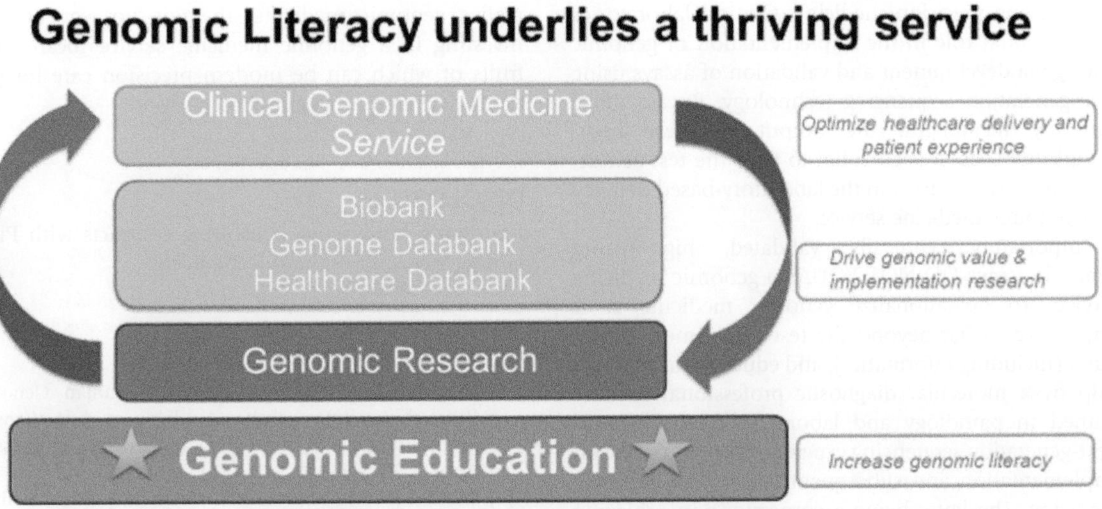

FIG. 11 Genomic literacy. A genomic medicine service can certainly optimize health care delivery and the patient experience. Genomic testing in the clinical laboratory generates rich data that drive genomic-based research which has significant potential to drive policy change related to the practice and adoption of precision medicine. However, of foundational importance, not only to facilitate implementation but also to foster sustained adoption of genomic medicine, is "genomic literacy". The latter requires a sustained commitment to genomic education.

beyond molecular diagnostics, the potential value of which is not to be underestimated.

Lastly, of foundational importance, not only to facilitate implementation but also to foster sustained adoption of genomic medicine, is "genomic literacy" [20]. *Implementation* of genomic medicine is a multifaceted process that occurs in a "precision medicine ecosystem". It requires building applications and procedures and onboarding supportive technology for clinical use in the practice of precision medicine. As the implementation of genomic medicine is resource intensive and may be viewed as disruptive, it is reasonable to expect that as the level of genomic literacy among the stakeholders increases, so does the efficiency of implementation. Yet implementation can still occur without widespread genomic literacy among potential stakeholders. *Adoption* of genomic medicine on the other hand happens when pertinent members of the ecosystem *use* genomic information and services to practice precision medicine. For adoption to occur, genomic literacy is essential.

Raising the level of genomic literacy is complex [21]. The education necessary to do so should be a *sustained* effort best delivered in a localized fashion whereby educational champions are adequately supported in this role and professional rapport can be established. Having a clinical service can certainly optimize health care delivery and the patient experience. The testing in the clinical laboratory generates rich data and can drive genomic-based research and hopefully drive reimbursement and policy decisions. However, return on investment to implement genomic medicine can only truly occur when there is adoption of genomics in clinical practice and the latter is founded upon genomic literacy across stakeholders (Fig. 11). It should be mentioned that payers should also be considered as stakeholders in genomic medicine, the adoption of which is best served when the educational champion also proactively engages with payers to educate not only about the clinical assay but importantly around assay delivery. It is therefore worthwhile and necessary to identify a champion of institutional genomic literacy. When genomic testing is delivered in the context of a genomic medicine service as described herein, molecular diagnostic professionals with expertise that bridges non-molecular facets of the laboratory and clinic are very well-poised to champion genomic education.

SUMMARY

Precision medicine describes a health care delivery model that goes beyond genomics to optimize health care provided to individual patients [3,22]. Yet clinical-grade genomic information is a key component of achieving precision medicine. Clinical laboratories play a central role in the implementation of genomic testing via development and validation of assays using next-generation sequencing technology. But to make clinically meaningful the output of these high-complexity tests, it is essential to view the test as one, albeit important, factor in the laboratory-based delivery of a genomic medicine service.

Importantly, clinically validated, high-quality genomic assays DO NOT EQUAL a genomic medicine service. To operationalize genomic medicine, it is imperative to "go beyond the test". Specimen, procedural (including informatics), and educational stewardship by a molecular diagnostic professional broadly trained in pathology and laboratory medicine with next-generation sequencing expertise is key to successful implementation and subsequent *adoption* of genomic medicine. The latter being a cornerstone in achieving the health care delivery model of precision medicine.

First and foremost, it is important to consider and define the local "precision medicine ecosystem". Genomic medicine requires collective, transdisciplinary resolve but the realization of collective resolve and operationalizing a genomic medicine service requires a champion. After establishing this framework, it is prudent to engage key stakeholders and obtain commitment from leadership since the latter is foundational for the implementation of genomics into health care.

Currently, the value of molecular diagnostic professionals in realizing the return on investment in genomic testing is generally under-recognized. These professionals are poised to champion the value-added components of a genomic medicine service as addressed herein. Much of the value lies in the informed design of care pathways supportive beyond an assay and the effort to increase genomic literacy within the precision medicine ecosystem. However, the current system does not incentivize the efforts necessary to perform these service-related duties.

The first step in resolving this fundamental system-based challenge requires awareness of the points addressed in this article. Significant work related to each facet of a genomic medicine service is currently underway and the field at large can benefit from more focused reports on related outcomes of such efforts. Lastly, it bears repeating that informatics and education underpin all efforts in precision medicine. There is an ever-present struggle between insourcing genomic analysis and thereby investing in the distributed model of genomics, versus sending this work out and thereby investing in a centralized model of genomics. Although the latter may seem like an "easier" solution, to truly realize genomic medicine, there is no way around investing in a genomic medicine service locally, the fruits of which can be modern precision care for patients delivered in an equitable fashion.

DISCLOSURE

I currently hold active consulting contracts with PierianDx, Merck, Bayer, and Genentech.

REFERENCES

[1] Genomics and medicine. National Human Genome Research Institute website. Available at: https://www.genome.gov/health/Genomics-and-Medicine [Accessed April 3, 2021].

[2] Table of pharmacogenomic biomarkers in drug labeling. U.S. Food and Drug Administration website. 2021. Available at: https://www.fda.gov/drugs/science-and-research-drugs/table-pharmacogenomic-biomarkers-drug-labeling [Accessed April 3, 2021].

[3] Ginsburg GS, Phillips KA. Precision medicine: from science to value. Health Aff (Millwood) 2018;37(5):694–701.

[4] Sireci AN, Patel JL, Joseph L, et al. Molecular pathology economics 101: an overview of molecular diagnostics coding, coverage, and reimbursement a report of the association for molecular pathology. J Mol Diagn 2020;22(8):975–93.

[5] Hsiao SJ, Mansukhani MM, Carter MC, et al. The history and impact of molecular coding changes on coverage and reimbursement of molecular diagnostic tests: transition from stacking codes to the current molecular code set including genomic sequencing procedures. J Mol Diagn 2018;20(2):177–83.

[6] Wolf J, Seto T, Han J, et al. Capmatinib in *MET* exon 14-mutated or *MET*-amplified non-small-cell lung cancer. N Engl J Med 2020;383(10):944–57.

[7] NCCN Clinical Practice Guidelines in Oncology Non-Small Cell Lung Cancer, NCCN Evidence Blocks Version 4.2021. National Comprehensive Cancer Network website. 2021. Available at: https://www.nccn.org/professionals/physician_gls/pdf/nscl_blocks.pdf [Accessed April 4, 2021].

[8] Awad M. Impaired c-Met receptor degradation mediated by *MET* exon 14 mutations in non-small-cell lung cancer. J Clin Oncol 2016;34(8):879–81.

[9] Frampton GM, Ali SM, Rosenzweig M, et al. Activation of MET via diverse exon 14 splicing alterations occurs in multiple tumor types and confers clinical sensitivity to MET inhibitors. Cancer Discov 2015;5(8):850–9.

[10] Davies KD, Aprille L, Lawrence CA, et al. DNA-based versus RNA-based detection of *MET* exon 14 skipping events in lung cancer. J Thorac Oncol 2019;14(4):737–41.

[11] Benayed R, Offin M, Mullaney K, et al. High yield of RNA sequencing for targetable kinase fusions in lung adenocarcinomas with no mitogenic driver alteration detected by DNA sequencing and low tumor mutation burden. Clin Cancer Res 2019;25(15):4712–22.

[12] Johnston KM, Sheffield BS, Yip S, et al. Comprehensive genomic profiling for non-small-cell lung cancer: health and budget impact. Curr Oncol 2020;27(6):569–77.

[13] Signorovitch J, Zhou Z, Ryan J, et al. Budget impact analysis of comprehensive genomic profiling in patients with advanced non-small cell lung cancer. J Med Econ 2019; 22(2):140–50.

[14] The personalized medicine report, 2020: opportunity, challenges, and the future. Personalized Medicine Coalition website. Available at: http://www.personalizedmedicinecoalition.org/Userfiles/PMC-Corporate/file/PMC_The_Personalized_Medicine_Report_Opportunity_Challenges_and_the_Future.pdf [Accessed April 10, 2021].

[15] Ascierto PA, Bifulco C, Palmieri G, et al. Preanalytic variables and tissue stewardship for reliable next-generation sequencing (NGS) clinical analysis. J Mol Diagn 2019; 21(5):756–67.

[16] Balla A, Hampel KJ, Sharma MK, et al. Comprehensive validation of cytology specimens for next-generation sequencing and clinical practice experience. J Mol Diagn 2018;20(6):812–21.

[17] Clinical Informatics. American Medical Informatics Association website. Available at: https://www.amia.org/applications-informatics/clinical-informatics#:~:text=Clinical%20Informatics-,Clinical%20Informatics%20is%20the%20application%20of%20informatics%20and%20information%20technology,clinical%20informatics%20and%20operational%20informatics &text=Clinical%20Informatics%20is%20concerned%20with%20information%20use%20in%20health%20care%20by%20clinicians [Accessed April 10, 2021].

[18] Roy S, LaFramboise WA, Nikiforov YE, et al. Next-generation sequencing informatics: challenges and strategies for implementation in a clinical environment. Arch Pathol Lab Med 2016;140(9):958–75.

[19] Sepulveda JL, Young DS. The ideal laboratory information system. Arch Pathol Lab Med 2013;137(8): 1129–40.

[20] Hurle B, Citrin T, Jenkins JF, et al. What does it mean to be genomically literate?: National Human Genome Research Institute Meeting Report. Genet Med 2013; 15(8):658–63.

[21] Bangash H, Kullo IJ. Implementation science to increase adoption of genomic medicine: an urgent need. J Pers Med 2021;11(1):19.

[22] National Research Council, Committee on A Framework for Developing a New Taxonomy of Disease. Toward precision medicine: building a Knowledge Network for Biomedical research and a New Taxonomy of Disease. Washington DC: National Academies Press; 2011.

Advances in Molecular Pathology 4 (2021) 187–198
ADVANCES IN MOLECULAR PATHOLOGY

Cell-free Nucleic Acids in Cancer

Current Approaches, Challenges, and Future Directions

Liron Barnea Slonim, MD, Kathy A. Mangold, PhD, Mir B. Alikhan, MD, Nora Joseph, MD, Kalpana S. Reddy, MD, Linda M. Sabatini, PhD, Karen L. Kaul, MD PhD*
Department of Pathology and Laboratory Medicine, NorthShore University HealthSystem, 2650 Ridge Avenue, Evanston, IL 60201

KEYWORDS
• Cell-free DNA • ctDNA • Companion diagnostics • PCR • Early detection • Liquid biopsy

KEY POINTS

- Tumors shed fragmented DNA and nucleic acids into the blood, generally during apoptosis.
- Technical advances now allow highly sensitive detection of tumor genomic alterations in a background of normal DNA.
- Cell-free DNA is a potential new tool for the clinical assessment of human tumors resistance.

Histologic and cytologic evaluation of tissue and cells remains the mainstay of cancer diagnosis and assessment, though pathologists have long worked to develop novel and improved approaches. Indeed, many biopsy and tissue sampling protocols, new immunostains, and other molecular assays have been implemented over the years to improve cancer detection and management. Recent technologic advances have allowed the evaluation of genomic change in tumor-derived nucleic acids found in blood samples, opening the door to a potentially extremely impactful and minimally invasive method for the detection and characterization of cancer.

Cell-free DNA (cfDNA) has been used for clinical purposes for a decade or more; noninvasive prenatal testing (NIPT) has become routine for screening at 10 to 12 weeks gestation [1,2]. cfDNA enters the blood following apoptosis—of normal cells, inflammatory cells, cells from the placenta, or tumor cells. Initial applications of NIPT focused on the detection of numeric chromosomal abnormalities such as trisomy 21, but more sensitive methods such as next-generation sequencing allow detection of other genetic abnormalities as well. The proportion of fetal DNA in maternal blood during pregnancy is at least tenfold greater than circulating tumor DNA (ctDNA) when present; however, NIPT has in many respects paved the way for current efforts in the detection and characterization of cell-free tumor DNA.

Although tumor-derived DNA can enter the bloodstream following cellular necrosis or by active secretion, the majority appears to arise from apoptosis, based on the size correspondence to nucleosomes [3,4]. The typical fragment size approximates 166 bp, though smaller and larger fragments can also be recovered. Newer analytical approaches are ideal for these smaller fragments.

Different tumor types show variable release of cfDNA fragments, which has a great impact on the clinical sensitivity of these tests. Bladder, colorectal, gastroesophageal, and ovarian cancers show the highest amount of plasma cfDNA, whereas little is detectable from glioma and thyroid tumors [5]. Furthermore, detection of cfDNA rises with the stage tumor [5]. The impact of other factors such as timing, treatment, and various histologic features remains unknown.

*Corresponding author, *E-mail address:* kkaul@northshore.org

https://doi.org/10.1016/j.yamp.2021.07.007
2589-4080/21/

PREANALYTICAL REQUIREMENTS

Successful liquid biopsy analysis starts in the preanalytical phase. This includes use of the appropriate specimen, proper collection and processing, and storage [3,6,7] to provide sufficient cfDNA or RNA for analysis. Many biofluids (sputum, CSF, and more) can be used as liquid biopsy specimens [8,9], but blood is the most common source. Early studies used serum samples instead of plasma because of a greater yield of total cfDNA, but the fraction of ctDNA is actually less because of DNA release from leukocytes during blood clotting; most studies therefore favor plasma [10,11]. Cellular lysis should be avoided during blood collection using proper phlebotomy technique [7,12]. Frozen whole blood is not acceptable because of hemolysis.

The biofluid should be processed quickly [12]; standard EDTA tubes can be used for plasma if processing will occur within 6 hours (optimally 1–3 hr); longer delays result in hemolysis and lymphocyte lysis as well as reduced plasma volume [7]. Specialized tubes containing stabilizers can extend the preprocessing time up to 14 days (3 days optimum) [11–15]. Within these time limits, several studies showed equivalent ctDNA yield and variant allele frequency (VAF) when either EDTA or specialized tubes were used [7,11,14,16]. Although some analyses have reported success with very low plasma volume, 1 mL of plasma on average yields only 3000 whole genomic equivalents [17]. If a typical 10 mL blood draw yields 4 mL of plasma, a theoretic assay sensitivity of ~0.01% would detect only one ctDNA copy among 12,000 wild-type copies, corresponding to an ~1 cm^3 tumor, assuming that early-stage tumor is actively shedding ctDNA into the bloodstream. To increase the amount of ctDNA available for variant analysis, increasing the plasma input volume and minimizing the extraction volume optimizes the downstream ctDNA analysis without altering the VAF [15,17–19].

Processing blood samples begins with 2 centrifugation steps for at least 10 minutes each [7]. The first low *g* force centrifugation separates the plasma from cells without damaging the latter (200–2500 × *g*). The second centrifugation (1600–18,400 × *g*) reduces cellular genomic DNA in the final sample. No statistically significant changes between the varied *g* forces have been found for either cfDNA yield or VAF [16]. If necessary, a second high-speed centrifugation can be performed if single-spun samples were stored frozen to obtain useable cfDNA [20–22]. The spun plasma should be stored at −80°C with minimal freeze-thaws [12].

The final preanalytical step is cfDNA extraction. Although greater than 40 cfDNA extraction kits are available, the most used remains QIAamp Circulating Nucleic Acid Kit (Qiagen, Germantown, MD, USA) [7]. Note that cfDNA sizes obtained may differ between kits, and the significance of this is unknown [3,7,23,24]. Some extraction kits recover all DNA in the sample, including high molecular weight DNA from cellular lysis, protected DNA in tri-, di-, and mononucleosomes, or even less than 100 bp fragmented DNA, as well as smaller circulating mitochondrial DNA not protected by histones [25]. Most analyses rely on the ~166 bp fragments corresponding to protected DNA in mononucleosomes [4] with minimal extraction volumes to increase ctDNA concentrations [7]. The flexibility shown above in preanalytical steps will permit successful transfer to the clinical testing environment, but standardization will enhance downstream analyses [12].

TECHNICAL APPROACHES

Detection of ctDNA is challenging because of the presence of normal cfDNA and the need to discriminate normal from tumor, the low levels of ctDNA, and the need to quantify the mutant fragments in a sample [26]. Many strategies have been used and include both limited and broad candidate gene panels, and less commonly whole exome and whole genome approaches. Single or limited gene panels require less DNA and can detect mutations with good sensitivity [27]. Although sensitivity is an advantage, these methods may be limited in their ability to detect novel genomic changes. Broader ctDNA analysis includes large gene panels and exome- and genome-wide analysis of mutations [28], require more ctDNA and have lower sensitivity and therefore would be less useful for early stage and MRD situations. Select commercially available methods are described in Table 1.

Limited Target Analysis

Many limited target assays exist and are often PCR-based platforms concentrating on one or few targets, such as specific hotspot mutational variants in a small panel of genes in the context of a specific type of cancer (eg, *EGFR* in non-small cell lung cancer [NSCLC]; Table 1).

Digital PCR is an ultrasensitive, quantitative method to detect point mutations in ctDNA at low allele fractions. Digital PCR includes ddPCR and BEAMing; in both, the sample is split into nanoliter droplets, which partition parallel fluorescence-emitting PCR reactions

TABLE 1
Examples of commercially available ctDNA detection assays

Test name	Category	Targets	Purpose	Test specifications/ Technology
cobas® EGFR Mutation Test v2[a]	Multiplex real-time PCR	*EGFR* mutations: exon 19 deletions; L858R in exon 21; T790M in exon 20; G719X in exon 18; S768I in exon 20; exon 20 insertion mutations; L861Q in exon 21	Qualitative detection of defined mutations of *EGFR* in cfDNA from plasma in NSCLC patients and formalin-fixed, paraffin-embedded (FFPE)	Allele-specific PCR amplification and fluorescent detection.
therascreen PIK3CA RGQ PCR test[b]	Multiplex real-time PCR	*PIK3CA* gene mutations: Exon 7: C420R; Exon 9: E542K, E545A, E545D [1635G>T only], E545G, E545K, Q546E, Q546R; and Exon 20: H1047L, H1047R, H1047Y.	Qualitative PCR test for the detection of *PIK3CA* gene mutations ctDNA from plasma (or tumor FFPE) of patients with breast cancer	Fluorescent detection using mutation-specific PCR primers.
FoundationOne® Liquid CDx[c]	NGS (hybridization-based capture)	Substitutions, insertions, and deletions (indels) in 311 genes, rearrangements in 3 genes (*ALK, BRCA1, BRCA2*), and copy number variations in 3 genes (*BRCA1, BRCA2, ERBB2*).	FDA approved for detection of *BRCA1/ BRCA2* alterations in metastatic castration-resistant prostate cancer and patients with epithelial ovarian cancer; *EGFR* activating mutations (Exon 19 deletions and L858R) in patients with advanced and metastatic NSCLC; *ALK* rearrangements in NSCLC; *PIK3CA* mutations patients with breast cancer	A whole-genome indexed library is amplified from plasma cfDNA Hybridization-based capture of all coding exons of 309 genes with select intronic regions of 3 genes. Deep sequencing performed using the NovaSeq6000 platform. A subset of targeted regions in 75 genes is baited for added sensitivity.
Guardant360® CDx[d]	NGS (hybridization-based capture)	Single nucleotide variants, insertions and deletions in 55 genes, copy number amplifications in 2 genes (*ERBB2, MET*), and fusions in 4 genes (*ALK, NTRK1, RET, ROS1*)	FDA approved for identification of *EGFR* exon 19 deletions, *EGFR* L858R, and *EGFR* T790M in NSCLC patients	Barcoded library construction/ amplification from cfDNA, with NGS on the Illumina NextSeq 550. Alterations in 55 genes are reported.
Ion Torrent Oncomine[TM e]	NGS (amplicon-based method)	Five different tumor type–specific assays (10–12 genes) or a 52-gene pan-cancer assay, are available.	Focused disease specific (lung, breast, or colon cancer) or comprehensive pan-	For the pan-cancer assay, a single library is constructed from plasma cfDNA and RNA following

(*continued on next page*)

TABLE 1
(*continued*)

Test name	Category	Targets	Purpose	Test specifications/ Technology
		The latter covers >900 hotspots and insertion deletions, 96 fusions 12 copy number variants and MET exon 14 skipping	cancer genomic profiling	multiplex PCR. 272 amplicons are used, and sequencing is performed on the Ion GeneStudio S5. A quick 2-d turnaround time is enabled by this approach. Variants present at an allele frequency as low as 0.1% can be detected with a 20 ng DNA input.
Illumina TruSight™ Oncology 500 ctDNA[f]	NGS (hybridization-based capture)	Analysis of the full coding sequence of 523 genes for single nucleotide variants, insertions and deletions, copy number variants and fusions. Microsatellite instability and tumor mutational burden are also assessed	Pan-cancer comprehensive genomic profiling	This method combines UMIs for library construction. Sequencing is performed on the NovaSeq 6000. Error correction software (and UMI use) enable error rate reduction even at low VAFs. 30 ng of cfDNA are required. With 30 ng, the analytical sensitivity at 0.2% VAF is 82.59% at 15,000× raw coverage depth.
BIO-RAD ddPCR™ Mutation Detection Assays[g]	digital droplet PCR	Primers can be designed for over >400 mutations from the COSMIC database, >200 validated targets for detection of KRAS G12/G13, KRAS Q61, NRAS G12, NRAS G12/G13, NRAS Q61, BRAF V600 mutations and EGFR exon 19 deletions, with other designs available. Copy number variant detection for >700 variants and 60 targets available	Detection/quantification of genomic alterations including mutations and copy number variations. This test has multiple other applications (such as gene expression profiling, or DNA quantification before NGS)	Emulsion droplet amplification of cfDNA fragments fluorescence detection to quantify the amount of target DNA 5 ng of plasma cfDNA is required to detect a mutation present at 0.2%.

(*continued on next page*)

TABLE 1
(*continued*)

Test name	Category	Targets	Purpose	Test specifications/ Technology
OncoBEAM[h]	BEAM (beads, emulsion, amplification, magnetics), a form of digital PCR	Available formats: (tumor-specific) Acute myeloid leukemia glioma breast cancer colorectal cancer lung cancer, melanoma, pancreatic cancer, prostatic cancer Single gene tests: AKT1, ALK, AR, BRAF, EGFR, ESR1, IDH1 IDH2, KRAS, NRAS, PIK3CA, and ROS1. Multigene tests: AKT1, ESR1, PIK3CA; ALK-ROS; BRAF-EGFR-KRAS; BRAF-KRAS-NRAS; BRAF-NRAS; IDH1-IDH2.	Detection and quantification of mutations	cfDNA from plasma is multiplex amplified using primers of specific regions of interest. Amplicons are bead captured and further amplified using emulsion PCR. Fluorescent flow cytometric assessment of the proportions of WT/ mutant DNA. Reported sensitivity ranges from 0.1% to 0.02% depending on the specific assay and sample.

Abbreviation: UMIs, unique molecular identifiers.

[a] Administration UFaD. cobas EGFR Mutation Test v2. https://www.accessdata.fda.gov/cdrh_docs/pdf15/P150047A.pdf. Published 2016. Accessed April 28, 2021, 2021.

[b] Administration UFaD. therascreen PIK3CA RGQ PCR kit. https://www.accessdata.fda.gov/cdrh_docs/pdf19/P190004A.pdf. Published 2019. Accessed April 28, 2021, 2021.

[c] Administration UFaD. FoundationOne Liquid CDx (F1 Liquid CDx). https://www.accessdata.fda.gov/cdrh_docs/pdf20/P200016A.pdf. Published 2020. Accessed April 28, 2021, 2021.

[d] Administration UFaD. Guardant360CDx. https://www.accessdata.fda.gov/cdrh_docs/pdf20/P200010A.pdf. Published 2020. Accessed April 28, 2021, 2021.

[e] Thermo Fisher Scientific Inc. Ion Torrent Oncomine. https://www.thermofisher.com/order/catalog/product/A37664?SID=srch-srp-A37664#/A37664?SID=srch-srp-A37664. Accessed April 28, 2021, 2021.

[f] Illumina Inc. TruSight Oncology 500. https://www.illumina.com/products/by-type/clinical-research-products/trusight-oncology-500.html. Accessed April 28, 2021, 2021.

[g] Bio-Rad Laboratories Inc. ddPCR mutation detection assays, Validated. https://www.bio-rad.com/webroot/web/pdf/lsr/literature/10033487.pdf. Published 2015. Accessed April 28, 2021, 2021.

[h] Sysmex Inostics I. OncoBEAM: Benchmark-Setting Liquid Biopsy Technology. https://www.sysmex-inostics.com/sysmex-onco-beam-technology-overview. Accessed April 28, 2021, 2021.

each amplifying a single DNA molecule from the sample. Fluorescence is measured by flow cytometry [28,29].

Broader Genomic Analysis

NGS-based broad gene panel testing is widely performed using LDPs, kits from the main NGS platform providers Illumina (TruSight Oncology 500 ctDNA) and Ion-Torrent (Oncomine cfDNA) and by some commercial labs (eg, Guardant, Foundation One (see Table 1). Some NGS-based methods have incorporated further modifications to increase the sensitivity of ctDNA detection, as described below.

Cancer personalized profiling by deep sequencing (CAPP-seq) is a targeted NGS-based method in which patient-specific genomic alterations are first identified then sought in cfDNA. This method optimizes library preparation for low DNA input, allows tracking of multiple mutations per patient, and achieves low levels of detection [30]. The CAPP-Seq method has been used to assess plasma ctDNA in NSCLC for both disease monitoring and minimal residual disease detection with ctDNA detection rates [31]. The sensitivity can be further increased when combined with integrated digital error suppression, a computational error correction method that uses molecular barcoding and removes nonbiological background errors introduced during library preparation and sequencing for the efficient recovery of cfDNA molecules [32].

Targeted error correction sequencing (TEC-Seq) allows ultrasensitive evaluation of sequence changes in cfDNA using massively parallel sequencing directed at a panel of 58 cancer-related genes. This method has proven sensitive for early-stage colorectal, breast, lung, and ovarian cancer, in which somatic mutations were detected in 71%, 59%, 59%, and 68%, respectively, in the plasma of patients with stage I or II disease [33].

Safe-Seq is an NGS approach that incorporates unique molecular identifiers (UMIs or UIDs) to each DNA molecule in the sample to identify duplicate reads of that molecule. The use of UMIs allows for error correction and enables the detection and quantification of rare mutations, and this approach is now commonly used in cfDNA NGS platforms [34].

TAm-Seq (Tagged-amplicon deep sequencing) [35] is used for deep sequencing of genomic regions spanning thousands of bases from as little as a single copy of fragmented DNA. This technique uses a combination of short amplicons, two-step amplification, sample barcodes, and high-throughput PCR. Because the first-round amplicons are short, this method effectively amplifies even small amounts of fragmented DNA. The two-step amplification includes a limited-cycle preamplification step where all primer sets are used to capture the starting molecules present in the sample, followed by individual amplification specific for intended targets. This permits primer multiplexing which enables amplification and sequencing of relatively large genomic regions by tiling short amplicons without loss of fidelity. Duplicate sequencing of each sample is performed to avoid incorporation of PCR errors. Allele frequencies as low as 0.2% can be detected with this method with reported sensitivity and specificity of greater than 97% [35].

In addition to the aforementioned methods, enrichment steps used before NGS can be used to greatly improve ctDNA analysis yield. Multiplex PCR (mPCR) provides an alternative to capture hybridization for targeted NGS. This enrichment technique is used in the CancerSEEK platform and the Tracking Cancer Evolution Through Therapy (TRACERx) platform (Signatera) [36]. In this mPCR approach, each template molecule is uniquely labeled with a DNA barcode, minimizing errors and enabling the use of small amounts of cfDNA. The reaction is divided into multiple aliquots and the assay is performed independently on each replicate, thus increasing sensitivity and the signal-to-noise ratio [36].

Other Markers Found in Plasma

DNA methylation changes are implicated in carcinogenesis and tumor progression, and can be used as a biomarker detectable in ctDNA [37,38]. Most methods use bisulfite to convert nonmethylated cytosine residues to uracil. The target can then be sequenced and methylation can be assessed and compared to a standard [39]. This can be performed on a whole genome level (methylome), or for specific biologically relevant CpG islands [38,40]. Differential methylation patterns are also used for the enrichment of ctDNA to enhance sensitivity and specificity, such as the platform designed by GRAIL technologies [41].

MicroRNA (miRNA) expression profiles serve as biomarkers for prognosis or even classification of certain cancers [42–44]. Circulating free or exosomal miRNA or can be isolated from plasma and converted to complementary DNA (cDNA), followed by quantitative real-time PCR (qRT-PCR), allowing relative quantitation of miRNA expression. Although qRT-PCR is a common method for the detection of miRNA, other options include in situ hybridization, enzymatic luminescence miRNA assay and northern blotting, microarrays, NGS, and nanopore technology [45].

CLINICAL APPLICATIONS

The current investigation of ctDNA for clinically significant alterations is primarily focused on patients with late-stage malignancies for targeted treatment selection and monitoring of response to systemic therapy. However, other applications, such as detection of early recurrence and emerging treatment resistance before imaging-detectable relapse, have great potential. Even more promising and challenging is the identification of ctDNA within an asymptomatic population for screening and initial detection of early-stage cancers [3,46,47]. These applications are summarized in Table 2.

Screening and Early Detection of Cancer

A major goal in cancer management is early identification, and cfDNA offers great potential as a screening tool [48,49]. Numerous studies have demonstrated detectable cfDNA in early-stage disease, before the presence of symptoms, and up to 2 years before cancer diagnosis [3]. However, high sensitivity and specificity is reported only in patients with a known diagnosis of cancer; testing an asymptomatic patient population with no known cancer history has proven to be more challenging because of the limited amount of cfDNA in the circulation. Ideally, ctDNA screening will be effective in detecting occult cancer, and incorporated into routine clinical care without unnecessary and invasive follow-up testing.

The CancerSeek assay profiles mutations in ctDNA from 16 genes and 9 protein biomarkers in a novel assay that has shown promise in stage I-III cancers for which traditional screening tests are not available, including ovary, liver, stomach, pancreas, esophagus, colorectal, and lung. CancerSEEK detected the majority of cancers along with tissue of origin, with sensitivities ranging from 69% to 98% and specificity greater than 99% [36]. This assay has been used in large screening study [36] of women with no history of cancer (DETECT-A); patients with positive results were referred for PET-CT [50]. A follow-up clinical trial (ASCEND) is underway to address issues of sensitivity and specificity, as well as tissue of origin identification [46].

Similarly, GRAIL Technologies has applied their methylation-based techniques to interrogate plasma ctDNA from solid and hematologic malignancies. The Circulating Cell-free Genome Atlas Consortium (CCGA) [41] recently published promising results on the detection and localization of multiple early- and late-stage cancers. Currently, there are several ongoing large-scale clinical trials using GRAILs multiplexed methylation-based assays to identify early cancers as part of general population-based screening programs [51].

Other ctDNA approaches to screen asymptomatic patients include the DNA evaluation of fragments for early interception (DELFI) platform [52], Epi proColon, an FDA-approved colorectal cancer screening test detecting methylation status of *SEPT9* promoter in blood [53], the LUNG Cancer Likelihood in Plasma (Lung-CLiP) assay [54] and CAncer Personalized Profiling by deep Sequencing (CAPP-Seq) to name a few [31].

Guiding Treatment

Currently, the most established clinical use for liquid biopsies is guiding first-line or subsequent systemic therapy in patients with metastatic tumors. ctDNA analysis is becoming the standard of care for patients with certain tumors, particularly NSCLC. Current NCCN recommendations for NSCLC directly address cfDNA testing, and support the use of cfDNA when a tissue biopsy is medically unsafe or if there is insufficient tissue

TABLE 2
Clinical Applications of Cell-free Nucleic Acid

Applications	Use/Impact	Advantages	Disadvantages
Screening/Early Detection	Routine screen for cf-NA in healthy individuals	• Earlier intervention • Help identify tissue of origin • May select patients for imaging	• Need low false positives • Risk of false negatives • Possible tumor localization • Cost
Diagnostics & Staging	Clarify diagnosis in suspect cases (eg, Lung nodule) Potential adjunct to traditional staging	• Can aid diagnosis in cases with limited tissue or access	• Tissue-based testing remains the gold standard
Prognostic & Predictive Markers	May aid therapy choice and planning	• Can aid diagnosis in cases with limited tissue or access	• Tissue-based testing is the gold standard
Monitoring for: • Therapeutic response • MRD • Recurrence	Longitudinal testing for therapy response, resistance, early relapse	• Earlier detection of disease • May reduce imaging • Tracking clonal evolution • Detection of emerging resistance • Improved outcome?	• Need more definitive data to show improved outcomes

for molecular testing and a follow-up tissue-based assay will be performed if no significant variants are identified (NCCN NSCLC v4.2021) [55]. However, the guidelines also state that cfDNA should not be used for the diagnosis of NSCLC.

Both FDA-approved and lab-developed assays are used to guide first or second-line systemic therapy for solid tumors. The Cobas EGFR mutation test v2 was the first liquid biopsy assay approved by the FDA as a companion diagnostic test to identify EGFR mutations in patients with advanced-stage NSCLC being considered for erlotinib (EGFR TKI therapy) [56]. The Guardant360 CDx assay has been approved for treatment decisions for any solid malignancy after positive results from the NILE study [57,58]. Based on results from the SOLAR-1 trial, PIK3CA RGQ PCR (Therascreen) assay is FDA approved for patients with HR+/HER2- advanced/metastatic breast cancer who progress after prior aromatase inhibitor therapy [59]. Foundation One Liquid CDx interrogates 324 genes and has been approved to identify druggable targets for advanced stage/metastatic disease in patients with solid tumors. Lastly, Resolution HRD is a cfDNA assay being developed to detect homologous recombination deficiency (HRD) in patients with metastatic castration-resistant prostate cancer who could benefit from PARP inhibitor therapy [60]. Although ctDNA analysis has been incorporated into routine clinical practice, it is important to note that a significant proportion of patients may have insufficient ctDNA, even with late-stage cancers, or alterations outside the scope of these assays [5].

Monitoring disease progression, early identification of relapse and drug resistance

Serial ctDNA sampling may be useful in monitoring disease, early detection of relapse, and determining when adjuvant in treatment is necessary. For example, ctDNA has been used to monitor patients with breast cancer after surgery, and positive results were highly correlated with metastatic relapse months later [61]. In further studies, surveillance of early-stage treated breast cancer patients for patient-specific mutations in ctDNA detected molecular relapse nearly a year before clinical signs [62]. Similarly, Signatera, a custom test for treatment monitoring and MRD assessment, generates a patient-specific "tumor signature" from whole exome sequencing of the primary tumor and matched normal control, which is then used to monitor plasma ctDNA [63]. A positive test predicted relapse with a positive predictive value (PPV) of over 98% across multiple solid tumors [64,65]. This technology can also be used to select patients for immune checkpoint blockade [66].

In addition, the development of resistance and emergence of subclones can be identified using cfDNA [67]. However, ctDNA alone is not yet used for routine monitoring of treatment response; while ctDNA can detect progression earlier than imagining, improved clinical outcomes have not yet been demonstrated following treatment decisions based on changes in ctDNA. In several tumor types, evaluation of ctDNA is currently used for patients who show clinical signs of relapse and progression when a tissue biopsy is either insufficient or cannot be tolerated [47].

Challenges in the Implementation of Cell-free Nucleic Acid Testing

Challenges in interpretation

ctDNA testing is complex, and interpretation of the results poses additional challenges. The results, if not understood correctly, can lead to considerable confusion among pathologists, clinicians, and patients. This necessitates that the report is clear with respect to the limitations of the analysis and what unexpected results may indicate.

Implications of a negative test result must be clearly understood; the negative predictive value can be as low as 60% depending on the tumor type, the clinical context, and timing of the test [68]. Conversely, a positive result seen during screening of healthy patients may be a harbinger of future malignancy, though these may occur more than 10 years later [18].

Another cause of misleading positive results stems from the detection of pathogenic mutations arising in myeloid cells, detected in cfDNA analysis. The most common would be clonal hematopoiesis of indeterminate potential (CHIP) [69], and related changes such as age-related clonal hematopoiesis [70]. These often involve mutations in *DNMT3A*, *TET2*, *ASXL1*, and even *TP53*, which would indicate an increased risk of development of myeloid neoplasms such as myelodysplastic syndrome. Patients with such mutations are also at increased risk of developing cardiovascular disease [71]. The allele frequencies in which these mutations are present, as well as the total number of mutations, factors into the risk of developing disease [72].

CHIP-like mutations may be detected in emerging therapy-related myeloid neoplasms (t-MNs). These are aggressive diseases in patients treated with radiation and/or chemotherapy and may develop months or years after completion of treatment. This is an important consideration when monitoring patients for residual solid tumor following therapy. Mutations in what are thought of as myeloid-related genes can be present

TABLE 3
Current Efforts to Develop Guidelines in cfDNA Testing

Project	Group	Reference
American Society Clinical Oncology and the College of American Pathologists, Joint Review	ASCO-CAP	[78]
Blood profiling atlas consortium, analytical variables working group	BloodPAC	[76]
Innovative Medicines Initiative Consortium	CANCER-ID	[79]
International Liquid Biopsy Standardization Alliance	ILSA	[80]
Multi-stakeholder invitational workshop		[77]

in solid tumors, such as DNMT3A [73]. In addition, mutations in TP53 are also common in myeloid neoplasms, particularly t-MNs. These factors must be taken into account when interpreting positive results from ctDNA testing that involves these gene targets.

Challenges in standardization

Lastly, as molecular oncology evolves at break-neck speed, it is challenging to rapidly establish guidelines to standardize the performance and interpretation of cfDNA molecular analysis. Owing to multiple strategies used for cfDNA analysis, there is lack of standardization across workflows, and sometimes a lack of concordance between assays [74,75]. Concordance studies have also been flawed by the timing of sample collection and other issues. Lack of concordance is most problematic at low allele fractions.

Multiple groups have convened to outline best practices and set guidelines (Table 3) for clinical implementation of cfDNA analysis [76–80]. There are also numerous publications on individual laboratory validation efforts [81,82]. Standardization should also address the intended use. Qualitative assays would have different validation protocols than quantitative panels. Further technologic advances (molecular barcoding, digital PCR strategies) may improve quantification efforts in the future [83,84].

Efforts are underway to help develop cancer-specific guidelines [80] to aid clinicians and pathologists in the use of these tests, though keeping such guidelines up to date will be challenging [78]. If there is near universal adaptation of guidelines, cfDNA testing can become more uniform and reliable for patient care.

Challenges in reimbursement

Cost of testing and reimbursement are necessary considerations as well. As with any test, the laboratory must weigh the practical benefits of bringing ctDNA testing in-house against the cost of sending the test to a reference laboratory. The technical challenges and bioinformatics requisite for such complex testing can be a substantial effort and expense.

Regardless of where the test is performed, reimbursement for ctDNA testing has increased from 2015 for both private payer and Medicare coverage [85]. Data from both coverage determinations favor cancer-specific approvals, such as coverage for NSCLC testing. However, the overall trend is toward coverage of pan-cancer panels, allowing testing for a significant subset of patients with cancer. In addition, there are draft and future local coverage determinations that would cover non–FDA-approved cfDNA testing [85].

Part of the challenge of cfDNA use is assessing the overall cost-benefit of the testing. One study focusing on screening for early cancer determined that as the cost of testing reaches $200, there is an overall benefit [85]. Others have shown that monitoring post-treatment may not be cost-effective [86]. As cost declines and the potential clinical impact of the test becomes more certain, payers will increasingly provide coverage, all promising for the widespread use of cfDNA testing over a range of tumor types.

SUMMARY

Since the first observation of cfDNA in blood samples in 1948 [87], great strides have been made in the biology, detection and clinical applications of this analyte. The tremendous improvements in our technical capabilities leading to greater analytical sensitivity, coupled with a growing understanding of the source and biology of ctDNA, will pave the way for the further advances needed. A clear understanding of factors affecting the release of ctDNA will help us understand how to best use this biomarker in various tumors and different clinical scenarios. In time, the use of ctDNA will be a valuable tool, used across the full range of clinical applications in patients with cancer.

CLINICS CARE POINTS

- Many technical approaches now exist to interrogate cell-free DNA from tumors in plasma.
- Cell-free DNA approaches are becoming standard for the assessment of drug resistance.
- Ongoing studies are needed to establish the role of cfDNA in early detection and monitoring of cancer.

DISCLOSURE

The authors have nothing to disclose.

REFERENCES

[1] American College of Obstetrics and Gynecologists' Committee on Practices: Bulletins-Obstetrics, American College of Obstetrics and Gynecologists' Committee on Genetics, Society of Maternal-fetal Medicine. Screening for Fetal Chromosomal Abnormalities: ACOG Practice Bulletin, Number 226. Obstet Gynecol 2020;136(4): e48–69.
[2] Lo YM, Corbetta N, Chamberlain PF, et al. Presence of fetal DNA in maternal plasma and serum. Lancet 1997; 350(9076):485–7.
[3] Bronkhorst AJ, Ungerer V, Holdenrieder S. The emerging role of cell-free DNA as a molecular marker for cancer management. Biomol Detect Quantif 2019;17:100087.
[4] Snyder MW, Kircher M, Hill AJ, et al. Cell-free DNA Comprises an In Vivo Nucleosome Footprint that Informs Its Tissues-Of-Origin. Cell 2016;164(1–2):57–68.
[5] Bettegowda C, Sausen M, Leary RJ, et al. Detection of circulating tumor DNA in early- and late-stage human malignancies. Sci Transl Med 2014;6(224):224ra224.
[6] Bronkhorst AJ, Ungerer V, Holdenrieder S. Comparison of methods for the isolation of cell-free DNA from cell culture supernatant. Tumour Biol 2020;42(4): 1010428320916314.
[7] Ungerer V, Bronkhorst AJ, Holdenrieder S. Preanalytical variables that affect the outcome of cell-free DNA measurements. Crit Rev Clin Lab Sci 2020;57(7):484–507.
[8] Fettke H, Kwan EM, Azad AA. Cell-free DNA in cancer: current insights. Cell Oncol 2019;42(1):13–28.
[9] Peng M, Chen C, Hulbert A, et al. Non-blood circulating tumor DNA detection in cancer. Oncotarget 2017;8(40): 69162–73.
[10] Lampignano R, Kloten V, Krahn T, et al. Integrating circulating miRNA analysis in the clinical management of lung cancer: Present or future? Mol Aspects Med 2020; 72:100844.
[11] Schneegans S, Luck L, Besler K, et al. Pre-analytical factors affecting the establishment of a single tube assay for multiparameter liquid biopsy detection in melanoma patients. Mol Oncol 2020;14(5):1001–15.
[12] Greytak SR, Engel KB, Parpart-Li S, et al. Harmonizing Cell-Free DNA Collection and Processing Practices through Evidence-Based Guidance. Clin Cancer Res 2020;26(13):3104–9.
[13] Sorber L, Zwaenepoel K, Jacobs J, et al. Specialized Blood Collection Tubes for Liquid Biopsy: Improving the Pre-analytical Conditions. Mol Diagn Ther 2020;24(1): 113–24.
[14] van Dessel LF, Beije N, Helmijr JC, et al. Application of circulating tumor DNA in prospective clinical oncology trials - standardization of preanalytical conditions. Mol Oncol 2017;11(3):295–304.
[15] van Dessel LF, Martens JWM, Lolkema MP. Fundamentals of liquid biopsies in metastatic prostate cancer: from characterization to stratification. Curr Opin Oncol 2020;32(5):527–34.
[16] Risberg B, Tsui DWY, Biggs H, et al. Effects of Collection and Processing Procedures on Plasma Circulating Cell-Free DNA from Cancer Patients. J Mol Diagn 2018; 20(6):883–92.
[17] Bronkhorst AJ, Ungerer V, Holdenrieder S. Early detection of cancer using circulating tumor DNA: biological, physiological and analytical considerations. Crit Rev Clin Lab Sci 2019;1–17.
[18] Alborelli I, Generali D, Jermann P, et al. Cell-free DNA analysis in healthy individuals by next-generation sequencing: a proof of concept and technical validation study. Cell Death Dis 2019;10(7):534.
[19] de Kock R, Deiman B, Kraaijvanger R, et al. Optimized (Pre) Analytical Conditions and Workflow for Droplet Digital PCR Analysis of Cell-Free DNA from Patients with Suspected Lung Carcinoma. J Mol Diagn 2019; 21(5):895–902.
[20] Barrett AN, Thadani HA, Laureano-Asibal C, et al. Stability of cell-free DNA from maternal plasma isolated following a single centrifugation step. Prenat Diagn 2014;34(13):1283–8.
[21] Cavallone L, Aldamry M, Lafleur J, et al. A Study of Pre-Analytical Variables and Optimization of Extraction Method for Circulating Tumor DNA Measurements by Digital Droplet PCR. Cancer Epidemiol Biomarkers Prev 2019;28(5):909–16.
[22] Swinkels DW, Wiegerinck E, Steegers EA, et al. Effects of blood-processing protocols on cell-free DNA quantification in plasma. Clin Chem 2003;49(3):525–6.
[23] Beije N, Martens JWM, Sleijfer S. Incorporating liquid biopsies into treatment decision-making: obstacles and possibilities. Drug Discov Today 2019;24(9): 1715–9.
[24] van Dessel LF, Vitale SR, Helmijr JCA, et al. High-throughput isolation of circulating tumor DNA: a

comparison of automated platforms. Mol Oncol 2019;13(2):392–402.

[25] Diefenbach RJ, Lee JH, Kefford RF, et al. Evaluation of commercial kits for purification of circulating free DNA. Cancer Genet 2018;228-229:21–7.

[26] Diaz LA Jr, Bardelli A. Liquid biopsies: genotyping circulating tumor DNA. J Clin Oncol 2014;32(6):579–86.

[27] Heitzer E, Haque IS, Roberts CES, et al. Current and future perspectives of liquid biopsies in genomics-driven oncology. Nat Rev Genet 2019;20(2):71–88.

[28] Elazezy M, Joosse SA. Techniques of using circulating tumor DNA as a liquid biopsy component in cancer management. Comput Struct Biotechnol J 2018;16:370–8.

[29] Hindson BJ, Ness KD, Masquelier DA, et al. High-throughput droplet digital PCR system for absolute quantitation of DNA copy number. Anal Chem 2011;83(22):8604–10.

[30] Chaudhuri AA, Chabon JJ, Lovejoy AF, et al. Early Detection of Molecular Residual Disease in Localized Lung Cancer by Circulating Tumor DNA Profiling. Cancer Discov 2017;7(12):1394–403.

[31] Newman AM, Bratman SV, To J, et al. An ultrasensitive method for quantitating circulating tumor DNA with broad patient coverage. Nat Med 2014;20(5):548–54.

[32] Newman AM, Lovejoy AF, Klass DM, et al. Integrated digital error suppression for improved detection of circulating tumor DNA. Nat Biotechnol 2016;34(5):547–55.

[33] Phallen J, Sausen M, Adleff V, et al. Direct detection of early-stage cancers using circulating tumor DNA. Sci Transl Med 2017;9(403):eaan2415.

[34] Abbosh C, Birkbak NJ, Swanton C. Early stage NSCLC - challenges to implementing ctDNA-based screening and MRD detection. Nat Rev Clin Oncol 2018;15(9):577–86.

[35] Forshew T, Murtaza M, Parkinson C, et al. Noninvasive identification and monitoring of cancer mutations by targeted deep sequencing of plasma DNA. Sci Transl Med 2012;4(136):136ra168.

[36] Cohen JD, Li L, Wang Y, et al. Detection and localization of surgically resectable cancers with a multi-analyte blood test. Science 2018;359(6378):926–30.

[37] Guo S, Diep D, Plongthongkum N, et al. Identification of methylation haplotype blocks aids in deconvolution of heterogeneous tissue samples and tumor tissue-of-origin mapping from plasma DNA. Nat Genet 2017;49(4):635–42.

[38] Zeng H, He B, Yi C, et al. Liquid biopsies: DNA methylation analyses in circulating cell-free DNA. J Genet Genomics 2018;45(4):185–92.

[39] Legendre C, Gooden GC, Johnson K, et al. Whole-genome bisulfite sequencing of cell-free DNA identifies signature associated with metastatic breast cancer. Clin Epigenet 2015;7:100.

[40] Wen L, Li J, Guo H, et al. Genome-scale detection of hypermethylated CpG islands in circulating cell-free DNA of hepatocellular carcinoma patients. Cell Res 2015;25(11):1250–64.

[41] Liu MC, Oxnard GR, Klein EA, et al. Sensitive and specific multi-cancer detection and localization using methylation signatures in cell-free DNA. Ann Oncol 2020;31(6):745–59.

[42] He FC, Meng WW, Qu YH, et al. Expression of circulating microRNA-20a and let-7a in esophageal squamous cell carcinoma. World J Gastroenterol 2015;21(15):4660–5.

[43] Lan H, Lu H, Wang X, et al. MicroRNAs as potential biomarkers in cancer: opportunities and challenges. Biomed Res Int 2015;2015:125094.

[44] Markou A, Liang Y, Lianidou E. Prognostic, therapeutic and diagnostic potential of microRNAs in non-small cell lung cancer. Clin Chem Lab Med 2011;49(10):1591–603.

[45] de Planell-Saguer M, Rodicio MC. Detection methods for microRNAs in clinic practice. Clin Biochem 2013;46(10–11):869–78.

[46] Detecting Cancers Earlier Through Elective Plasma-based CancerSEEK Testing (ASCEND). 2021. Available at: https://clinicaltrials.gov/ct2/show/NCT04213326. [Accessed 28 April 2021].

[47] Ignatiadis M, Sledge GW, Jeffrey SS. Liquid biopsy enters the clinic - implementation issues and future challenges. Nat Rev Clin Oncol 2021;18(5):297–312.

[48] Kalinich M, Haber DA. Cancer detection: Seeking signals in blood. Science 2018;359(6378):866–7.

[49] Liu MC. Transforming the landscape of early cancer detection using blood tests-Commentary on current methodologies and future prospects. Br J Cancer 2021;124(9):1475–7.

[50] Lennon AM, Buchanan AH, Kinde I, et al. Feasibility of blood testing combined with PET-CT to screen for cancer and guide intervention. Science 2020;(6499):369.

[51] GRAIL Clinical Research Program. 2020. Available at: https://grail.com/clinical-studies/. [Accessed 28 April 2001].

[52] Cristiano S, Leal A, Phallen J, et al. Genome-wide cell-free DNA fragmentation in patients with cancer. Nature 2019;570(7761):385–9.

[53] Potter NT, Hurban P, White MN, et al. Validation of a real-time PCR-based qualitative assay for the detection of methylated SEPT9 DNA in human plasma. Clin Chem 2014;60(9):1183–91.

[54] Chabon JJ, Hamilton EG, Kurtz DM, et al. Integrating genomic features for non-invasive early lung cancer detection. Nature 2020;580(7802):245–51.

[55] Network NCC. NCCN Guidelines Non-Small Cell Lung Cancer v4.2021. 2021. Available at: https://www.nccn.org/professionals/physician_gls/pdf/nscl.pdf. [Accessed 28 April 2021].

[56] Malapelle U, Sirera R, Jantus-Lewintre E, et al. Profile of the Roche cobas(R) EGFR mutation test v2 for non-small cell lung cancer. Expert Rev Mol Diagn 2017;17(3):209–15.

[57] Aggarwal C, Rolfo CD, Oxnard GR, et al. Strategies for the successful implementation of plasma-based NSCLC genotyping in clinical practice. Nat Rev Clin Oncol 2021;18(1):56–62.

[58] Leighl NB, Page RD, Raymond VM, et al. Clinical Utility of Comprehensive Cell-free DNA Analysis to Identify

Genomic Biomarkers in Patients with Newly Diagnosed Metastatic Non-small Cell Lung Cancer. Clin Cancer Res 2019;25(15):4691–700.

[59] Andre F, Ciruelos E, Rubovszky G, et al. Alpelisib for PIK3CA-Mutated, Hormone Receptor-Positive Advanced Breast Cancer. N Engl J Med 2019;380(20):1929–40.

[60] Teyssonneau D, Margot H, Cabart M, et al. Prostate cancer and PARP inhibitors: progress and challenges. J Hematol Oncol 2021;14(1):51.

[61] Garcia-Murillas I, Schiavon G, Weigelt B, et al. Mutation tracking in circulating tumor DNA predicts relapse in early breast cancer. Sci Transl Med 2015;7(302): 302ra133.

[62] Garcia-Murillas I, Chopra N, Comino-Mendez I, et al. Assessment of Molecular Relapse Detection in Early-Stage Breast Cancer. JAMA Oncol 2019;5(10):1473–8.

[63] Abbosh C, Birkbak NJ, Wilson GA, et al. Phylogenetic ctDNA analysis depicts early-stage lung cancer evolution. Nature 2017;545(7655):446–51.

[64] Christensen E, Birkenkamp-Demtroder K, Sethi H, et al. Early Detection of Metastatic Relapse and Monitoring of Therapeutic Efficacy by Ultra-Deep Sequencing of Plasma Cell-Free DNA in Patients With Urothelial Bladder Carcinoma. J Clin Oncol 2019;37(18):1547–57.

[65] Coombes RC, Page K, Salari R, et al. Personalized Detection of Circulating Tumor DNA Antedates Breast Cancer Metastatic Recurrence. Clin Cancer Res 2019;25(14): 4255–63.

[66] Bratman SV, Yang SYC, Iafolla MAJ, et al. Personalized circulating tumor DNA analysis as a predictive biomarker in solid tumor patients treated with pembrolizumab. Nat Cancer 2020;1(9):873–81.

[67] Parikh AR, Leshchiner I, Elagina L, et al. Liquid versus tissue biopsy for detecting acquired resistance and tumor heterogeneity in gastrointestinal cancers. Nat Med 2019;25(9):1415–21.

[68] Cavallone L, Aguilar-Mahecha A, Lafleur J, et al. Prognostic and predictive value of circulating tumor DNA during neoadjuvant chemotherapy for triple negative breast cancer. Sci Rep 2020;10(1):14704.

[69] Steensma DP, Bejar R, Jaiswal S, et al. Clonal hematopoiesis of indeterminate potential and its distinction from myelodysplastic syndromes. Blood 2015;126(1):9–16.

[70] Jaiswal S, Fontanillas P, Flannick J, et al. Age-related clonal hematopoiesis associated with adverse outcomes. N Engl J Med 2014;371(26):2488–98.

[71] Jaiswal S, Natarajan P, Silver AJ, et al. Clonal Hematopoiesis and Risk of Atherosclerotic Cardiovascular Disease. N Engl J Med 2017;377(2):111–21.

[72] Gondek LP, DeZern AE. Assessing clonal haematopoiesis: clinical burdens and benefits of diagnosing myelodysplastic syndrome precursor states. Lancet Haematol 2020;7(1):e73–81.

[73] Zhang W, Xu J. DNA methyltransferases and their roles in tumorigenesis. Biol Res 2017;5:1.

[74] Kuderer NM, Burton KA, Blau S, et al. Comparison of 2 Commercially Available Next-Generation Sequencing Platforms in Oncology. JAMA Oncol 2017;3(7):996–8.

[75] Stetson D, Ahmed A, Xu X, et al. Orthogonal Comparison of Four Plasma NGS Tests With Tumor Suggests Technical Factors are a Major Source of Assay Discordance. JCO Precision Oncol 2019;(3):1–9.

[76] Godsey JH, Silvestro A, Barrett JC, et al. Generic Protocols for the Analytical Validation of Next-Generation Sequencing-Based ctDNA Assays: A Joint Consensus Recommendation of the BloodPAC's Analytical Variables Working Group. Clin Chem 2020;66(9):1156–66.

[77] IJzerman MJ, de Boer J, Azad A, et al. Towards Routine Implementation of Liquid Biopsies in Cancer Management: It Is Always Too Early, until Suddenly It Is Too Late. Diagnostics 2021;11(1):103.

[78] Merker JD, Oxnard GR, Compton C, et al. Circulating Tumor DNA Analysis in Patients With Cancer: American Society of Clinical Oncology and College of American Pathologists Joint Review. J Clin Oncol 2018;36(16): 1631–41.

[79] Weber S, Spiegl B, Perakis SO, et al. Technical Evaluation of Commercial Mutation Analysis Platforms and Reference Materials for Liquid Biopsy Profiling. Cancers (Basel) 2020;12(6).

[80] Connors D, Allen J, Alvarez JD, et al. International liquid biopsy standardization alliance white paper. Crit Rev Oncol Hematol 2020;156:103112.

[81] Verma S, Moore MW, Ringler R, et al. Analytical performance evaluation of a commercial next generation sequencing liquid biopsy platform using plasma ctDNA, reference standards, and synthetic serial dilution samples derived from normal plasma. BMC Cancer 2020;20(1): 945.

[82] Fettke H, Steen JA, Kwan EM, et al. Analytical validation of an error-corrected ultra-sensitive ctDNA next-generation sequencing assay. BioTechniques 2020; 69(2):133–40.

[83] Johansson G, Andersson D, Filges S, et al. Considerations and quality controls when analyzing cell-free tumor DNA. Biomol Detect Quantif 2019;17:100078.

[84] Yu Q, Huang F, Zhang M, et al. Multiplex picoliter-droplet digital PCR for quantitative assessment of EGFR mutations in circulating cell-free DNA derived from advanced non-small cell lung cancer patients. Mol Med Rep 2017;16(2):1157–66.

[85] Douglas MP, Gray SW, Phillips KA. Private Payer and Medicare Coverage for Circulating Tumor DNA Testing: A Historical Analysis of Coverage Policies From 2015 to 2019. J Natl Compr Canc Netw 2020;18(7):866–72.

[86] Sanchez-Calderon D, Pedraza A, Mancera Urrego C, et al. Analysis of the Cost-Effectiveness of Liquid Biopsy to Determine Treatment Change in Patients with Her2-Positive Advanced Breast Cancer in Colombia. Clin Outcomes Res 2020;12:115–22.

[87] Mandel P, Metais P. Nuclear Acids In Human Blood Plasma. C R Seances Soc Biol Fil 1948;142(3–4):241–3.

Advances in Molecular Pathology 4 (2021) 199–204
ADVANCES IN MOLECULAR PATHOLOGY

Tumor Mutational Burden Calculation and Microsatellite Instability Detection in Clinical Next-Generation Sequencing Assays

Ashkan Bigdeli, ALM[a,b,*], Amanda Oran, PhD[a], Robyn Sussman, PhD[a]
[a]Division of Precision and Computational Diagnostics, Department of Pathology & Laboratory Medicine, Hospital of the University of Pennsylvania, 3020 Market Street, Suite 220, Philadelphia, PA 19104, USA; [b]Drexel University, School of Biomedical Engineering, Science and Health Systems, 2141 Chestnut Street, Philadelphia, PA 19104, USA

KEYWORDS
• TMB • MSI • ICB • Immune checkpoint blockade • Microsatellite instability • Tumor mutational burden
• Clinical NGS validation

KEY POINTS
- TMB and MSI are important biomarkers for use of immune checkpoint blockade therapies in multiple malignancies.
- Filtration strategies are critical to achieving concordance between TMB from WES and targeted panels.
- Cohort selection is an important aspect of clinical validation and implementation for the detection of TMB and MSI.
- Determining the ability to call MSI from targeted gene panels and available methods and thresholds when doing so.

CHECKPOINT BLOCKADE THERAPY, TUMOR MUTATIONAL BURDEN, AND MICROSATELLITE INSTABILITY

Immune checkpoint blockade (ICB) therapy uses antibodies to target molecules including cytotoxic T-lymphocyte-associated protein 4, programmed cell death 1 (PD-1), or its ligand (PD-L1). The inhibition of these immunologic checkpoints has been shown to prevent the termination of and restore the exhaustion of antitumor T cells in a subset of solid tumors [1]. Resulting ICB therapies have proven to be an effective treatment strategy for regressing these cancers, and six immune checkpoint inhibitors have been approved by the Food and Drug Administration backed by robust supporting evidence provided by the National Comprehensive Cancer Network [2,3].

Given the demonstrated efficacy of ICB therapies, effective biomarker detection is essential in clinical diagnostics. Tumor mutational burden (TMB) and microsatellite instability (MSI) are two biomarkers for sensitivity to ICB therapies and durable remission in multiple malignancies [4,5]. TMB can be evaluated using DNA next-generation sequencing (NGS), and while polymerase chain reaction (PCR)-specific methods are available for the detection of MSI, NGS remains an attractive option as clinicians can obtain data on several tumor profiling variations including, but not limited to, small variations, copy number, TMB, and MSI.

TMB is an estimation of the number of variants that can potentially translate into "nonself" tumor-specific epitopes or neoantigens, and the calculation of TMB can be concisely defined as the number of coding mutations per mega base (muts/Mb) of the genome. This is

*Corresponding author, *E-mail addresses:* Ashkan.Bigdeli@pennmedicine.upenn.edu; Twitter: @ashkbig (A.B.)

https://doi.org/10.1016/j.yamp.2021.07.008
2589-4080/21/

most effectively measured using whole exome sequencing (WES) and tumor-normal match paired informatic analysis to produce a refined call set of somatic variations that accurately represent the antigen landscape of the tumor in question. If the number of these variations is sufficiently high and immune regulators are suppressed through ICB, tumors may no longer be able to escape immune surveillance.

High MSI (MSI-H) is characterized by a deficiency in DNA mismatch repair (dMMR) resulting in the accumulation of insertions and/or deletions (indels) in short tandem repeat regions that are typically 1 to 9 base pairs in length. Immunohistochemistry (IHC) for the mismatch repair proteins MLH1, MSH2, MSH6, and PMS2 can be used as a surrogate for MSI detection, with loss of expression suggesting MSI-H and sensitivity to ICB. While MSI has been shown in several cancers at varying frequencies, it has been correlated to survival in colorectal cancers [6], and the FDA recently approved an immunotherapy drug in adult and pediatric solid tumor patients with an MSI-H indication [7].

Here, we seek to review laboratory and algorithmic practices that may prove useful in detecting these biomarkers from existing assays being used in laboratories providing NGS for clinical cancer diagnostics. With the gold standard of TMB requiring WES, and MSI algorithms relying heavily on the comparative distribution of NGS reads at MSI loci, a unique set of challenges arise for laboratories providing clinical diagnostics through targeted gene panels. Laboratories often trade sequencing landscape for greater depth of coverage and detection sensitivity with samples at a higher DNA degradation and lower input concentration. For a variety of reasons associated with costs and logistics, these same laboratories often omit a matched normal sample, compounding challenges that we address when validating TMB and MSI algorithms using cancer-associated targeted gene NGS panels in the absence of a matched normal.

TUMOR MUTATIONAL BURDEN ALGORITHMS

Chalmer and colleagues [8] demonstrated the ability to accurately estimate TMB using a 315-gene panel covering ~1.1 Mb of the genome, and in doing so, they provided an effective framework for the validation of TMB using targeted panels when validation against WES is possible. Given the clinical efficacy of immunotherapy, laboratories may be able to stretch the bounds of the exome sampled if measured TMB concordance to WES can be conclusively demonstrated. As such, we outline several algorithmic considerations when validating TMB stratification in solid tumors for clinical reporting.

To accurately infer TMB using targeted NGS without a matched normal sample, one must account for both normal contamination and bias introduced when working with a subset of the genome preselected for cancer-associated variations. In addition, the removal of artifactual mutations introduced during sample preparation and sequencing as well as an understanding of the baseline mutation rate of a given assay are paramount in correlating targeted NGS assays to WES.

An effective strategy for eliminating technical artifacts associated with NGS is the use of a Panel of Normals (PON) as outlined in the Genome Analysis Toolkits best practices for somatic mutation calling [9]. Normal samples should be those known to have no somatic alterations and with a primary purpose of capturing technical artifacts in mutation calling; the sequencing of these normal samples should occur with the same reasonable variability that one would encounter in a clinical laboratory. To mitigate technical artifacts observed during sequencing, normal samples should be distributed across all sequencers being used to implement the clinical workflow.

Artifacts resulting from the fixation of formalin in formalin-fixed paraffin-embedded (FFPE) tissues must also be mitigated. As these types of artifacts are not reproducible, a pipelined process must be implemented, and as such, The Cancer Genome Atlas' implementation of GATK's OxoG filtration was used for the removal of FFPE artifacts [10]. Non-FFPE samples were unaffected when processed using this method, allowing for a single-sample agnostic informatics workflow (Fig. 1).

At this stage in processing, the call-set should be limited to real biological events, and the filtration of these events to form a representation of the tumor neoantigen landscape focuses primarily on suspected germline variations. To this end, gnomAD population allele frequency and count, in tandem with observed allelic frequencies, serve as a valid filtration metric. While unable to capture germline events with the same efficacy as a matched normal sample, the usage of a PON, gnomAD filtration, and variants at suspected germline frequencies can serve as a valuable surrogate [11].

The remaining variations should be ready for validation and parameter tuning against an orthogonally validated WES sample set of 59 or more samples per Association for Molecular Pathology (AMP) and College of American Pathologists (CAP) [12] recommendations. If the error rate of the assay is known [13], and/or

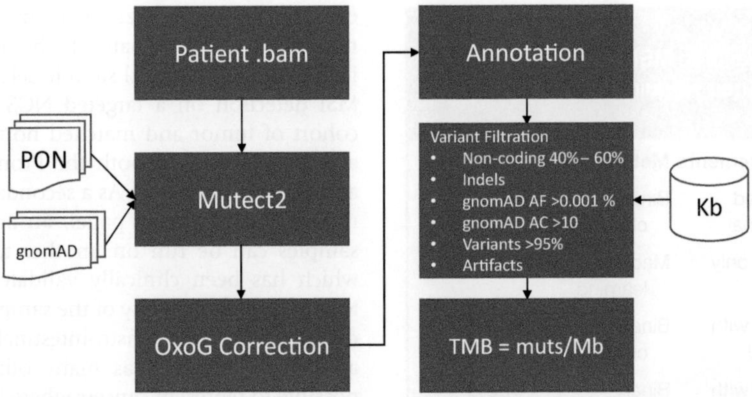

FIG. 1 Outline of sample agnostic informatic pipelining to call TMB from targeted cancer-associated gene panels in the absence of a matched normal companion diagnostic.

if an internal knowledge base of previously classified variations is available, it should be used in the tuning of filtration against WES sequencing. Panel size is the greatest barrier in the validation of TMB from targeted NGS, and the FDA noted that panels under 0.6 MB [14] show dramatic increases in variance. Sequencing panels covering less than 0.6 MB should report variance when compared to WES through a confidence interval informing clinicians of the lower and upper bounds of the TMB call.

MICROSATELLITE INSTABILITY DETECTION

Several algorithms exist for the detection of MSI from NGS data (Table 1), but the primary strategy in the detection of MSI should focus on the availability of accessible targets in an NGS panel. Small gene panels that focus only on the coding regions of cancer-associated genes are unlikely to inherently contain enough regions to be statistically confident when calling MSI. As such, it is critical that the assay development process be mindful in either (1) assessing enough of the genome to contain enough valid sites for MSI or (2) have specific targets for MSI included just as one would for gene-specific targets.

To determine if an assay can effectively call MSI from the available protein-coding regions, the targets of the assay should be screened for both repeat and low-complexity regions. One method to achieve this is to download repeat regions from a resource such as the University of California, Santa Cruz (UCSC) genome browser [15] and evaluate, most easily through .bed file intersection, if the assay in question has enough callable MSI loci. While there is no known lower limit for callable MSI loci, there seems to be a thresholding range of 3.5% to 40% of MSI loci available showing instability [5,16–18]. Several methods can also be cleanly pipelined with previously derived normal samples serving as a baseline for which MSI-H samples can be called (MSIsensor2, mSINGS, MSI-Colon Core, Nowak method). It is recommended that these values be validated with concordance assessment against IHC-confirmed MSI-H samples. If panel size limits the number of callable MSI sites, the loci included in the Bethesda/National Cancer Institute (NCI) panel can be included within the panel design [16]. These loci (BAT-25, BAT-26, NR-21, NR-22, and NR-24) have been the gold standard in MSI detection for over 20 years, and while NGS has allowed for the calling of MSI through additional targets [5], the inclusion of these sites should be sufficient when dealing with limited genomic space.

VALIDATION OF MICROSATELLITE INSTABILITY DETERMINATION AND TUMOR MUTATIONAL BURDEN CALCULATION

As discussed previously, the most reliable way to calculate TMB is via WES of tumor and matched normal samples because all exons are analyzed for the presence of nonsynonymous variants [19]. By having all exons of a tumor sequenced, as well as its matched normal tissue, one can readily determine the absolute number of somatic mutations per Mb of the exome. However, WES poses several challenges to a clinical laboratory including cost, turnaround time, and limited access to

TABLE 1
A Partial List of Available MSI-Detection Methods Using NGS, and Their Requirements and Thresholds

Algorithm	Requirements	Method	Threshold
MSIsensor	Matched normal	Binary classification	>3.5%
MSIsensor2	Tumor only	Machine learning	>20%
MSI-Colon Core	Tumor with PON	Binary classification	>40%
mSINGS	Tumor with PON	Binary classification	>20%
Cortest-Ciriano	Matched normal	Random forest	MSI>0.4
Nowak method	Tumor only	Binary classification	40 muts/MB

samples. As a more attainable alternative, many clinical laboratories are more commonly turning to targeted panels for determination of TMB [20–23]. The appropriate specimens to include for validation of TMB calculation on a targeted NGS panel should predominantly be a cohort of tumor and matched normal samples which have had WES performed in a Clinical Laboratory Improvement Amendments (CLIA) laboratory. If obtaining 59 samples, as recommended by the AMP and CAP guidelines for validation of NGS-based oncology panels [12], poses a challenge to the laboratory, a secondary cohort of tumor-only samples can be run on another clinically validated targeted NGS panel that provides a TMB score. Concordance rates compared to both the WES results and targeted panel calling TMB can be determined as part of the validation.

There are currently two standard methods for MSI detection and knowing dMMR status: PCR for microsatellite regions followed by capillary electrophoresis [24,25] and IHC for MMR proteins [26], respectively. However, variants in the MMR genes can cause loss of MMR protein function without loss of protein expression. The MSI Analysis System, Version 1.2 (Promega, Madison WI) is the gold standard for MSI detection via PCR. This method amplifies the DNA of tumor and matched normal samples by PCR with fluorescently labeled primers at the five standard Bethesda/NCI loci [5]. After PCR, the amplified fragments are separated based on size via capillary electrophoresis. The size of fragments present in the tumor DNA are compared with the size of fragments in the matched normal DNA to designate whether instability is present in the tumor. The ideal sample selection for validating MSI detection on a targeted NGS panel would be a cohort of tumor and matched normal samples which are characterized by both the Promega assay for MSI and by IHC for dMMR. As a secondary source of confirmation for a targeted panel, an additional cohort of samples can be run on another targeted NGS panel which has been clinically validated for detection of MSI. While the majority of the samples used in the validation can be from gastrointestinal (GI) tumors, it is advisable to include as many other tumor types as possible to represent cancers where MSI is less common [27,28], with the aim of obtaining at least 59 data points, as suggested by the AMP guidelines [12]. Owing to the difficulty in obtaining the appropriate specimen types, if a laboratory is unable to reach 59, they should use as many samples as available.

For the validation of MSI detection via NGS, sample results should be compared to the appropriate orthogonal methods. MSI detection is a qualitative test which provides a status, in contrast to a typical NGS quantitative test. Accuracy and analytical specificity of MSI detection can be determined by comparing the number of MSI-H cases called by the NGS algorithm compared with the number of MSI-H cases determined by the Promega PCR assay. Any cases with MSI-H status on the Promega assay can be considered true positives. To determine the accuracy of the NGS test, the percentage of true positives which the panel also deemed MSI-H can be calculated. In addition to comparison with PCR, the laboratory can also investigate the correlation of NGS results to dMMR status determined by IHC. However, it is understood that there may be MSI-H cases which were not identified as dMMR because of the possibility that a genetic variant may cause loss of protein function and therefore contribute to MSI but does not exhibit loss of protein expression [26,29]. Additional support for the performance of the panel can be from another MSI detection assay such as the Blocker Displacement Amplification assay [30,31] currently in development by NuProbe.

Similarly, TMB status (high or low) as called by an NGS panel should be compared to TMB status determined by orthogonal assays. Although TMB assays provide a quantitative score, they can be considered qualitative tests in the context of therapy guidance. A score of greater than 10 mutations per Mb from an FDA-cleared assay is designated as TMB high (TMB-H) [32,33], based on the KEYNOTE-158 study [34] which led to FDA approval of PD-1 inhibitor pembrolizumab for the treatment of solid tumors with high TMB. To confirm that the NGS assay is accurate, the TMB status should be compared to TMB that was calculated using WES from a tumor-normal pair. As an alternative to WES, results can be compared to a TMB status determined on a secondary orthogonal method such as another targeted panel [8,19,35]. For additional confirmation of the targeted panel performance, the numerical TMB scores determined by the different assays can be compared.

To determine the analytical specificity of either assay, the percentage of total positive NGS calls which were expected from the orthogonal methods can be calculated. The laboratory can also include nontumor samples in the validation to ensure confidence that in samples without somatic variants, there is no evidence of MSI, and the TMB score is 0. Demonstration of the validity of an assay can be achieved by the use of reference standards which have been well characterized and confirmed with documentation from the provider. While reference standards with predetermined TMB scores are available for purchase, these can be cost-prohibitive for many academic clinical laboratories. As an alternative, one can use clinical samples that have been well characterized. For example, substitute a reference standard with a sample being used as a clinical control on an orthogonal assay. Positive and negative control samples will have been included in many replicates of the orthogonal assay and therefore will have many confirmatory data points. One way to address the validation criteria for the lower limit of detection is by diluting tumor samples with matched normal samples. The tumor percentage of the original sample should be estimated by an anatomic pathologist. This can provide an estimate of the lowest tumor percentage at which the assay can reliably determine TMB or MSI status. By providing the aforementioned examples, we have addressed how a clinical laboratory can validate laboratory developed tests for the determination of MSI and calculation of TMB using a targeted NGS panel.

In summary, validation of both TMB score and MSI detection in a targeted NGS panel requires appropriate sample sourcing, experimental design, and bioinformatics algorithms. Including these in a clinical NGS panel enables clinical decision-making for ICB therapy from a single test that is already being ordered on a tumor sample. Particularly for tumor types that are less likely to be MSI-H or TMB-H, including these as part of a broader NGS panel enables rare tumors that are MSI-H or TMB-H from less commonly high histologies to be treated using ICB in a testing algorithm that is cost-effective and efficient.

CLINICS CARE POINTS

- Clinical importance of biomarker detection for ICB therapies
- Clinical validation design of TMB and MSI
- Clinical implementation of TMB and MSI algorithms

DISCLOSURE

The authors have nothing to disclose.

REFERENCES

[1] Korman AJ, Peggs KS, Allison JP. Checkpoint blockade in cancer immunotherapy. Adv Immunol 2006;90:297–339.

[2] Hargadon KM, Johnson CE, Williams CJ. Immune checkpoint blockade therapy for cancer: an overview of FDA-approved immune checkpoint inhibitors. Int Immunopharmacol 2018;62:29–39.

[3] Vaddepally RK, Kharel P, Pandey R, et al. Review of indications of FDA-approved immune checkpoint inhibitors per NCCN guidelines with the level of evidence. Cancers (Basel) 2020;12(3):738.

[4] Goodman AM, Kato S, Bazhenova L, et al. Tumor mutational burden as an independent predictor of response to immunotherapy in diverse cancers. Mol Cancer Ther 2017;16(11):2598–608.

[5] Baudrin LG, Deleuze JF, How-Kit A. Molecular and computational methods for the detection of microsatellite instability in cancer. Front Oncol 2018;8:621.

[6] Nojadeh JN, Behrouz Sharif S, Sakhinia E. Microsatellite instability in colorectal cancer. EXCLI J 2018;17:159–68.

[7] Chang L, Chang M, Chang HM, et al. Microsatellite instability: a predictive biomarker for cancer immunotherapy. Appl Immunohistochem Mol Morphol 2018;26(2):e15–21.

[8] Chalmers ZR, Connelly CF, Fabrizio D, et al. Analysis of 100,000 human cancer genomes reveals the landscape of tumor mutational burden. Genome Med 2017;9(1):34.

[9] Van der Auwera GA, Carneiro MO, Hartl C, et al. From FastQ data to high confidence variant calls: the Genome Analysis Toolkit best practices pipeline. Curr Protoc Bioinformatics 2013;43(1110):11.10.1–11.10.33.

[10] DNA-seq analysis pipeline. GDC Docs. Available at: https://docs.gdc.cancer.gov/Data/Bioinformatics_Pipelines/DNA_Seq_Variant_Calling_Pipeline/. Accessed May 6, 2021.

[11] Li MM, Datto M, Duncavage EJ, et al. Standards and guidelines for the interpretation and reporting of sequence variants in cancer: a joint consensus recommendation of the Association for Molecular Pathology,

American Society of Clinical Oncology, and College of American Pathologists. J Mol Diagn 2017;19(1):4–23.
[12] Jennings LJ, Arcila ME, Corless C, et al. Guidelines for validation of next-generation sequencing-based oncology panels: a joint consensus recommendation of the Association for Molecular Pathology and College of American Pathologists. J Mol Diagn 2017;19(3):341–65.
[13] Ma X, Shao Y, Tian L, et al. Analysis of error profiles in deep next-generation sequencing data. Genome Biol 2019;20:50.
[14] Fda.gov. 2021. Available at: https://www.fda.gov/media/141990/download. Accessed May 11, 2021.
[15] Kent WJ, Sugnet CW, Furey TS, et al. The human genome browser at UCSC. Genome Res 2002;12(6):996–1006.
[16] Umar A, Boland CR, Terdiman JP, et al. Revised bethesda guidelines for hereditary nonpolyposis colorectal cancer (lynch syndrome) and microsatellite instability. J Natl Cancer Inst 2004;96:261–8.
[17] Bonneville R, Krook MA, Chen HZ, et al. Detection of microsatellite instability biomarkers via next-generation sequencing. Methods Mol Biol 2020;2055:119–32.
[18] Niu B, Ye K, Zhang Q, et al. MSIsensor: microsatellite instability detection using paired tumor-normal sequence data. Bioinformatics 2014;30:1015–6.
[19] Chan TA, Yarchoan M, Jaffee E, et al. Development of tumor mutation burden as an immunotherapy biomarker: utility for the oncology clinic. Ann Oncol 2019;30(1):44–56.
[20] Budczies J, Allgäuer M, Litchfield K, et al. Optimizing panel-based tumor mutational burden (TMB) measurement. Ann Oncol 2019;30(9):1496–506.
[21] Budczies J, Kazdal D, Allgäuer M, et al. Quantifying potential confounders of panel-based tumor mutational burden (TMB) measurement. Lung Cancer 2020;142:114–9.
[22] Büttner R, Longshore JW, López-Ríos F, et al. Implementing TMB measurement in clinical practice: considerations on assay requirements. ESMO Open 2019;4(1):e000442.
[23] Heydt C, Rehker J, Pappesch R, et al. Analysis of tumor mutational burden: correlation of five large gene panels with whole exome sequencing. Sci Rep 2020;10(1):11387.
[24] Gallon R, Sheth H, Hayes C, et al. Sequencing-based microsatellite instability testing using as few as six markers for high-throughput clinical diagnostics. Hum Mutat 2020;41(1):332–41.
[25] Luchini C, Bibeau F, Ligtenberg MJL, et al. ESMO recommendations on microsatellite instability testing for immunotherapy in cancer, and its relationship with PD-1/PD-L1 expression and tumour mutational burden: a systematic review-based approach. Ann Oncol 2019;30(8):1232–43.
[26] Sobocińska J, Kolenda T, Teresiak A, et al. Diagnostics of mutations in MMR/*EPCAM* genes and their role in the treatment and care of patients with lynch syndrome. Diagnostics (Basel) 2020;10(10):786.
[27] Hause RJ, Pritchard CC, Shendure J, et al. Classification and characterization of microsatellite instability across 18 cancer types [published correction appears in Nat Med. 2017;23 (10):1241] [published correction appears in Nat Med. 2018 Apr 10;24(4):525]. Nat Med 2016;22(11):1342–50.
[28] Bonneville R, Krook MA, Kautto EA, et al. Landscape of microsatellite instability across 39 cancer types. JCO Precis Oncol 2017;2017:PO.17.00073.
[29] Gilson P, Merlin JL, Harlé A. Detection of microsatellite instability: state of the art and future applications in circulating tumour DNA (ctDNA). Cancers (Basel) 2021;13(7):1491.
[30] Wu LR, Chen SX, Wu Y, et al. Multiplexed enrichment of rare DNA variants via sequence-selective and temperature-robust amplification [published correction appears in Nat Biomed Eng. 2017 Dec;1(12):1005]. Nat Biomed Eng 2017;1:714–23.
[31] Gambin T, Liu Q, Karolak JA, et al. Low-level parental somatic mosaic SNVs in exomes from a large cohort of trios with diverse suspected Mendelian conditions. Genet Med 2020;22(11):1768–76.
[32] Strickler JH, Hanks BA, Khasraw M. Tumor mutational burden as a predictor of immunotherapy response: is more always better? Clin Cancer Res 2021;27(5):1236–41.
[33] Hellmann MD, Ciuleanu TE, Pluzanski A, et al. Nivolumab plus ipilimumab in lung cancer with a high tumor mutational burden. N Engl J Med 2018;378(22):2093–104.
[34] Marabelle A, Fakih M, Lopez J, et al. Association of tumour mutational burden with outcomes in patients with advanced solid tumours treated with pembrolizumab: prospective biomarker analysis of the multicohort, open-label, phase 2 KEYNOTE-158 study. Lancet Oncol 2020;21(10):1353–65.
[35] Garofalo A, Sholl L, Reardon B, et al. The impact of tumor profiling approaches and genomic data strategies for cancer precision medicine. Genome Med 2016;8(1):79.

COVID-19

Advances in Molecular Pathology 4 (2021) 205–216
ADVANCES IN MOLECULAR PATHOLOGY

A PENNdemic Year in Review

Sarah E. Herlihy, PhD*, Caren Gentile, MS
Department of Pathology and Laboratory Medicine, Molecular Pathology Laboratory, Hospital of the University of Pennsylvania, 7 Maloney Building, 3400 Spruce Street, Philadelphia, PA 19104, USA

KEYWORDS
- Severe acute respiratory virus coronavirus 2 (SARS-CoV-2) • COVID-19 • Clinical development
- Pandemic response

KEY POINTS

- A dedicated clinical development team is advantageous and allows flexibility during an emergency so that clinical work can continue uninterrupted.
- Supply chain restrictions required laboratories to validate multiple tests for severe acute respiratory syndrome coronavirus 2 (SARS-CoV-2) detection to provide redundancy in testing and allow for flexibility based on clinical urgency.
- A comprehensive SARS-CoV-2 screening program can allow secondary institutions to reopen safely.
- Although surveillance-based sequencing can provide important information for public health initiatives, the clinical utility of sequencing individuals remains unclear.

INTRODUCTION

The novel coronavirus severe acute respiratory syndrome coronavirus 2 (SARS-CoV-2) was first identified in Wuhan, China in December 2019 as the causative agent of the worldwide spread of coronavirus disease 2019 (COVID-19). By March 2021, greater than 120 million cases have been identified worldwide with approximately 25% of all cases occurring in the United States [1]. In addition, one-fifth of the total global deaths, which currently top more than 2.5 million, have occurred in the United States [1]. Several major cities, including the Philadelphia region, have been hard hit by COVID-19. Since the beginning of the pandemic, there have been 135,632 confirmed cases and 3333 deaths accounting for ~14% and ~13% of cases and deaths, respectively, in Pennsylvania [2,3].

In Philadelphia, like many cities across the nation, clinical laboratories faced unprecedented struggles and unpredictable changes while being at the forefront of the pandemic response. Although clinical testing challenges varied (limited vendor assays, Food and Drug Administration [FDA] regulations, supply chain disruptions on all aspects of the testing supplies, collection logistics, and personnel issues), over the course of the pandemic, the need for a swift response was imperative. This article highlights how a dedicated clinical development team (CDT), at a major academic institute in Philadelphia, was able to successfully navigate the shifting landscape of the COVID-19 pandemic while allowing clinical SARS-CoV-2 patient testing to continue and expand uninterrupted.

THE FIRST PHASE: NAVIGATING THE EMERGENCY

When the World Health Organization declared COVID-19 a global pandemic on March 11, 2020, clinical laboratories across the United States had already been hard at work, and Philadelphia had confirmed its first positive case 2 days previously [3,4]. Two months before that, the CDT, a group dedicated to molecular clinical test validation, had begun discussions with the

*Corresponding author, *E-mail address:* Sarah.herlihy@pennmedicine.upenn.edu

https://doi.org/10.1016/j.yamp.2021.06.007
2589-4080/21/

faculty of the Molecular Pathology and Microbiology Laboratories regarding the response to increasing SARS-CoV-2 infections. An expanded COVID-19 research and development task force (CoV R&D) was developed in late February that consisted of faculty and fellows from the Molecular Pathology and Microbiology Laboratories, Pathology and Laboratory Medicine administrative staff, laboratory managers, and 2 members of the CDT from the Hospital of the University of Pennsylvania (HUP). A daily meeting was adopted to discuss operations and acute issues, regulatory guidelines, supply chain disruptions, guide the evolution of testing (new methods, specimen types, and media, and so forth), and review recently published literature. Members of CoV R&D participated in overlapping departmental and health system task force meetings in order to maintain awareness of the big picture as well as interact with operational and logistical teams across the enterprise of PennMedicine's 6 hospitals.

The sole responsibility of the CDT is to bring new clinical molecular testing in house and maintain all current molecular testing platforms. Consequently, the CDT has intimate knowledge of the assay development and verification process, including both the technical and the regulatory aspects, which allowed the rapid deployment of 7 SARS-CoV-2 testing methods in the first 8 weeks of our pandemic response, two of which were implemented in the Microbiology Laboratory, with the remaining deployed in the Molecular Pathology Laboratory. Assays were distributed based on the existing platforms in each laboratory and the technical expertise of the staff (ie, more manual or pipetting heavy assays in the Molecular Pathology Laboratory). The CoV R&D discussed and planned all verification studies to be consistent with the fluctuating regulatory guidelines. Because the Microbiology Laboratory does not have a dedicated development team, the tasks performed by the CDT became the responsibility of the fellow and the faculty laboratory director, who were already stretched thin.

New assay development can be disruptive to clinical testing, and when technologists are required to split their time, development work gets sidelined, as patient care is their primary responsibility. A CDT can quickly adapt to the changing needs of the health system and laboratory, and this allowed assay verifications and the supportive paperwork associated with implementing clinical testing, such as, but not limited to, verification documents, standard operating procedures, report interpretations, and maintenance log templates, to be completed on an abbreviated timeline. This was accomplished by pivoting assay development priorities; at the beginning of the pandemic, multiple non-COVID development projects were being juggled by the CDT, but by early February, all efforts completely shifted to development of SARS-CoV-2 testing in accordance with regulatory guidance. Having a dedicated development team allowed SARS-CoV-2 testing capacity to scale up to meet the increasing clinical needs without sacrificing patient testing. In addition, it provided the framework for coordinating decentralized rapid testing across our then 6 hospital health system.

An unexpected outcome of the CoV R&D was that it provided a support system and a mechanism for assessing the overall well-being of all laboratory technologists, faculty, and staff. During a pandemic, many individuals experience heightened levels of stress, insomnia, alcohol and drug misuse, and symptoms of posttraumatic stress disorder [5]. In addition, health care workers often face stigma, because of working in a high-risk environment, which can have a negative effect on their psychological health and increase their risk of burnout, anxiety, and depression. Health care workers are hit especially hard because of extended working hours and social isolation that emergency situations create. This pandemic has had a profound effect on laboratory workers [5]. It is common for technologists to work with repetitive motion injuries, have feelings of guilt when they leave samples behind for the following shift, become instrument-troubleshooting experts, and experience emotional exhaustion from the never-ending specimen backlog [6]. Daily CoV R&D meetings provided an outlet to bring feedback from the technologists to laboratory administration and opportunities to work through difficulties.

THE SECOND PHASE: BUILDING A TESTING STRATEGY

Uniquely, during the COVID-19 pandemic, supply chain shortages of reagents and instrumentation were pivotal in method choice. The extent of disruption spanned all aspects of testing with deficiencies in collection kits, instrumentation, assay reagents and consumables, and personal protective equipment (PPE). In an April 2020 survey published by the Association of Molecular Pathology (AMP), 85% of respondents reported disruptions to supply chains, which caused either a delay in testing or a decrease in testing volume; by the August survey, this number was up to 93% [7,8]. Academic medical centers and community hospitals were disproportionately affected by shortages of testing kits compared with commercial reference laboratories [7,8]. Hospital laboratories are inherently different from commercial reference laboratories. From early on, it was evident that assay-specific shortages would require hospital laboratories to implement multiple testing platforms for redundancy in testing and the flexibility to accommodate both rapid and routine testing to respond to various clinical scenarios. In the same April AMP survey, 57% of respondents from academic medical centers or community hospitals were running 3 or more assays compared with only 20% of commercial reference laboratories [8]. By August, these numbers jumped to 80% and 30%, for academic and commercial laboratories, respectively [7].

As manufacturers developed new assays, they were vetted by the CoV R&D to determine if implementation was necessary and feasible. Tests to implement were chosen based on the technical feasibility, projected daily capacity, cost, Emergency Use Authorization (EUA) approval status, the availability of instrumentation and reagents as well as alignment with the clinical needs of the 6 hospitals in our health system. CDT members maintained efficiency by dividing the laboratory and clerical work based on each member's strengths.

The timeline for clinical SARS-CoV-2 assay development is shown in Fig. 1A. On March 3, validation studies for the ePlex SARS-CoV-2 (GenMark Diagnostics, Carlsbad, CA) assay began while the assay was still under review for EUA, and by March 12, the first of many SARS-CoV-2 tests was performed. Although our theoretic testing capacity (based on instrument capacity) was several hundred per day, supply chain issues on test kits further limited the actual capacity to ~20 per day. Therefore, only the sickest patients and health care exposures from Occupational Medicine were tested following approval by hospital Infection Control. Hospital visitation was restricted, and multiple staff hotlines were set up 1 day following SARS-CoV-2 testing go-live to handle inquiries regarding clinical situations and staff questions about infection control, PPE, supplies, operational issues, and testing. By March 15, hospital visitation was completely suspended, and the laboratory was already hard at work bringing in new assay platforms for additional testing, which was complicated by supply chain shortages and regulatory oversight. The next day, statewide mitigations went

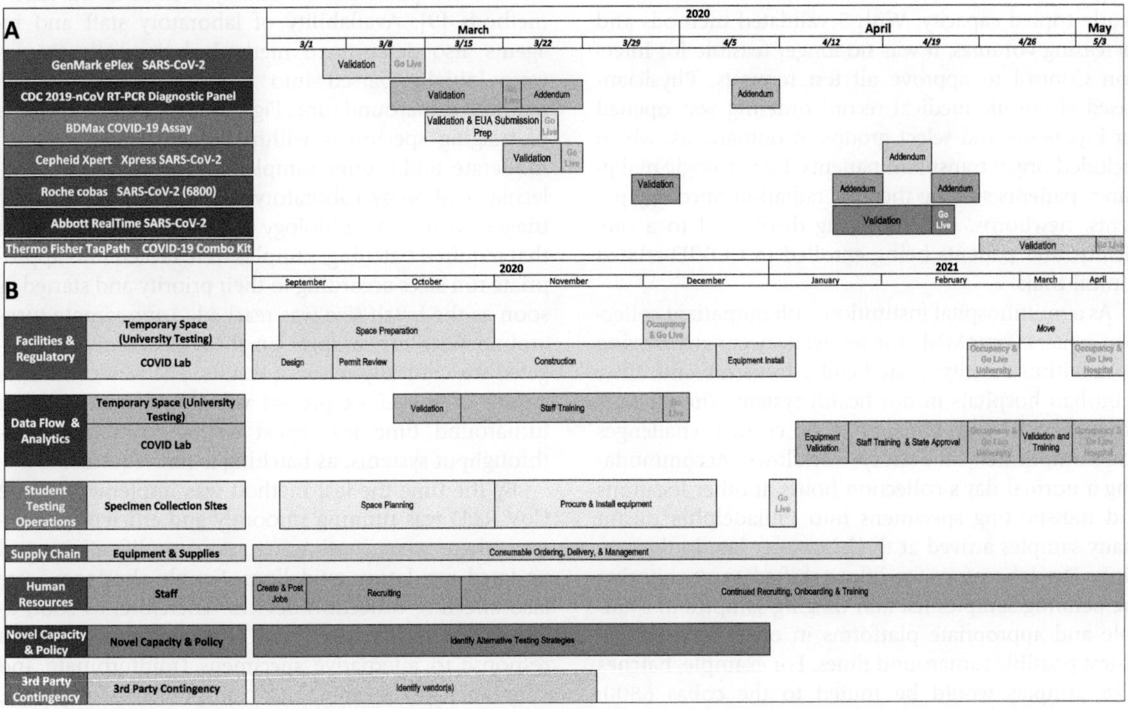

FIG. 1 Timelines for development and Project Quaker. (*A*) The timeline for initial clinical assay development from March to May 2020 in the Molecular Pathology and Microbiology Laboratories. (*B*) Timelines for Project Quaker from implementation of work groups to go-live of all clinical testing (September 2020 to April 2021).

into effect, and the confirmed cases in the Philadelphia region numbered 52 [2].

One week later, the CDT completed validation of the second method, the Centers for Disease Control and Prevention (CDC) 2019-nCoV Real-Time RT-PCR Diagnostic Panel (Atlanta, GA, USA). The next week, 2 tests, a laboratory-developed test (LDT) using the BD Max platform (BD Molecular Diagnostics, Franklin Lakes, NJ, USA) and the GeneXpert SARS-CoV-2 (Cepheid, Sunnyvale, CA, USA), went live within days of each other in the Microbiology Laboratory. The BDMax LDT was validated using archived residual specimens following the FDA's Molecular Diagnostic Template for Laboratories. The BDMax LDT assay was reviewed and approved for EUA by the FDA. The Cepheid platform was implemented at all hospitals in the health systems to address rapid community-based testing while centralizing routine testing at HUP. These 3 platform additions expanded theoretic instrument capacity, but all test requests were still being triaged through Infection Control because of continued supply chain shortages of assay kits, which limited capacity to ~200 tests per day. The subsequent week, the high-throughput cobas 6800/8800 SARS-CoV-2 assay (Roche Diagnostics, Indianapolis, IN, USA) was validated and nearly tripled capacity. With 5 validated methods and increasing volumes, it was no longer feasible for Infection Control to approve all test requests. Physician-based electronic medical record ordering was opened for inpatients and select groups of outpatients, which included organ transplant patients, hematologic malignancy patients starting therapy, radiation oncology patients, newborns, patients being discharged to a care facility, and patients being enrolled in COVID-related clinical trials.

As a multihospital institution with outpatient collection centers, PennMedicine received specimens arriving from within the city, tented collection sites, and other suburban hospitals in our health system. The logistics of collection and transportation created challenges and complicated laboratory workflows. Accommodating a normal day's collection hours at other locations and transporting specimens into Philadelphia meant many samples arrived at the laboratory late in the evening. The laboratory workflow shifted to monitoring the pending samples list and triaging samples to available and appropriate platforms in order to meet the fastest possible turnaround times. For example, batches $\geq$48 samples would be routed to the cobas 6800; batches under 48 would be routed to either the CDC assay or the ePlex or sent to the Microbiology Laboratory for testing on the BD Max with all urgent testing still occurring in the Microbiology Laboratory. By April 21, our sixth assay, the Real*Time* SARS-CoV-2 (Abbott Molecular Inc, Des Plaines, IL, USA) was live, bringing our daily testing capacity to more than 1000 tests per day at HUP. Shortly thereafter, the seventh method, TaqPath COVID-19 Combo Kit (Thermo Fisher, Waltham, MA, USA), was validated. Both of the newest assays improved triage for batched workflows within the laboratory.

Each assay was successfully implemented, allowing patient testing to expand concurrently. Gradually, the increased testing capacity facilitated the hospital to reopen at full capacity once the Governor lifted hospital admissions to non-COVID cases. With a testing capability of approximately 3000 tests per day (for both symptomatic and asymptomatic), testing was opened to all departments in the health system, and triaging workflows were adjusted accordingly. Because comparison studies showed that the analytical sensitivity of 6 of our 7 methods had similar limits of detection, samples could be stratified by clinical urgency without concern for loss of detection (Table 1) [9]. Following manufacturer workflow modifications, as described in the table legend, all 7 assays had similar limits of detection [9]. Table 1 compares chosen quality metrics of the first 7 methods [9]. Availability of laboratory staff and reagents also determined method choice. All samples were initially parsed into 4 groups based on the required turnaround time. Fig. 2 outlines the operations of triaging specimens within 2 laboratories. Urgent, moderate, and routine samples were triaged in the Molecular Pathology Laboratory, and STAT samples were triaged in the Microbiology Laboratory. For methods that required batching, samples were racked into appropriate run sizes according to their priority and started as soon as the batch size was reached. Approximate turnaround time for samples on these platforms was targeted for clinically relevant results. The random access nature of the ePlex proved valuable for minimizing turnaround time for repeat testing from our high-throughput systems, as batching is not required.

By the time the last method was implemented, the CoV R&D was running smoothly and efficiently; however, there were continuous assay modifications and updated regulatory guidelines. Supply shortages were also affecting collection devices. Therefore, as soon as testing was established, the CDT needed to have a swift response to alternative specimens (midturbinate and anterior nares swabs) and transport media (saline, phosphate-buffered saline, and so forth) as reagent supply and testing needs evolved. In addition, the CDT handled all validation related to changes in EUA

TABLE 1
Selected Quality Metrics for 7 Severe Acute Respiratory Syndrome Coronavirus 2 Methods (Top) and 5 Methods Added Later (Bottom)

Method	Batch Size	Approximate Assay Time (h)	Ease of Use	Technologists to Run Efficiently	Laboratory Assistants to Run Efficiently	Cost per Reaction	Approximate Laboratory-Established Sensitivity (Copies/mL)
Abbott RealTime SARS-CoV-2	Up to 94	8	Moderate	1.5	N/A	$$	50
Cepheid Xpert Xpress SARS-CoV-2	1	0.83	Easy	1	N/A	$$$	100
GenMark ePlex SARS-CoV-2	1	1.75	Easy	1	N/A	$$$$	10,000[a]
Roche cobas SARS-CoV-2 (6800)	Up to 94	4	Moderate	1	1	$	500
Thermo Fisher TaqPathCOVID-19 Combo Kit	Up to 94	3.5	Difficult	2	N/A	$$	100
BDMax COVID-19 Assay (EUA LDT)	Up to 22	2.5	Easy	1	N/A	$$	1000
CDC 2019-nCoV RT-PCR Diagnostic Panel	Up to 29	7	Difficult	2	N/A	$	500
Additional added platforms							
Roche cobas SARS-CoV-2 & Influenza A/B (Liat)	1	0.20	Easy	1	N/A	$$$	Not assessed
DiaSorin Simplexa COVID-19 Direct	Up to 8	1.75	Easy	1	N/A	$$$	Not assessed
Fluidigm AdvantaDx SARS-CoV-2 RT-PCR Assay	Up to 186	5.5–8[b]	Difficult[b]	1–2	2	$	Not assessed
Thermo Fisher Amplitude Solution TaqPath COVID-19 High-Throughput Combo Kit	Up to 376	5	Moderate	2	2	$	Not assessed
Roche cobas SARS-CoV-2 (8800)	Up to 94	4	Moderate	2	1–2	$	Not assessed

Assay time accounts for preprocessing time, instrument time, and resulting. Sample collection, transport, and accessioning time are considered equivalent and are not included. The Roche 6800/8800, Amplitude, and Fluidigm platforms can be started in a staggered manner to increase throughput. The time to result staggered runs is decreased. Staff is split into laboratory assistants who perform the preprocessing steps, if included, and technologists, who perform the analytical and postanalytical steps. Analytical sensitivity was evaluated on the first 7 methods with a dilution series (50,000–1000 copies/mL) of quantified positive archived clinical specimens generated with pooled negative samples. Positive samples were quantitated on a CDC-based methodology with a standard curve generated using synthetic RNA of the SARS-CoV-2 N gene. Dilutions under 1000 cp/mL were evaluated on selected methods based on the stated limit of detection. The 5 additional platforms were implemented after comparison studies were completed.

Abbreviation: N/A, not applicable.

[a] Following workflow modifications, the ePlex SARS-CoV-2 had comparable sensitivity levels to the other assays.

[b] Fluidigm assay time and ease of use are dependent on the use of robotics, which both shorten the length of the assay and reduce the technical difficulties.

Modified from Gentile C, Richard-Greenblatt, M, Fink, J, et al. A Practical Comparison of Seven Molecular SARS-CoV-2 Methods. Paper presented at: Association for Molecular Pathology Annual Meeting 2020; November 16-20, 2020; with permission.

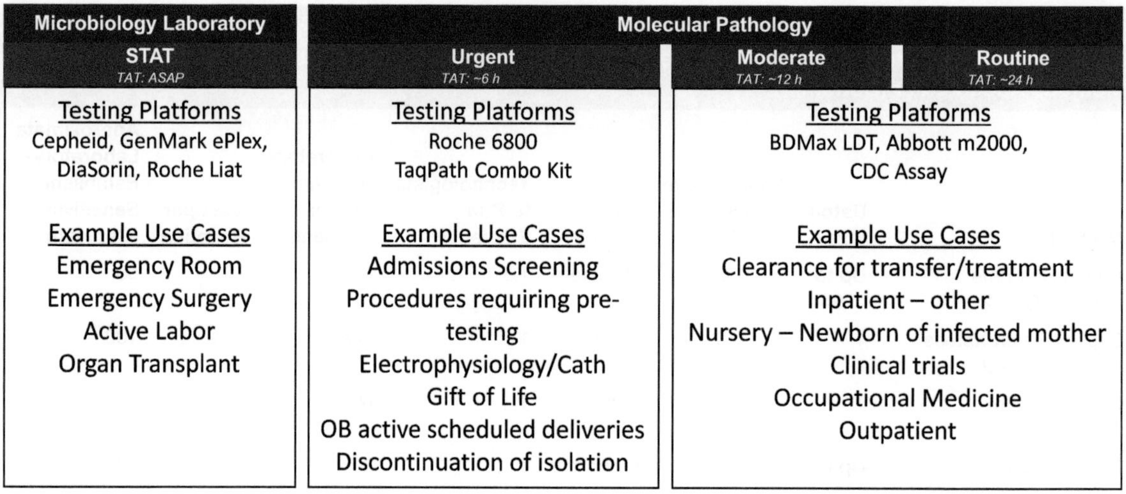

FIG. 2 Example workflow schematic when using multiple methods for testing. Outline of how testing was deployed across multiple laboratories to serve patients with various clinical needs. Figure does not include the new methods deployed at the COVID Testing Laboratory. ASAP, as soon as possible; OB, obstetrics; STAT, immediately (from the Latin "statim"); TAT, turnaround time.

manufacturer's instructions for use, such as a modified workflow for the ePlex that removed the use of the sample delivery device, a new internal control volume for the Abbott Real*Time* assay, and new vortexing and centrifugation requirements, new extraction reagent manufacturer, and new analysis workflows for the Thermo Fisher TaqPath assay. These smaller validations were handled in a similar manner as the assay validations: working together as a team while catering to each member's strengths and allowing clinical SARS-CoV-2 testing to continue uninterrupted. Because of the prominent role the CDT plays in training, the team provided onsite training at HUP for one of the suburban entities on the Thermo Fisher TaqPath assay to support routine testing at that entity.

Following the initial implementations and even with an additional 2 platforms (DiaSorin Simplexa and Roche Liat), it was clear that the capacity for testing was limited by the both the methods and the technologist time required. The next phase of SARS-CoV-2 testing was expanding both the testing capacity and the staffing to better serve the health system's patients and the Philadelphia community, including the UPenn faculty, staff, and students. The solution was Project Quaker: 2 high-throughput COVID-19 testing laboratories for both swab and saliva testing. Timelines for Project Quaker are shown in Fig. 1B. Again, the CDT took an active role in vetting the instrumentation, including robotics, designing the laboratory space, and validating the new assays, while maintaining regulatory compliance. The CDT's role allowed existing swab-based testing to continue in the Molecular Pathology and Microbiology Laboratories.

THE THIRD PHASE: EXPANSION

By midyear 2020, with the testing and supply chain more stabilized, the focus of many academic institutes became how to safely open universities. Closures during the 2020 spring semester brought financial losses to institutions [10]. Psychological impacts of closure on faculty, staff, and students were evident by studies showing moderate to severe scores for anxiety, depression, and stress during the spring semester [11,12]. Academic centers needed to balance the financial pressure and continued strain on mental health with the safety of reopening. The Philadelphia area boasts 80 secondary education institutes, many of which reside in the dense urban setting. Therefore, considerations extend beyond the vulnerable members of the university to those within the surrounding community [10,13,14]. An analytical modeling study found that an effective screening design, robust testing supplies, results management strategy, and compliance to mitigation efforts were crucial to successful university openings and keeping the community safe [13]. A decision tree analysis by members of our institution determined the ideal testing strategy to both mitigate infection rates and minimize inaccurate results [15]. Reopening designs incorporated the testing strategy and infection control measures that would need to be in place to bring students back to campus safely.

Regulations on the testing programs complicated operational planning. The FDA and CDC differentiate screening and surveillance of SARS-CoV-2. Surveillance and screening both permit broad population testing, but where surveillance can only be reported as an aggregate data, screening results are reported on an individual level to allow isolation and contact tracing to further reduce spread [16,17]. Although the Molecular Pathology Laboratory was able to support UPenn student testing during the fall 2020 semester, this was not a durable solution nor could the capacity encompass all university testing at the effective screening rate [15]. UPenn partnered with Penn Medicine, with expertise in clinical testing, to develop a screening strategy for reopening and sustaining a safe learning environment designated PennCares. Fig. 3 shows the structure and diversity of the Project Quaker team to oversee both the PennCares testing program design and the expansion of hospital SARS-CoV-2 testing. Under the guidance of both university and hospital administration, specialty workstreams developed comprehensive operations for a spring 2021 opening. Campuses that remained open during fall 2020 cited that this integrative planning proved beneficial to mitigate spread [18].

The result of this multidisciplinary approach was the PennCares testing program using the EUA saliva-based platform manufactured by Fluidigm paired with Perkin Elmer Janus G3 liquid handlers to automate technically challenging steps. The PennCares program incorporates what Paltiel and colleagues [13] described as essential components to a screening program: ease of collection along with an accurate, cost-effective, and scalable testing method that could be turned around in a short amount of time. Members of the university community are screened 1 to 3 times per week depending on their risk categorization. The laboratory maintains a turnaround time of 24 hours or less for timely isolation and contact tracing of positive persons. During the spring semester thus far, the positivity rate among university screening tests has remained low, only spiking higher than 1.2% during 3 weeks in January, but positivity always remained below the percent positivity in Philadelphia [3,19]. Two of the high positivity weeks coincided with move-in weeks, indicating that students

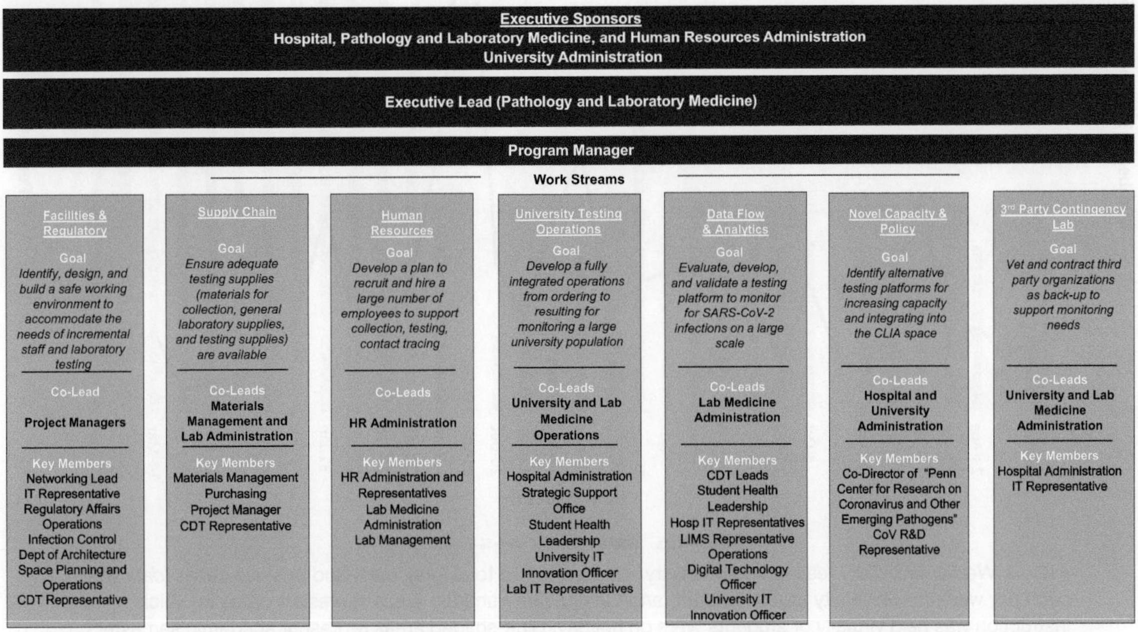

FIG. 3 Structure of Project Quaker. Individual workstream teams were co-led with a particular goal to be accomplished. A project manager and executive lead oversaw the progress of each workstream weekly. The executive lead acted as a liaison between the stakeholders and the workstreams. Hosp, hospital; HR, human resources; IT, information technology; LIMS, Laboratory Information Management System.

were arriving on campus with existing infection. The third week with high positivity was 2 weeks after move-in, reflecting some initial noncompliance. Noncompliance, as outlined in agreements signed by students before returning to campus, was met with violation citations, which spiked in January, and steadily decreased thereafter [19]. Cumulative testing and positivity rates over the 2020 to 2021 academic year are presented in Fig. 4 [19]. Overall, implementation of SARS-CoV-2 monitoring has been successful at UPenn and throughout campuses across the United States.

Key struggles to the implementation of Project Quaker centered on the Human Resources workstream ranging from recruiting to training. With numerous clinical laboratories filling the testing demand for SARS-CoV-2, the pools of technical staff qualified to perform high complexity testing were limited. The candidate pool was expanded by splitting the preanalytical and analytical/postanalytical responsibilities into 2 well-defined roles, the laboratory assistant and the medical technologist. This splitting of responsibilities permitted hiring of laboratory assistants to perform preanalytical tasks, such as specimen accessioning and processing, as these are not considered high complexity by the FDA. An advantage of the laboratory assistant position was that hired persons could also staff specimen collection sites, building redundancy with cross-training. To obtain the large number of required staff, Penn partnered with the West Philadelphia Skills Initiative (WPSI) to hire 50 laboratory assistants for the expansion of university and hospital testing. WPSI is a

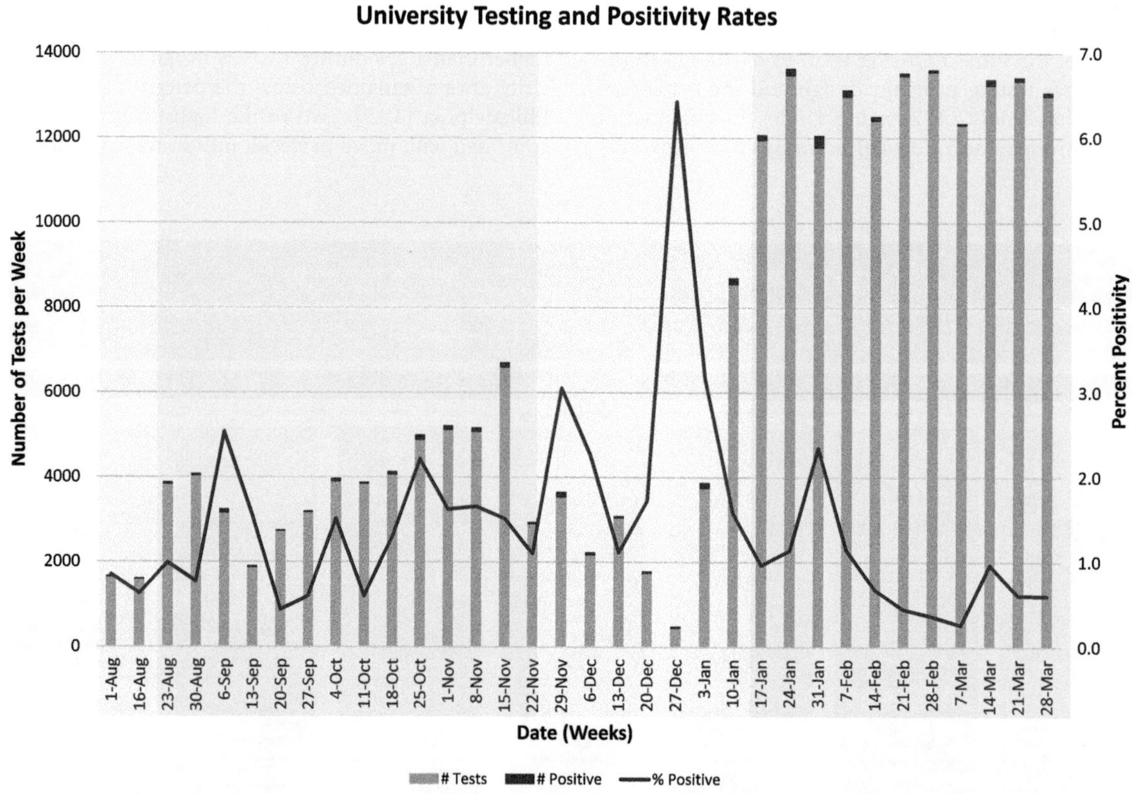

FIG. 4 Weekly university testing and positivity. The number of total (*gray bars*) and positive cases (*dark blue bars*) per week for university students, staff, and faculty. Gray-shaded areas represent dates in which instruction was held virtually or students were on holiday. Blue-shaded areas represent academic semesters. During the fall semester, classes were held virtually, but testing was available. During the spring 2021 semester, testing was mandated 1 to 3 times per week depending on the population risk category. The percent positivity is shown as a red line. (*Data from* COVID-19 Dashboard. University of Pennsylvania. https://coronavirus.upenn.edu/content/dashboard. Published 2021. Accessed 2021.)

program that helps link unemployed Philadelphians with employers through job-specific training models [20]. The partnership developed a 2-week training course, which all laboratory assistant candidates underwent before hire. This model of education and training became crucial to the success of the laboratory. Many of the new staff, both laboratory assistants and medical technologists alike, were in their first jobs and/or had not previously worked in a hospital or Clinical Laboratory Improvement Amendments (CLIA) laboratory environment. As such, job-specific education and training were developed and overseen by the CDT, which now included 2 recently gained full-time employees and several part-time volunteers. Instructional courses covering laboratory regulations (College of American Pathologists [CAP]/CLIA), basic virology, molecular biology, and SARS-CoV-2 diagnostics were required for staff. Additional assay-specific content, including instrumentation and maintenance, general and laboratory information systems workflows, assay performance characteristics, and analysis, was created. Knowledge retention was evaluated with content assessments. Without an experienced group of technologists to guide and train new staff, the CDT took on the role of trainers. Each new technologist began technical training with an in-house developed pipetting course and then assay-specific training, the length of which depended on the experience level of the person. Laboratory assistants and technologists were cleared for clinical work once the CDT deemed them competent in technical skills and assay-specific–based knowledge. We are not alone in recognizing the need for more robust and extensive training with such a new workforce. Recently, the CDC launched the OneLab initiative to develop training and strengthen learning communities to better prepare for emergency responses [21].

The coordinated efforts of Project Quaker greatly expanded SARS-CoV-2 testing capacities. Quality metrics for each of the expanded assays are shown in Table 1 [8]. Both UPenn and its population and the greater Philadelphia community have benefited. Mitigation of spread at the university level maintains a sense of security for the surrounding areas. Increased capacity at the hospital level allows expanded testing for the hospital, but also Philadelphians, hopefully curbing spread and threats of another wave.

THE FOURTH PHASE: LOOKING FORWARD

As the landscape of the SARS-CoV-2 pandemic is ever changing, the CoV R&D group continues to meet on a regular basis, albeit less frequently, to discuss workflow improvements, monitor regulatory policies, and forecast the fluctuating needs within the clinical laboratory. Although various topics, such as home collection, sample pooling, the utility of antigen and antibody testing, and the use of C_T values, are discussed, the recurrent debate is the utility of research and clinical sequencing.

SARS-CoV-2 has a mutation rate of 2.5 nucleotides per month [22]. The clinical utility of sequencing for SARS-CoV-2 variants for individual patients is unclear at the time of writing this article. The Centers for Medicare and Medicaid prohibits lineage identification from surveillance efforts outside of the CLIA laboratory to be returned to patients or clinicians [23]. It remains important to correlate any lineage and variant information closely with clinical presentations and epidemiologic data to inform public health decisions [24,25]. Although no approved variant-specific treatments are currently available, it is difficult to envision a large demand for clinical sequencing without them [26]. Limitations to implementing clinical grade sequencing include costs with no current reimbursement plan, scalability, and informatics [24]. Clinical laboratories themselves benefit from sequencing by rapidly identifying variants that affect polymerase chain reaction detection that have the potential to escape detection [24]. Several identified variant changes lie within the primer/probe regions of commercial nucleic acid amplification tests (NAAT) with known target disruption [27–30]. Tests relying on a single gene target are especially vulnerable; however, most NAATs minimize the risk with multiple target designs. Emerging variants also pose a risk to monoclonal antibody treatments [31–33]. Rapid identification of drug-resistant variants allows health care providers to modify treatments appropriately. As more research is completed and identified variants have known advantages and disadvantages for clinical care, it is possible that sequencing will move into the clinical laboratory setting. However, without a clear utility, clinical-grade sequencing remains minimal. Therefore, sequencing of positive specimens suspected to contain variants of concern often occurs in a research setting as surveillance.

In late 2020, the B.1.1.7 UK lineage spread rapidly throughout England after being identified as a variant of concern [34]. The United Kingdom's centralized sequencing surveillance program documented the quicker spread of B.1.1.7 compared with other circulating strains [35]. Stricter mitigation efforts in England, such as social distancing and a new lockdown, reduced the transmission advantage of the B.1.1.7 lineage [34]. Around the same time, the P.1 and B.1.351 lineages with like variants emerged synchronously [34]. More

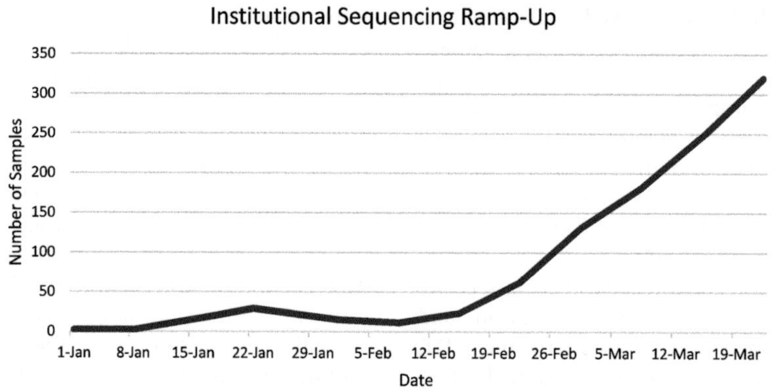

FIG. 5 Penn institutional sequencing. The ramp-up of sequencing efforts during 2021 with the goal of reaching 10% to 20% of all positive cases from the health system and university. A combination of biased and unbiased samples is included for public health initiatives, clinical laboratory quality assurance, and surveillance.

recently, the B.1.526 and B.1.427/429 were identified regionally in New York and California, respectively [36,37]. These discoveries highlighted the need for global lineage surveillance. Lineage and variant identification can inform public health authorities to circulating lineages in a region that have increased transmissibility or infectivity, can cause disease of greater severity, and can decrease treatment responses, and it can be used to identify origins, trace outbreaks, and monitor vaccine effectiveness [24]. Informed decisions, both locally and regionally, to improve protective measures, such as social distancing, gathering restrictions, and cleaning, may be guided by variant detection in monitored regions [22]. In addition, publicly available sequences may be used by manufacturers to pinpoint conserved regions of the genome for future vaccine targets [38]. Given the evolutionary trends of SARS-CoV-2, vaccine breakthrough and vaccine-driven virus evolution are anticipated [39,40]. For these reasons and others, the CDC, public health laboratories, and many institutions and developers have adopted a surveillance strategy, sequencing a percentage of the positive cases. These efforts are both decentralized and constrained in the United States [35,41]. A UPenn research laboratory, similar to efforts at other institutions, accommodates both unbiased surveillance and selective quality assurance and public health sequencing for hospital and university specimens [42]. As shown in Fig. 5, UPenn has been able to scale sequencing efforts over the past few months, but a limit to the capacity exists. Likewise, the GISAID public database shows a rapid increase in sequencing in the United States beginning in November [35]. The CDC has been seeking partnership with commercial diagnostic laboratories, clinical laboratories, and public health laboratories to expand sequencing capacity [43]. The importance of global surveillance intensifies to discover emerging lineages and moderate COVID-19 spread.

SUMMARY

The ability to quickly evolve clinical laboratory testing in a pandemic is essential to patient care. Here, a coordinated cross-disciplinary team and a dedicated CDT streamlined the validation process for SARS-CoV-2 detection implementation and expansion of capacity as well as aided in the design, building, and deployment of 2 new COVID-19 testing laboratories, in a rapidly changing environment. The expanded CDT also established and executed an enhanced training program for new employees. Both the CoV R&D and larger Project Quaker team supported all endeavors. Patient and university SARS-CoV-2 testing was uninterrupted even during expansion and relocation to the new laboratory, thus highlighting the important role of a dedicated CDT especially in the midst of an emergency.

ACKNOWLEDGMENTS

There are so many people to acknowledge for their work, dedication, and guidance over the past year. Our heartfelt thanks to all members of Project Quaker, the staff in Central Receiving, Molecular Pathology, Microbiology, and COVID Testing Laboratories, Frederic Bushman's lab at UPenn, and the members of CoV R&D for their commitment to the group's success.

A special thanks to Amy Trenton, Corey Rogers, Mike Feldman, and Vivianna Van Deerlin for their input on the manuscript and figures.

DISCLOSURE

The authors have nothing to disclose.

REFERENCES

[1] Dong E, Du H, Gardner L. An interactive web-based dashboard to track COVID-19 in real time. Lancet Infect Dis 2020;20(5):533–4.

[2] COVID-19 in Pennsylvania. Pennsylvania Department of Health; 2021. Available at: https://www.health.pa.gov/topics/disease/coronavirus/Pages/Coronavirus.aspx. Accessed April 9, 2021.

[3] Coronavirus disease 2019 (COVID-19): providing information and updates about COVID-19 in Philadelphia. Philadelphia Department of Health; 2021. Available at: https://www.phila.gov/programs/coronavirus-disease-2019-covid-19/. Accessed April 9, 2021.

[4] Opening remarks at the media briefing on COVID19 [press release]. Available at: https://www.who.int/director-general/speeches/detail/who-director-general-s-opening-remarks-at-the-media-briefing-on-covid-19—11-march-2020.

[5] Giorgi G, Lecca LI, Alessio F, et al. COVID-19-related mental health effects in the workplace: a narrative review. Int J Environ Res Public Health 2020;17(21):7857.

[6] Wu KL. 'Nobody sees us': testing-lab workers strain under demand. 2020. Available at: https://www.nytimes.com/2020/12/03/health/coronavirus-testing-labs-workers.html. Accessed April 8, 2021.

[7] Association for Molecular Pathology SARS-CoV-2 molecular testing: summary of August SARS-CoV-2 molecular testing survey. Association for Molecular Pathology; 2020. Available at: https://www.amp.org/advocacy/sars-cov-2-survey/.

[8] Association for Molecular Pathology SARS-CoV-2 Molecular Testing: Summary of April SARS-CoV-2 Molecular Testing Survey. Association for Molecular Pathology;2020.

[9] Gentile C, Richard-Greenblatt, M, Fink, J, et al. A practical comparison of seven molecular SARS-CoV-2 methods paper presented at: Association for Molecular Pathology Annual Meeting November 16-20, 2020.

[10] Wrighton MS, Lawrence SJ. Reopening colleges and universities during the COVID-19 pandemic. Ann Intern Med 2020;173(8):664–5.

[11] Odriozola-Gonzalez P, Planchuelo-Gomez A, Irurtia MJ, et al. Psychological effects of the COVID-19 outbreak and lockdown among students and workers of a Spanish university. Psychiatry Res 2020;290:113108.

[12] Dhar BK, Ayittey FK, Sarkar SM. Impact of COVID-19 on psychology among the university students. Glob Chall 2020;4(11):2000038.

[13] Paltiel AD, Zheng A, Walensky RP. Assessment of SARS-CoV-2 screening strategies to permit the safe reopening of college campuses in the United States. JAMA Netw Open 2020;3(7):e2016818.

[14] Tanabe KO, Hayden ME, Zunder B, et al. Identifying vulnerable populations at a university during the COVID-19 pandemic. J Am Coll Health 2021;1–4.

[15] Van Pelt A, Glick HA, Yang W, et al. Evaluation of COVID-19 testing strategies for repopulating college and university campuses: a decision tree analysis. J Adolesc Health 2021;68(1):28–34.

[16] Overview of testing for SARS-CoV-2 (COVID-19). Centers for Disease Control and Prevention; 2021. Available at: https://www.cdc.gov/coronavirus/2019-ncov/hcp/testing-overview.html. Accessed March 25, 2021.

[17] Screening for COVID-19: deciding which test to use when establishing testing programs. U.S. Food and Drug Administration; 2021. Available at: https://www.fda.gov/medical-devices/coronavirus-covid-19-and-medical-devices/screening-covid-19-deciding-which-test-use-when-establishing-testing-programs. Accessed March 25, 2021.

[18] Ryan BJ, Muehlenbein MP, Allen J, et al. Sustaining university operations during the COVID-19 pandemic. Disaster Med Public Health Prep 2021;1–24.

[19] COVID-19 dashboard. University of Pennsylvania; 2021. Available at: https://coronavirus.upenn.edu/content/dashboard. Accessed 2021.

[20] West Philadelphia Skills Initiative. Available at: https://philadelphiaskills.org/. Accessed April 7, 2021.

[21] CDC OneLab. Division of laboratory systems 2021. Available at: https://www.cdc.gov/labtraining/onelab.html. Accessed April 7, 2021.

[22] Meredith LW, Hamilton WL, Warne B, et al. Rapid implementation of SARS-CoV-2 sequencing to investigate cases of health-care associated COVID-19: a prospective genomic surveillance study. Lancet Infect Dis 2020;20(11):1263–71.

[23] CLIA SARS-CoV-2 variant testing frequently asked question. 2021. Available at: https://www.cms.gov/files/document/clia-sars-cov-2-variant.pdf?ACSTrackingID=USCDC_2146-DM52811&ACSTrackingLabel=Laboratory%20Update%3A%20CMS%20Posts%20FAQ%20for%20Reporting%20Sequencing%20Results%20for%20SARS-CoV-2%20Variants&deliveryName=USCDC_2146-DM52811. Accessed April 5, 2021.

[24] Harilal D, Ramaswamy S, Loney T, et al. SARS-CoV-2 whole genome amplification and sequencing for effective population-based surveillance and control of viral transmission. Clin Chem 2020;66(11):1450–8.

[25] Behrmann O, Spiegel M. COVID-19: from rapid genome sequencing to fast decisions. Lancet Infect Dis 2020;20(11):1218.

[26] Emergency Use Authorization. Available at: https://www.fda.gov/emergency-preparedness-and-response/mcm-legal-regulatory-and-policy-framework/emergency-use-authorization#coviddrugs. Accessed April 8, 2021.

[27] SARS-CoV-2 viral mutations: impact on COVID-19 tests. Available at: https://www.fda.gov/medical-devices/coronavirus-covid-19-and-medical-devices/sars-cov-2-viral-mutations-impact-covid-19-tests?utm_medium=email&utm_source=govdelivery. Accessed June 8, 2021.

[28] Artesi M, Bontems S, Gobbels P, et al. A recurrent mutation at position 26340 of SARS-CoV-2 is associated with failure of the e gene quantitative reverse transcription-PCR utilized in a commercial dual-target diagnostic assay. J Clin Microbiol 2020;58(10):e01598.

[29] Staff BTB. Thermo Fisher's COVID-19 tests: designed with virus mutations in mind, vol. 2021, 2020. Available at: https://www.thermofisher.com/blog/behindthebench/thermo-fishers-covid-19-tests-designed-with-virus-mutations-in-mind/?icid=fl-covid19mutations.

[30] Hasan MR, Sundararaju S, Manickam C, et al. A novel point mutation in the N gene of SARS-CoV-2 may affect the detection of the virus by reverse transcription-quantitative PCR. J Clin Microbiol 2021;59(4):e03278.

[31] FDA authorizes revisions to fact sheets to address SARS-CoV-2 variants for monoclonal antibody products under Emergency Use Authorization. Available at: https://www.fda.gov/drugs/drug-safety-and-availability/fda-authorizes-revisions-fact-sheets-address-sars-cov-2-variants-monoclonal-antibody-products-under. Accessed June 8, 2021.

[32] Taylor PC, Adams AC, Hufford MM, et al. Neutralizing monoclonal antibodies for treatment of COVID-19. Nat Rev Immunol 2021;21(6):382–93.

[33] Tada T, Dcosta BM, Zhou H, et al. Decreased neutralization of SARS-CoV-2 global variants by therapeutic anti-spike protein monoclonal antibodies. bioRxiv 2021.

[34] Volz E, Mishra S, Chand M, et al. Assessing transmissibility of SARS-CoV-2 lineage B.1.1.7 in England. Nature 2021.

[35] Callaway E. Multitude of coronavirus variants found in the US - but the threat is unclear. Nature 2021; 591(7849):190.

[36] Deng X, Garcia-Knight MA, Khalid MM, et al. Transmission, infectivity, and antibody neutralization of an emerging SARS-CoV-2 variant in California carrying a L452R spike protein mutation. medRxiv 2021.

[37] Annavajhala MK, Mohri H, Zucker JE, et al. A novel SARS-CoV-2 variant of concern, B.1.526, identified in New York. medRxiv 2021.

[38] Furuse Y. Genomic sequencing effort for SARS-CoV-2 by country during the pandemic. Int J Infect Dis 2021;103: 305–7.

[39] Domingo E, Perales C. The time for COVID-19 vaccination. J Virol 2021.

[40] Kennedy DA, Read AF. Monitor for COVID-19 vaccine resistance evolution during clinical trials. PLoS Biol 2020;18(11):e3001000.

[41] Wadman M. United States rushes to fill void in viral sequencing. Science 2021;371(6530):657–8.

[42] UNC surveillance report. UNC Contributing labs. Available at: http://unc.cov2seq.org/. Accessed April 8, 2021.

[43] Genomic surveillance for SARS-CoV-2 variants. National Center for Immunization and Respiratory Diseases (NCIRD), division of viral diseases. 2021. Available at: https://www.cdc.gov/coronavirus/2019-ncov/cases-updates/variant-surveillance.html. Accessed April 8, 2021.

Advances in Molecular Pathology 4 (2021) 217–229
ADVANCES IN MOLECULAR PATHOLOGY

Review of SARS-CoV-2 Antigen and Antibody Testing in Diagnosis and Community Surveillance

Robert D. Nerenz, PhD[1], Jacqueline A. Hubbard, PhD[*,1], Mark A. Cervinski, PhD
Department of Pathology and Laboratory Medicine, Dartmouth-Hitchcock Medical Center, 1 Medical Center Drive, Lebanon, NH 03756, USA

KEYWORDS
• COVID-19 • SARS-CoV-2 • Antigen • Antibody • Serology • Vaccine • Pfizer • Moderna

KEY POINTS

- SARS-CoV-2 antigen tests offer short turnaround time and high specificity but the lower sensitivity relative to nucleic acid testing increases the risk of further transmission by patients with false-negative antigen test results.
- Although numerous SARS-CoV-2 antibody detection methods exist, the lack of harmonization and correlation with neutralizing antibodies limits their clinical usefulness.
- SARS-CoV-2 antibody titers are higher after vaccination than after a natural infection, but antibody longevity and the frequency at which vaccine re-immunization will be needed remain unknown.

INTRODUCTION

The severe acute respiratory syndrome coronavirus 2 (SARS-CoV-2), identified as the cause of the coronavirus disease 2019 (COVID-19) global pandemic, is a single-stranded RNA virus belonging to the coronavirus family. It consists of structural spike proteins that interact with angiotensin-converting enzyme 2 receptors to infect host cells, nucleocapsid protein that encapsulates the RNA, and envelope protein that surrounds the nucleocapsid [1]. Commercially available antibody assays have predominantly been developed to target antibodies to either the spike or nucleocapsid proteins. Although the nucleocapsid protein is highly conserved and less susceptible to genetic variation, the spike protein is the target of neutralizing antibodies, which are hypothesized to correlate with immunity [2–5].

Despite public health efforts to encourage masking, social distancing, and surveillance testing, the SARS-CoV-2 virus continued to spread at an alarming rate. As a result, significant effort was dedicated to the development of vaccines against SARS-CoV-2. After rapid development and deployment, several manufacturers began clinical trials on their vaccine within just months of the sequencing of the SARS-CoV-2 virus [6]. All vaccines available at the time of this publication target the spike protein, and immunocompetent individuals who receive the vaccine develop only antispike antibodies. In contrast, after a natural infection, both antispike and antinucleocapsid antibodies are detectable. Additional longitudinal studies are required to determine the longevity of antibodies after a natural infection or vaccination.

[1] Authors contributed equally to this article.

*Corresponding author, *E-mail address:* Jacqueline.a.hubbard@hitchcock.org

https://doi.org/10.1016/j.yamp.2021.06.008
2589-4080/21/

The gold standard for diagnosing a SARS-CoV-2 infection is nucleic acid amplification testing with throat or nasopharyngeal swabs [6]. However, difficulty of sample collection, slow turnaround time owing to batch mode testing and limited instrument availability, and supply chain shortages for reagents and consumables limited the ability to produce quick diagnostic results in many laboratories. As a result, several manufacturers developed rapid antigen-based assays for the diagnosis of SARS-CoV-2. Although these tests offer several logistical advantages, including rapid identification of infected individuals and ease of implementation in a nonlaboratory setting, antigen testing is considered less sensitive than molecular diagnostic techniques. Furthermore, the performance may vary considerably depending on whether it is used to diagnose symptomatic individuals, or to screen for asymptomatic individuals [7].

The essential role of rapid and accurate clinical laboratory testing has been highlighted during the SARS-CoV-2 global pandemic. In this review, we discuss the design and performance characteristics of commercially available antibody platforms. We then review antibody response after natural infection and after vaccination, with an emphasis on development of the 3 vaccines currently authorized for use in the United States (Pfizer-BioNtech, Moderna, and Janssen Biotech, Inc). Finally, we consider the use of antigen testing as an alternative diagnostic tool to nucleic acid testing. Taken together, we emphasize the essential contributions of laboratory medicine professionals in the global effort to detect, contain, and eradicate SARS-CoV-2.

ANTIBODY TESTING

The appearance of and subsequent spread of SARS-CoV-2 has challenged health care systems on a global scale. The accurate and rapid detection of the SARS-CoV-2 virus has propelled the laboratory community, particularly molecular pathology and microbiology laboratories, into the spotlight. As the pandemic has grown and evolved, new assay modalities focusing on the human host's adaptive immune response to SARS-CoV-2 have become available.

By April of 2020 the US Food and Drug Administration (FDA) began to grant emergency use authorization (EUA) for a limited number of immunoassays designed to detect the presence of antibodies specific to the SARS-CoV-2 virus [8]. Importantly these serology tests are not designed to detect current infection with the SARS-CoV-2 virus, because the immunoglobulins specific to viral proteins may not have developed in the time between infection and symptom onset. Consequently, a diagnosis of active SARS-CoV-2 infection is best achieved using nucleic acid techniques, or via specific detection of SARS-CoV-2 viral proteins.

Despite these limitations, numerous in vitro diagnostic companies and clinical laboratories devoted considerable resources to develop serologic methods to detect SARS-CoV-2 specific IgM and IgG antibodies with the expectation that these assays may fill an unmet laboratory testing need.

Assay Format

At the time of this report, 52 assays have attained EUA from the FDA, with the exclusion of point-of-care lateral flow immunoassays and laboratory developed tests. These EUA SARS-CoV-2 serology assays fall into 2 general methodologic categories, antibody isotype specific, and nonspecific or total immunoglobulin assays (Fig. 1, Table 1). Within the isotype-nonspecific and -specific categories, there are also methodologic differences in the antigen immobilization scheme used, with assays using microparticle or paramagnetic/magnetic particles predominating over the more traditional microwell- or plate-based formats.

Given the close homology of SARS-CoV-2 proteins with those of other coronaviruses, including the SARS-CoV-1 virus that caused the more limited SARS outbreak between 2002 and 2004, there was concern that serology assays would be subject to frequent false-positive results owing to prior exposure to related human coronaviruses (HCoV). The spike proteins of the related betacorona viruses infecting humans display varying degrees of sequence homology (SARS-CoV-1 = 76%, Middle Eastern respiratory syndrome [MERS]-CoV = 42%, HCoV-OC43 = 30%, and HCoV-HKU1 = 29%). Although HCoV-OC43 and HCoV-HKU1 are endemic and seroprevalence is high, the sequence differences in spike proteins between them and SARS-CoV-2 are sufficient to prevent measurable or significant cross-reactivity [9]. Although there is predicted to be intermediate cross-reactivity between spike antibodies to SARS-CoV-1 and MERS-CoV for SARS-CoV-2 spike serology assays, the low seroprevalence for these 2 coronaviruses cause them to be less of a concern [10].

The low cross-reactivity for spike proteins from human betacoronaviruses was a welcomed discovery, and this feature also extends to assays targeting the SARS-CoV-2 nucleocapsid protein. Although the nucleocapsid protein of the closely related SARS-CoV-1 virus and MERS-CoV display homology with SARS-CoV-2, the amino acid sequence differences between SARS-CoV-2

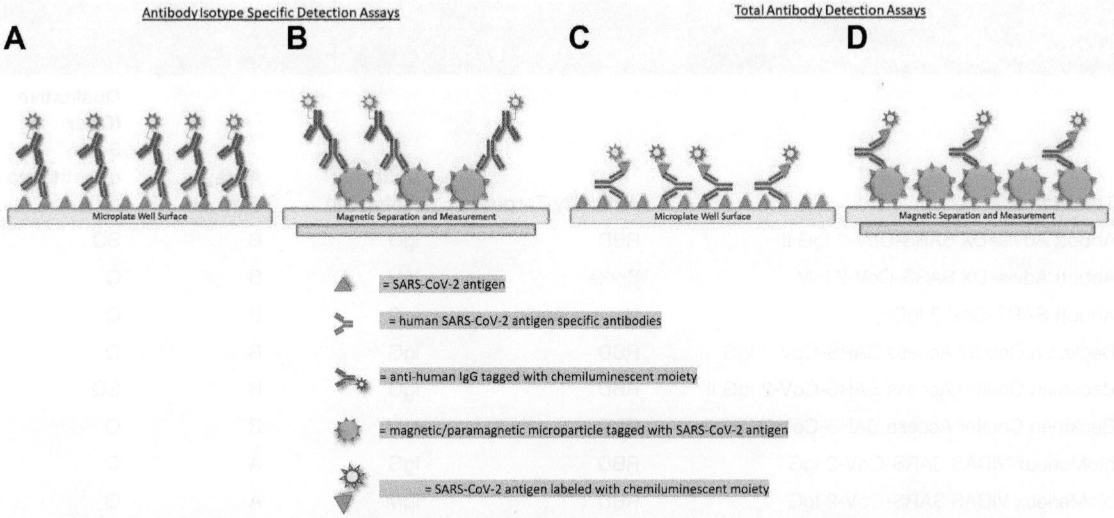

FIG. 1 SARS-CoV-2 serology assays fall into 2 distinct groups, those that are antibody isotype specific (**A, B**), and those that are total antibody assays that cannot distinguish between IgA, IgG, and IgM antibody isotype (**C, D**). The assays also differ in regards to separation technology with SARS-CoV-2 antigen immobilized on a microwell or microtiter plate (A, C), or a paramagnetic or magnetic microparticle (**B, D**).

nucleocapsid and the other endemic coronaviruses [11–13] are sufficient to limit predicted cross-reactivity.

Data from subsequent publications examining available serologic assays from in vitro diagnostic manufacturers has confirmed these predictions. These publications demonstrated very low false-positive rates across multiple test manufacturers and platforms by testing sera from either well-characterized SARS-CoV-2 polymerase chain reaction (PCR)-negative patients, or samples collected before December 2019, the generally accepted date associated with SARS-CoV-2 spread [14–17].

These articles also characterized the persistence of antibody up to 200 days after a positive SARS-CoV-2 PCR test result [15]. When the data of these publications are normalized to the number of days after a positive SARS-CoV-2 PCR test, the in vitro diagnostic platforms examined (Table 2) display sensitivities ranging from 75% to 99% [14–17].

Further, these articles also provide indirect evidence as to the clear lack of usefulness in diagnosing active SARS-CoV-2 infection. The sensitivity for detecting a specific antibody response at approximately 7 days after a positive SARS-CoV-2 PCR result ranged from 58% to 96%. This wide range in sensitivity is surprising, particularly in that the same platform in one publication displayed a sensitivity of 59% between 3 and 7 days post positive PCR result, whereas in another the sensitivity was reported as 96% for samples collected less than 7 days after a positive PCR test [15,17]. One possible explanation for the discrepancy in sensitivity is a difference in time between symptom onset and performance of the PCR test.

Serology Correlation with Neutralizing Antibody Titer

Of the numerous hurdles limiting the clinical usefulness of SARS-CoV-2 serology testing are the lack of assay harmonization or international standardization, as well as the currently sparse data correlating serology antibody result with neutralizing antibody titer. In 2 recent publications, this question of correlation of serology result to neutralizing titer was examined [18,19]. Both publications demonstrated that a positive correlation exists between automated serology assay signal and neutralizing antibody titer. The limitation of these studies is that neither article contains data from quantitative or semiquantitative serology assays, but rather rely on the ratio of assay signal to a positive calibrator or cut-off signal.

In the publication by Tang and colleagues [19], the authors demonstrate that at a neutralizing titer of 1:64, the positive percent agreement (PPA) for the Abbott, Roche, and Euroimmun assays are 96%, 100%, and 92%, respectively, when using the manufacturers' specified positive ratio thresholds. At the

TABLE 1
SARS-CoV-2 Serology Assays

Test Name	Antibody Target	Antibody Isotype(s)	Assay Format[d]	Qualitative (Q) or Semi-quantitative (SQ)
Abbott AdviseDX SARS-CoV-2 IgG II	RBD	IgG	B	SQ
Abbott AdviseDX SARS-CoV-2 IgM	Spike	IgM	B	Q
Abbott SARS-CoV-2 IgG[a]	Nucleocapsid	IgG	B	Q
Beckman Coulter Access SARS-CoV-2 IgG	RBD	IgG	B	Q
Beckman Coulter Access SARS-CoV-2 IgG II	RBD	IgG	B	SQ
Beckman Coulter Access SARS-CoV-2 IgM II	RBD	IgM	B	Q
bioMerieux VIDAS SARS-CoV-2 IgG	RBD	IgG	A	Q
bioMerieux VIDAS SARS-CoV-2 IgG	RBD	IgM	A	Q
Bio-Rad Platelia SARS-CoV-2 Total Ab	Nucleocapsid	IgA, IgG, IgM	C	Q
DiaSorin Liaison SARS-CoV-2 IgM	RBD	IgM	B	Q
DiaSorin Liaison SARS-CoV-2 S1/S2 IgG	S1 and S2	IgG	B	Q
Diazyme DZ-Lite SARS-CoV-2 IgG	Nucleocapsid and spike	IgG	B	Q
Diazyme DZ-Lite SARS-CoV-2 IgM	Nucleocapsid and spike	IgM	B	Q
Euroimmun Anti-SARS-CoV-2	S1	IgG	A	Q
IDS SARS-CoV-2 IgG	Nucleocapsid and spike	IgG	B	Q
Inova Diagnostics, QUANTA Flash SARS-CoV-2 IgG	Nucleocapsid and spike	IgG	B	SQ
Luminex xMAP SARS-CoV-2 Multi-Antigen IgG Assay	S1, RBD, nucleocapsid	IgG	B	Q
Ortho-Clinical Diagnostics VITROS Anti-SARS-CoV-2 IgG	Spike	IgG	A	Q
Ortho-Clinical Diagnostics VITROS Anti-SARS-CoV-2 Total	Spike	IgA, IgG, IgM	C	Q
Phadia AB ELIA SARS-CoV-2-Sp1 IgG	Spike	IgG	A	SQ
Roche Elecsys Anti-SARS-CoV-2	Nucleocapsid	IgA, IgG, IgM	D	Q
Roche Elecsys Anti-SARS-CoV-2 s	Spike	IgA, IgG, IgM	D	SQ
Siemens Healthcare Diagnostics SARS-COV-2 IgG[b]	RBD	IgG	B	SQ
Siemens Healthcare Diagnostics SARS-CoV-2 Total[b]	RBD	IgA, IgG, IgM	D	SQ

(continued on next page)

TABLE 1
(*continued*)

Test Name	Antibody Target	Antibody Isotype(s)	Assay Format[d]	Qualitative (Q) or Semi-quantitative (SQ)
Siemens Healthcare Diagnostics Dimension/Dimension EXL SARS-CoV-2 IgG[c]	RBD	IgG	Other	SQ
Siemens Healthcare Diagnostics Dimension/Dimension EXL SARS-CoV-2 Total[c]	RBD	IgA, IgG, IgM	Other	Q
Thermo Fisher OmniPATH COVID-19	Spike	IgA, IgG, IgM	C	Q
Zeus Scientific ELISA SARS-CoV-2 IgG	Spike and nucleocapsid	IgG	A	Q
Zeus Scientific ELISA SARS-CoV-2 Total	Spike and nucleocapsid	IgA, IgG, IgM	C	Q

Abbreviations: RBD, receptor binding domain; S1, S1 domain of SARS-CoV-2 spike protein; S2, S2 domain of SARS-CoV-2 spike protein.
[a] Abbott Alinity i SARS-CoV-2 and Abbott ARCHITECT SARS-CoV-2 use the same assay format and are shown here in one row.
[b] Siemens ADIVA Centaur and Atellica assays utilize the same assay format and are show here in one row per assay format (IgG vs Total Immunoglobulin).use
[c] Siemens Dimension and Dimension EXL SARS-CoV-2 assays use the LOCI (luminescent oxygen channeling assay) technology not depicted in Fig. 1.
[d] Assay format described in Figure 1.

manufacturer specified positive thresholds the negative predictive agreement of the 3 were 50%, 70%, and 47%, respectively. The authors also calculated assay-specific ideal ratios for the 3 assays which slightly decreased the PPA, but increased the negative predictive agreement for each assay.

In an article by Suhandynata and colleagues [20], the authors examined the PPA between 3 commercially

TABLE 2
In Vitro Diagnostic Platform Performance Characteristics

Assay Manufacturer	Sensitivity (%)	References
Abbott SARS-CoV-2 IgG	81[a]–99	(Poore et al, [15] 2021; Tang et al, 2020)
Beckman Coulter Access SARS-CoV-2 IgG	78	(Poore et al, [15] 2021)
Diazyme DZ-Lite SARS-CoV-2 IgG	96	(Suhandynata et al, [16] 2020)
Euroimmun Anti-SARS-CoV-2	75[a]	(Tang et al, [17] 2020)
Roche Elecsys Anti-SARS-CoV-2	87–96	(Poore et al, [15] 2021; Suhandynata et al., 2020)

[a] Sensitivity defined as positive serology result at either *≥14 d or ≥15 d after a positive SARS-CoV-2 PCR result.

available serology assays as well as a neutralization assay titer of 50. Samples testing positive on both the Diazyme and Roche assays or the Diazyme and Abbott assays had PPA values of 79.2% and 78.4%, respectively. Unfortunately, owing to the methodologic differences between the 2 articles, a direct comparison of data is not possible.

These early studies correlating automated serology assay signal with the neutralization titer are encouraging; however, additional studies using semiquantitative or quantitative assays are needed to determine if a universal threshold indicating immunity is possible.

ANTIBODY RESPONSE

Early publications supported a classic viral response pattern after infection with SARS-CoV-2 [21,22]. In this model, IgM antibodies are first detected within 1 week after infection, and IgG antibodies develop several days after that. Instead, IgG antibodies to SARS-CoV-2 appear before or at the same time as IgM antibodies [23,24]. In the classic viral response model, IgG antibodies were predicted to increase over time, peak around 1 month after an infection, and remain detectable for 1 to 6 years [22]. Although antibody longevity may not be confirmed for several years, many research groups have investigated the time to initial antibody detection and ongoing studies are monitoring antibody response over time.

Determining antibody seroconversion rates after a SARS-CoV-2 infection can be difficult because the exact day of infection is often unknown. The window period between infection and the presence of detectable antibodies ranged from less than 4 days to several weeks after a confirmed infection [16,23–27]. Seroconversion kinetics may also depend on disease severity. People with mild or asymptomatic infections generally had a weaker immune response than those with symptomatic or severe infection [23,26]. However, it has also been reported that asymptomatic patients seroconvert more quickly compared with those are who are symptomatic [27]. Interindividual variation combined with the novelty of the SARS-CoV-2 virus have contributed to an incomplete understanding of the humoral response.

As described elsewhere in this article, the antibody response pattern over time varies widely with the analytical platform being used [14–17]. However, differing antibody trends are at least partially attributed to whether antinucleocapsid or antispike antibodies are being monitored. Previous reports have demonstrated that, although nucleocapsid antibodies continue to increase over time, antibodies to the spike protein begin to decrease within 1 to 4 months after symptom onset [15,28,29]. This phenomenon has been observed on several different test platforms. Despite this finding, antibodies to both the spike and nucleocapsid antibodies remain detectable for several months after infection. Future studies should continue to monitor the longevity of antibodies to both the nucleocapsid and spike proteins after natural infection.

Neutralizing antibodies can block infection by the SARS-CoV-2 virus. Because the spike protein engages angiotensin-converting enzyme 2 receptors to initiate infection, antibodies to the spike protein have been theorized to correlate with antibody neutralization [5,19,20]. After a natural infection, spike antibodies were moderately associated (R^2 = 0.46) with neutralizing antibody titers but suffered from a poor negative percent agreement [19]. Interestingly, the correlation between antinucleocapsid antibodies with neutralizing antibodies was assay dependent, but ranged from a coefficient of determination of 0.29 to 0.47. After vaccination, antibodies to the spike protein also exhibited a moderate association (R^2 = 0.39) with neutralizing titers [20]. Current vaccinations only elicit a humoral response against the spike protein of SARS-CoV-2 and, therefore, would not have any association with nucleocapsid antibody response.

As a result of the COVID-19 global pandemic, vaccine development through multinational collaborations has occurred at an unprecedented rate. Antibody response after vaccination will be an important consideration when establishing reimmunization intervals. At the time of this publication, all vaccines currently granted EUA by the World Health Organization target the spike protein and, therefore, only elicit antispike antibodies. In these cases, vaccination status should be monitored with an antispike assay. However, there are vaccines currently under development that contain live, attenuated, or inactivated virus that would induce both a nucleocapsid and spike antibody response, similar to a natural infection [30]. In these cases, vaccination antibody response could be monitored with either an antispike or antinucleocapsid assay and would remain indistinguishable from a natural infection. Currently available vaccines result in antibody titers that exceed those seen after a natural infection [31–33]. Although this robust response is promising, antibody longevity after vaccination remains unknown and may vary with vaccine technology. Understanding how each vaccine works will be an important consideration when monitoring antibody titers to determine reimmunization frequency.

COVID-19 VACCINES

After the COVID-19 outbreak in December 2019, the entire genomic sequence of SARS-CoV-2 was published in January 2020. By March 2020, vaccines were developed, shipped to appropriate testing sites, and early phase clinical and preclinical trials were underway. As of June 2021, nearly 300 vaccine candidates were under clinical or preclinical development [30]. These vaccines use a variety of technologies, including adenovirus vectors, viral-like particles, inactivated or attenuated virus, and synthetic DNA or RNA. Dosing schemes range from 1 to 3 doses given over zero to 56 days. Although more than a dozen vaccines have already been cleared for emergency use by the World Health Organization, only 3 vaccines were granted FDA EUA status for use in the United States. These vaccines are manufactured by Pfizer-BioNTech, Moderna, and Janssen Biotech, Inc.

Pfizer-BioNTech Vaccine

Pfizer-BioNTech produced 2 RNA-based vaccines formulated in lipid nanoparticles. The first, BNT162b1, encoded a trimerized SARS-CoV-2 receptor-binding domain of the spike glycoprotein whereas the second, BNT162b2, encoded a membrane-anchored full-length spike glycoprotein stabilized in the prefusion conformation [31,34,35]. During phase I clinical trials, immunogenicity and safety were monitored for various dosing paradigms of BNT162b1 and BNT162b2. Although both vaccines were found to be effective and exhibited tolerability profiles similar to other messenger RNA (mRNA)-based vaccines [36], BNT162b2 had a milder systemic reactogenicity profile while exhibiting a similar antibody response to BNT162b1. Both vaccines exhibited a strong dose-dependent response, and the 2-dose series of 30 μg BNT162b2 vaccine was selected as the candidate to advance to phase II and III clinical trials [31].

The Pfizer-BioNTech BNT162b2 vaccine was submitted for EUA to the FDA on November 20, 2020 [37]. The vaccine series consisted of 2 doses given 21 days apart. The submission included data from ongoing clinical trials consisting of 44,000 participants and the vaccine was found to be 95% effective at preventing SARS-CoV-2 infection with no major safety concerns identified. On December 11, 2020, this became the first COVID-19 vaccine to receive EUA clearance from the FDA in the United States. In May 2021, the FDA expanded the EUA to allow for vaccination in children as young as 12 years of age.

Moderna Vaccine

Similar to Pfizer-BioNTech BNT162b2, the Moderna mRNA-1273 vaccine is also a lipid nanoparticle–encapsulated mRNA-based vaccine encoding a stabilized prefusion trimer of the spike glycoprotein. In early clinical trials, participants received 2 injections of either a 25, 100, or 250 μg dose 28 days apart [32,38]. Two doses were deemed necessary to elicit sufficient pseudovirus neutralizing activity. The median antibody response was similar between the 100 μg and 250 μg dose groups but the 100 μg dose group had a more favorable reactogenicity profile. Therefore, the 100 μg dose was chosen to advance into additional clinical trials.

Moderna submitted the mRNA-1273 COVID-19 vaccine (2 doses of 100 μg, administered 1 month apart) to the FDA for EUA on November 30, 2020, for adults 18 years of age or older [39]. The phase III clinical trials consisted of 30,400 participants and demonstrated a greater than 94% efficacy at preventing COVID-19 [40]. Adverse reactions were reported frequently, but were considered mild, with injection site arm pain, fatigue, and headache being the most common. One week after Pfizer-BioNTech, the Moderna mRNA-1272 vaccine was issued EUA from the FDA for use in adults on December 18, 2020.

Janssen Biotech, Inc, Vaccine

The Janssen Biotech, Inc (Johnson & Johnson) Ad26.COV2.S vaccine is an adenovirus vector encoding a variant of the SARS-CoV-2 spike protein. Beginning in July 2020, Janssen conducted multicenter phase I clinical trials with doses of 5×10^{10} or 1×10^{10} viral particles per milliliter given as a single dose or on a 2-dose schedule [33,41]. All dosing schemes had an acceptable safety and reactogenicity profile and more than 90% of participants demonstrated the presence of both S-binding and neutralizing antibodies after a single dose of either potency vaccine. Interestingly, adverse events were more common after the first dose, a finding that contrasted both the Pfizer-BioNTech and Moderna mRNA-based vaccines [33]. Although a second vaccine dose exhibited slightly increased immunogenicity, Janssen recognized the logistical advantages of a single-dose vaccine and decided to proceed with a single dose of the 1×10^{10} viral particles per milliliter vaccine in phase III clinical trials. This decision was further supported by nonhuman primate studies that demonstrated complete or near-complete protection against SARS-COV-2 [42]. More recently, it was discovered that the Ad26.COV2.S vaccine may offer some protection against other SARS-CoV-2 variants of concern [43].

Janssen Biotech, Inc, submitted the Ad26.COV2.S single dose vaccine consisting of 5×10^{10} viral particles for EUA by the FDA on February 4, 2021 [44]. Phase III clinical trials of more than 40,000 participants demonstrated that this vaccine was both safe and at least 66%

effective in preventing the development of COVID-19 in adults 18 years of age or older. On February 27, 2021, the FDA issued an EUA for the Janssen the Ad26.COV2.S single dose vaccine, making it the third approved for use in the United States. However, on April 23, 2021, the FDA amended the EUA to include information about the rare occurrence of cerebral venous sinus thrombosis in women after vaccination.

As more vaccines are developed, it will become increasingly important to monitor reactogenicity and immunogenicity in addition to efficacy. Differences in immune response and frequency of adverse events may help to personalize vaccine selection, with potent vaccines preferred in individuals who may produce a suboptimal immune response, and single-dose vaccines preferred for those who are prone to adverse reactions after vaccination.

SARS-CoV-2 ANTIGEN TESTING

Nucleic acid amplification tests detecting the presence of SARS-CoV-2 RNA are considered the gold standard for the diagnosis of symptomatic patients by the Centers for Disease Control and Prevention [45]. Although these assays offer optimal sensitivity and specificity, their implementation can be hindered by the limited availability of reagents or other consumables, they require capital investment in the necessary instrumentation, and they must be performed by specialized and highly trained laboratory personnel. Owing to the centralized nature of this testing model, results are often returned several hours or days after specimen collection, complicating efforts to limit further viral spread.

To overcome these limitations, several manufacturers have developed rapid, lateral flow devices that detect SARS-CoV-2 antigen (typically the nucleocapsid protein) in nasal or nasopharyngeal swabs with results available in 15 to 30 minutes. Briefly, viral proteins present on the test swab are suspended by mixing in a buffer solution, which is transferred to the test cartridge. Labeled antibodies bind to the viral protein of interest and the buffer-suspended antibody–antigen complex migrates through an internal membrane toward the test and control lines. The test line consists of a capture antibody attached to the solid phase that recognizes a different epitope on the viral protein, immobilizing the antigen detector–antibody complex and forming a visible line. Any unbound detector antibody flows past the test line and accumulates at the control line, indicating a valid test. Result interpretation varies by device, but typically follows 1 of 2 models. In the first, after the introduction of patient sample, each device is placed into a reader that evaluates the signal intensity at the test and control lines and produces a digital "detected" or "not detected" result. In the second, test and control line signal intensity is evaluated visually after a manufacturer-defined incubation period. Result interpretation outside of this window can lead to erroneous results.

Although these rapid antigen devices are not considered the gold standard for SARS-CoV-2 diagnosis, they may offer several advantages, including limited expense, capacity for rapid implementation without extensive infrastructure, short turnaround time, and high specificity in populations with a high prevalence of disease. At the time of release for clinical use, the performance of these devices was largely unknown beyond the manufacturers' validation studies described in the package inserts. However, after implementation in a variety of clinical settings, several recent publications have described the performance characteristics of rapid antigen tests relative to concurrently performed nucleic acid testing as the reference method.

BinaxNOW

The Abbott BinaxNOW COVID-19 antigen card is a lateral flow device granted EUA by the FDA in August 2020. Results are interpreted visually between 15 and 30 minutes after the introduction of the resuspended patient sample to the test card. Analytical sensitivity has been estimated to fall between 4 and 8×10^4 copies per swab, roughly approximating a generic reverse transcriptase (RT)-PCR cycle threshold value of 29 to 30 [46].

One study compared the performance of the BinaxNOW lateral flow antigen test to the Thermo Fisher TaqPath COVID-19 Combo kit in 2645 asymptomatic students at the University of Utah using 2 concurrent nasal swabs self-collected by study participants under the supervision of trained, nonmedical personnel [47]. Antigen testing was performed at the collection site by trained nonmedical personnel while RT-PCR testing was performed at a reference laboratory. SARS-CoV-2 RNA was detected by RT-PCR in 1.7% of the study participants. Relative to RT-PCR, the BinaxNOW antigen test demonstrated a sensitivity of 53.3% and a specificity of 100%.

A second study summarized the performance of the BinaxNOW antigen device relative to the Clinical Research Sequencing Platform (CRSP) SARS-CoV-2 RT-PCR assay in specimens collected at a drive-through community testing site in Massachusetts [7]. Two nasal swabs were collected from each participant by trained medical personnel, with 1 swab used to perform BinaxNOW testing on-site in a dedicated testing tent while the other swab was sent to an off-site reference laboratory for RT-PCR testing. In this study population, 974 of 1380 adults (71%) and 829 of 928 children (89%) were asymptomatic. Among symptomatic participants, the BinaxNOW device demonstrated a sensitivity of 96.5% in adults and 84.6% in children (ages 7–17 years) and a specificity of 100% in both age groups. Among asymptomatic participants, the sensitivity was 70.2% in adults and 65.5% in children and the specificity was 99.6% in adults and 99.0% in children.

A third study compared the BinaxNOW antigen device to either the CDC or Fosun SARS-CoV-2 RT-PCR assay using concurrently collected nasal (antigen) and nasopharyngeal (RT-PCR) samples from participants in 2 community testing centers in Pima County, Arizona [48]. Antigen testing was performed on site according to the manufacturer's instructions and RT-PCR testing was performed within 24 to 48 hours at an off-site laboratory. Of the 3419 participants, 827 (24.2%) reported at least 1 symptom consistent with SARS-CoV-2 infection. SARS-CoV-2 RNA was detected in 161 participants (4.7%): 113 of 827 were symptomatic (13.7%) and 48 of 2592 were asymptomatic (1.9%). In symptomatic participants presenting within 7 days of symptom onset, the sensitivity and specificity of the BinaxNOW device were 71.1% and 100%, respectively. In asymptomatic participants, the sensitivity and specificity were 35.8% and 99.8%, respectively.

Sofia

The Quidel Sofia SARS-CoV-2 lateral flow antigen assay was granted EUA in May 2020 and is intended for use within 5 days of symptom onset. Results are introduced into a device reader that reports digital results as positive or negative between 15 and 30 minutes.

One study performed on 2 college campuses in Wisconsin compared the performance of the Sofia antigen device to either the Centers for Disease Control and Prevention or Thermo Fisher TaqPath COVID-19 Combo RT-PCR assays [49]. At University A, all persons tested for screening or diagnostic purposes were eligible to participate in the study. At University B, participation was limited to only those quarantined after a known COVID-19 exposure. Two concurrent nasal swabs were collected from participants in both groups (medical personnel collect at University A, self-collect at University B). Limited information was provided regarding the logistics of antigen test performance, with the authors indicating only that testing was performed according to the manufacturer's instructions. Of the 1098 participants, 227 (20.7%) reported at least 1 symptom; 871 (79.3%) were asymptomatic. Overall RT-PCR positivity was 5.2% (40 symptomatic and 17 asymptomatic participants). The sensitivity, specificity, positive predictive value, and negative predictive value were 80.0%, 98.9%, 94.1%, and 95.9%, respectively, in the symptomatic group and 41.2%, 98.4%, 33.3%, and 98.8%, respectively, in the asymptomatic group.

A second study evaluated the performance of the Sofia antigen device in the emergency department of a tertiary medical center in Los Angeles, California [50]. Paired nasal (antigen) and nasopharyngeal (RT-PCR) specimens were collected by medical personnel for all patients admitted to the hospital through the emergency department. RT-PCR testing was performed using the Fulgent COVID-19 assay and antigen testing was performed on-site in the emergency department. Of the 2039 participants, 307 (15.1%) reported at least 1 symptom. SARS-CoV-2 RNA was detected in 68 of 307 symptomatic participants (22.1%) and 81 of 1732 asymptomatic participants (4.7%). Relative to RT-PCR, the sensitivity and specificity of the Sofia antigen test were 72.1% and 98.7%, respectively, in the symptomatic group and 60.5% and 99.5%, respectively, in the asymptomatic group.

A third study evaluated the performance of the Sofia antigen device relative to the Hologic Aptima SARS-CoV-2 TMA assay in symptomatic individuals presenting to an urgent care center in West Bend, Wisconsin [51]. Concurrently collected nasal (antigen) and nasopharyngeal samples (TMA) were collected by medical staff in the urgent care center, with both specimens sent to a clinical laboratory for testing. SARS-CoV-2 RNA was detected in 18% of symptomatic patients seen in the clinic in the month before the implementation of antigen testing and this positivity rate remained constant throughout the study period. Of the 298 patients tested within 5 days of symptom onset, the sensitivity, specificity, positive predictive value, and negative predictive value were 82.0%, 100%, 100%, and 96.5%, respectively. Of the 48 patients tested more than 5 days after symptom onset, antigen test performance decreased, with a sensitivity, specificity, positive predictive value, and negative predictive value of 54.5%, 97.3%, 85.7%, and 87.8%, respectively.

Becton Dickinson Veritor

The Becton Dickinson (BD) Veritor lateral flow antigen device was granted EUA in July 2020 and is intended for use with nasal swabs collected from patients suspected of SARS-CoV-2 infection within 5 days of symptom onset. Results are generated by a cartridge reader at least

15 minutes after introduction of the sample to the test device and are reported qualitatively as positive or presumptive negative.

One study evaluated the performance of the BD Veritor device relative to the Simplexa COVID-19 Direct EUA RT-PCR assay in paired nasal (antigen) and nasopharyngeal (RT-PCR) samples from 1384 patients with known SARS-CoV-2 exposure within 5 days of symptom onset presenting to a hospital system in Winston-Salem, North Carolina [52]. Antigen testing was performed at the site of collection according to the manufacturer's instructions, whereas RT-PCR testing was performed in a central laboratory. SARS-CoV-2 RNA was detected in 116 of 1384 specimens (8.4%). Relative to RT-PCR, the BD Veritor demonstrated a sensitivity, specificity, positive predictive value, and negative predictive value of 66.4%, 98.8%, 83.7%, and 97.0%, respectively.

A second study with 2 parts evaluated the BD Veritor relative to the Lyra RT-PCR assay in concurrently collected nasal (antigen) and nasopharyngeal or oropharyngeal swabs (RT-PCR) in 251 symptomatic individuals within 7 days of symptom onset presenting to 21 geographically diverse study locations (part 1) [53]. RT-PCR testing was performed at a commercial reference laboratory and antigen testing was performed at a laboratory operated by the device manufacturer. SARS-CoV-2 RNA was detected in 38 of 251 part 1 study participants (15.1%). In participants with 2 or more symptoms, the sensitivity, specificity, positive predictive value, and negative predictive value were 88%, 100%, 100%, and 97.3%, respectively. In participants with 1 symptom, values were 67%, 100%, 100%, and 97.7%, respectively. In part 2, concurrently collected nasal swabs from 377 symptomatic participants at 5 study sites were tested at an off-site commercial reference laboratory on the BD Veritor and Sofia devices according to the manufacturer's instructions. Using the Sofia device as the reference method, the BD Veritor demonstrated a sensitivity and specificity of 97.4% and 98.1%, respectively.

Effectiveness of Antigen Testing in Controlling Viral Spread

Many have advocated for the implementation of serial SARS-CoV-2 antigen testing to facilitate rapid identification of infected individuals and permit timely self-quarantine to prevent further viral spread. Although antigen testing is consistently less sensitive than molecular diagnostic techniques, the short turnaround time and capacity for repeated testing may support efforts at viral containment more effectively than single sample nucleic acid testing with a long turnaround time. To date, relatively few studies have tested this hypothesis.

One publication describing the implementation of the Sofia antigen device in routine monitoring of intercollegiate athletes documented 2 separate SARS-CoV-2 outbreaks attributed to false-negative antigen test results [54]. In outbreak A, 32 confirmed cases were traced to contact during a team meeting with a single infectious individual whose antigen test result was negative on the morning of the meeting. Viral RNA sequences were closely related, supporting transmission from a single individual to the other team members. The authors note that viral transmission was not interrupted until the implementation of RT-PCR testing, which led to the identification of an additional 21 confirmed SARS-CoV-2 infections, 18 of which were not detected by concurrent antigen testing. In outbreak B, 12 confirmed cases were documented in 2 teams competing against each other, all of whose participants received negative antigen test results on the day of competition. Viral RNA sequences were closely related and distinctly different from strains circulating in one of the teams' communities, supporting transmission from one team to the other.

Antigen Conclusions

To decrease the rates of viral transmission, SARS-CoV-2 diagnostic test methods must be analytically accurate, accessible, and reported in a timely and effective manner. Antigen methods generate rapid results and their high specificity and positive predictive value allows SARS-CoV-2–positive individuals to quickly self-isolate, minimizing the risk of further viral spread. However, the lower sensitivity of antigen testing relative to nucleic acid methods increases the likelihood of further transmission in high interaction environments by individuals with false-negative antigen results. With this limitation in mind, confirmation of negative antigen results by nucleic acid testing is recommended, particularly in patient populations with a high disease prevalence.

In addition to the test method used, the environment in which testing is performed is a primary determinant of the effectiveness of SARS-CoV-2 testing efforts. The majority of studies evaluating antigen test performance described dedicated testing spaces staffed by trained operators with no other competing responsibilities. Little is known about how antigen devices perform when implemented in patient care settings with testing performed by clinical personnel who are also actively caring for patients. The limited available data using the BD Veritor device suggest improved performance in a controlled laboratory setting relative to an active patient care environment [52,53]. However, this observation is complicated by differences in reference method and disease prevalence in the study populations.

SUMMARY

Laboratory medicine professionals play an integral role in the global response to SARS-CoV-2 through the development and implementation of test methods to identify infected individuals and monitor the immune response to vaccination and natural infection. SARS-CoV-2 antibody test methods can be used to confirm past infection and, pending further correlation with neutralizing antibody assays, may help to guide personalized vaccine selection or the establishment of revaccination intervals. Antigen test methods offer rapid turnaround time and improved access to testing as well as high specificity, but their limited sensitivity requires confirmation of negative results by nucleic acid testing, particularly in populations with high disease prevalence.

CLINICS CARE POINTS

- Antigen tests exhibit lower sensitivity relative to nucleic acid testing and increase the risk of further transmission by patients with false-negative antigen results.
- SARS-CoV-2 antibody test methods lack harmonization and correlation with neutralizing antibodies, limiting their clinical usefulness.
- Current vaccines result in higher antibody titers than natural infection, and antibodies made after vaccination should be monitored with antispike antibody assays.

DISCLOSURE

The authors have nothing to disclose.

REFERENCES

[1] Park SE. Epidemiology, virology, and clinical features of severe acute respiratory syndrome -coronavirus-2 (SARS-CoV-2; Coronavirus Disease-19). Clin Exp Pediatr 2020; 63(4):119–24.

[2] Dutta NK, Mazumdar K, Gordy JT. The nucleocapsid protein of SARS–CoV-2: a target for vaccine development. J Virol 2020;94(13). https://doi.org/10.1128/JVI.00647-20.

[3] Cong Y, Ulasli M, Schepers H, et al. Nucleocapsid protein recruitment to replication-transcription complexes plays a crucial role in coronaviral life cycle. J Virol 2020; 94(4). https://doi.org/10.1128/JVI.01925-19.

[4] Burbelo PD, Riedo FX, Morishima C, et al. Detection of nucleocapsid antibody to SARS-CoV-2 is more sensitive than antibody to spike protein in COVID-19 patients. J Infect Dis 2020. https://doi.org/10.1093/infdis/jiaa273.

[5] Garcia-Beltran WF, Lam EC, Astudillo MG, et al. COVID-19-neutralizing antibodies predict disease severity and survival. Cell 2021;184(2):476–88.e11.

[6] Esbin MN, Whitney ON, Chong S, et al. Overcoming the bottleneck to widespread testing: a rapid review of nucleic acid testing approaches for COVID-19 detection. RNA 2020. https://doi.org/10.1261/rna.076232.120 rna.076232.120.

[7] Pollock NR, Jacobs JR, Tran K, et al. Performance and implementation evaluation of the Abbott BinaxNOW Rapid antigen test in a high-throughput drive-through community testing site in Massachusetts. J Clin Microbiol 2021; 59(5). https://doi.org/10.1128/JCM.00083-21.

[8] Health C for D and R. EUA Authorized Serology Test Performance. FDA. 2021. Available at: https://www.fda.gov/medical-devices/coronavirus-disease-2019-covid-19-emergency-use-authorizations-medical-devices/eua-authorized-serology-test-performance. Accessed June 16, 2021.

[9] Hicks J, Klumpp-Thomas C, Kalish H, et al. Serologic cross-reactivity of SARS-CoV-2 with endemic and seasonal betacoronaviruses. J Clin Immunol 2021. https://doi.org/10.1007/s10875-021-00997-6.

[10] Jaimes JA, André NM, Chappie JS, et al. Phylogenetic analysis and structural modeling of SARS-CoV-2 spike protein reveals an evolutionary distinct and proteolytically sensitive activation loop. J Mol Biol 2020; 432(10):3309–25.

[11] Burbelo PD, Riedo FX, Morishima C, et al. Sensitivity in detection of antibodies to nucleocapsid and spike proteins of severe acute respiratory syndrome coronavirus 2 in patients with coronavirus disease 2019. J Infect Dis 2020;222(2):206–13.

[12] Gussow AB, Auslander N, Faure G, et al. Genomic determinants of pathogenicity in SARS-CoV-2 and other human coronaviruses. Proc Natl Acad Sci U S A 2020; 117(26):15193–9.

[13] Kang S, Yang M, Hong Z, et al. Crystal structure of SARS-CoV-2 nucleocapsid protein RNA binding domain reveals potential unique drug targeting sites. Acta Pharm Sin B 2020;10(7):1228–38.

[14] Hubbard JA, Geno KA, Khan J, et al. Comparison of two automated immunoassays for the detection of SARS-CoV-2 nucleocapsid antibodies. J Appl Lab Med 2021; 6(2):429–40.

[15] Poore B, Nerenz RD, Brodis D, et al. A comparison of SARS-CoV-2 nucleocapsid and spike antibody detection using three commercially available automated immunoassays. Clin Biochem 2021. https://doi.org/10.1016/j.clinbiochem.2021.05.011.

[16] Suhandynata RT, Hoffman MA, Kelner MJ, et al. Multiplatform comparison of SARS-CoV-2 serology assays for the detection of COVID-19. J Appl Lab Med 2020; 5(6):1324–36.

[17] Tang MS, Hock KG, Logsdon NM, et al. Clinical performance of two SARS-CoV-2 serologic assays. Clin Chem 2020;66(8):1055–62.

[18] Suhandynata RT, Hoffman MA, Huang D, et al. Commercial serology assays predict neutralization activity against SARS-CoV-2. Clin Chem 2021;67(2):404–14.

[19] Tang MS, Case JB, Franks CE, et al. Association between SARS-CoV-2 neutralizing antibodies and commercial serological assays. Clin Chem 2020. https://doi.org/10.1093/clinchem/hvaa211.

[20] Suhandynata RT, Bevins NJ, Tran JT, et al. SARS-CoV-2 serology status detected by commercialized platforms distinguishes previous infection and vaccination adaptive immune responses. medRxiv 2021. https://doi.org/10.1101/2021.03.10.21253299.

[21] Guo L, Ren L, Yang S, et al. Profiling early humoral response to diagnose novel coronavirus disease (COVID-19). Clin Infect Dis 2020;71(15):778–85.

[22] Galipeau Y, Greig M, Liu G, et al. Humoral responses and serological assays in SARS-CoV-2 infections. Front Immunol 2020;11. https://doi.org/10.3389/fimmu.2020.610688.

[23] Long Q-X, Liu B-Z, Deng H-J, et al. Antibody responses to SARS-CoV-2 in patients with COVID-19. Nat Med 2020; 1–4. https://doi.org/10.1038/s41591-020-0897-1.

[24] Suhandynata RT, Hoffman MA, Kelner MJ, et al. Longitudinal monitoring of SARS-CoV-2 IgM and IgG seropositivity to detect COVID-19. J Appl Lab Med 2020; jfaa079. https://doi.org/10.1093/jalm/jfaa079.

[25] Long Q-X, Tang X-J, Shi Q-L, et al. Clinical and immunological assessment of asymptomatic SARS-CoV-2 infections. Nat Med 2020;26(8):1200–4.

[26] Jiang C, Wang Y, Hu M, et al. Antibody seroconversion in asymptomatic and symptomatic patients infected with severe acute respiratory syndrome coronavirus 2 (SARS-CoV-2). Clin Transl Immunology 2020;9(9): e1182.

[27] Zhao J, Yuan Q, Wang H, et al. Antibody responses to SARS-CoV-2 in patients of novel coronavirus disease 2019. medRxiv 2020. https://doi.org/10.1101/2020.03.02.20030189 2020.03.02.20030189.

[28] Ibarrondo FJ, Fulcher JA, Goodman-Meza D, et al. Rapid decay of anti–SARS-CoV-2 antibodies in persons with mild Covid-19. N Engl J Med 2020. https://doi.org/10.1056/NEJMc2025179.

[29] Perreault J, Tremblay T, Fournier M-J, et al. Waning of SARS-CoV-2 RBD antibodies in longitudinal convalescent plasma samples within 4 months after symptom onset. Blood 2020;136(22):2588–91.

[30] COVID-19 vaccine tracker and landscape. Available at: https://www.who.int/publications/m/item/draft-landscape-of-covid-19-candidate-vaccines. Accessed June 14, 2021.

[31] Walsh EE, Frenck RW, Falsey AR, et al. Safety and immunogenicity of two RNA-based covid-19 vaccine candidates. N Engl J Med 2020;383(25):2439–50.

[32] Anderson EJ, Rouphael NG, Widge AT, et al. Safety and immunogenicity of SARS-CoV-2 mRNA-1273 vaccine in older adults. N Engl J Med 2020;383(25):2427–38.

[33] Sadoff J, Le Gars M, Shukarev G, et al. Interim results of a phase 1–2a trial of Ad26.COV2.S Covid-19 vaccine. N Engl J Med 2021. https://doi.org/10.1056/NEJMoa2034201.

[34] Sahin U, Muik A, Derhovanessian E, et al. COVID-19 vaccine BNT162b1 elicits human antibody and T H 1 T cell responses. Nature 2020;586(7830):594–9.

[35] Mulligan MJ, Lyke KE, Kitchin N, et al. Phase I/II study of COVID-19 RNA vaccine BNT162b1 in adults. Nature 2020;586(7830):589–93.

[36] Feldman RA, Fuhr R, Smolenov I, et al. mRNA vaccines against H10N8 and H7N9 influenza viruses of pandemic potential are immunogenic and well tolerated in healthy adults in phase 1 randomized clinical trials. Vaccine 2019;37(25):3326–34.

[37] Covid P-B. Vaccines and Related Biological Products Advisory Committee Meeting December 10, 2020. 53.

[38] Jackson LA, Anderson EJ, Rouphael NG, et al. An mRNA Vaccine against SARS-CoV-2 — Preliminary report. N Engl J Med 2020. https://doi.org/10.1056/NEJMoa2022483.

[39] Vaccines and Related Biological Products Advisory Committee December 17, 2020 Meeting Announcement - 12/17/2020 - 12/17/2020. FDA. 2021. Available at: https://www.fda.gov/advisory-committees/advisory-committee-calendar/vaccines-and-related-biological-products-advisory-committee-december-17-2020-meeting-announcement. Accessed June 15, 2021.

[40] Baden LR, El Sahly HM, Essink B, et al. Efficacy and safety of the mRNA-1273 SARS-CoV-2 vaccine. N Engl J Med 2021;384(5):403–16.

[41] Stephenson KE, Le Gars M, Sadoff J, et al. Immunogenicity of the Ad26.COV2.S vaccine for COVID-19. JAMA 2021;325(15):1535–44.

[42] Mercado NB, Zahn R, Wegmann F, et al. Single-shot Ad26 vaccine protects against SARS-CoV-2 in rhesus macaques. Nature 2020;586(7830):583–8. https://doi.org/10.1038/s41586-020-2607-z.

[43] Alter G, Yu J, Liu J, et al. Immunogenicity of Ad26.COV2.S vaccine against SARS-CoV-2 variants in humans. Nature 2021. https://doi.org/10.1038/s41586-021-03681-2.

[44] Covid J. Vaccines and Related Biological Products Advisory Committee Meeting February 26, 202. 62.

[45] CDC. Labs. Centers for Disease Control and Prevention. 2020. Available at: https://www.cdc.gov/coronavirus/2019-ncov/lab/resources/antigen-tests-guidelines.html. Accessed June 16, 2021.

[46] Perchetti GA, Huang M-L, Mills MG, et al. Analytical sensitivity of the Abbott BinaxNOW COVID-19 Ag

card. J Clin Microbiol 2021;59(3). https://doi.org/10.1128/JCM.02880-20.

[47] Okoye NC, Barker AP, Curtis K, et al. Performance characteristics of BinaxNOW COVID-19 antigen card for screening asymptomatic individuals in a university setting. J Clin Microbiol 2021;59(4). https://doi.org/10.1128/JCM.03282-20.

[48] Prince-Guerra JL, Almendares O, Nolen LD, et al. Evaluation of Abbott BinaxNOW rapid antigen test for SARS-CoV-2 Infection at two community-based testing sites - Pima County, Arizona, November 3-17, 2020. MMWR Morb Mortal Wkly Rep 2021;70(3):100–5.

[49] Pray IW, Ford L, Cole D, et al. Performance of an antigen-based test for asymptomatic and symptomatic SARS-CoV-2 testing at two university campuses - Wisconsin, September-October 2020. MMWR Morb Mortal Wkly Rep 2021;69(5152):1642–7.

[50] Brihn A, Chang J, OYong K, et al. Diagnostic performance of an antigen test with RT-PCR for the detection of SARS-CoV-2 in a hospital setting - Los Angeles County, California, June-August 2020. MMWR Morb Mortal Wkly Rep 2021;70(19):702–6.

[51] Beck ET, Paar W, Fojut L, et al. Comparison of the Quidel Sofia SARS FIA test to the hologic aptima SARS-CoV-2 TMA test for diagnosis of COVID-19 in symptomatic outpatients. J Clin Microbiol 2021;59(2). https://doi.org/10.1128/JCM.02727-20.

[52] Kilic A, Hiestand B, Palavecino E. Evaluation of performance of the BD Veritor SARS-CoV-2 chromatographic immunoassay test in patients with symptoms of COVID-19. J Clin Microbiol 2021;59(5). https://doi.org/10.1128/JCM.00260-21.

[53] Young S, Taylor SN, Cammarata CL, et al. Clinical evaluation of BD veritor SARS-CoV-2 point-of-care test performance compared to PCR-based testing and versus the Sofia 2 SARS antigen point-of-care test. J Clin Microbiol 2020;59(1). https://doi.org/10.1128/JCM.02338-20.

[54] Moreno GK, Braun KM, Pray IW, et al. SARS-CoV-2 transmission in intercollegiate athletics not fully mitigated with daily antigen testing. Clin Infect Dis 2021. https://doi.org/10.1093/cid/ciab343.

Advances in Molecular Pathology 4 (2021) 231–235
ADVANCES IN MOLECULAR PATHOLOGY

The Genomic Landscape of Severe Acute Respiratory Syndrome Coronavirus 2

Surveillance of Variants of Concern

M. Shaheen S. Malick, MD, Helen Fernandes, PhD*
Department of Pathology & Cell Biology, Columbia University Irving Medical Center, 630 West 168th Street, New York, NY 10032, USA

KEYWORDS
• Genomic surveillance • SARS-CoV-2 mutations/variants • Variants of concern • COVID-19 pandemic

KEY POINTS

- Severe acute respiratory syndrome coronavirus 2 variants or strains may have varying degrees of transmissibility, virulence, pathogenicity and response to vaccines.
- Monitoring and identifying variants is crucial to control the current pandemic.
- Vaccines developed for the wild-type virus may have decreased efficacy against some variants of concern.
- Global surveillance is important for public health initiatives.

Mutations are random events that naturally occur during replication of the error-prone viral genome. The host–pathogen interaction drives the selective pressure by which variants capable of escaping aspects of the natural and, perhaps, induced immunity subsequently start to dominate the circulating pool of infecting strains [1]. Rapid characterization and active monitoring of emerging variants to understand their potential impact on countermeasures against severe acute respiratory syndrome coronavirus 2 (SARS-CoV-2) is critical to the control of the pandemic. The Centers for Disease Control and Prevention (cdc.gov) has classified emerging variants into 3 categories based on the degree of impact of coronavirus disease-2019 (COVID-19) in the United States, namely, variants of interest, Variants of concern, and variants of high consequence (see https://www.cdc.gov/coronavirus/2019-ncov/cases-updates/variant-surveillance/variant-info.html for further details). Variants of concern have been in part responsible for the waves of infection that we see globally (Fig. 1).

There are several key reasons why genomic surveillance has now become crucial in the global efforts to manage the COVID-19 pandemic. Since late fall of 2020, 4 new SARS CoV-2 variants of concern emerged; the UK variant, known as 501Y.V1 or B.1.1.7; the South African variant known as 501Y.V2 or B.1.351; the 501Y.V3 or P.1 variant from Brazil; and most recently the B.1.617.2 variant in India. These variants share some common mutations but each has their own unique genomic landscape. On May 31 2021, the World Health organization elected to simplify the names of theses variants of concern with Greek alphabets. The 4 variants of concern are now alpha, beta, gamma, and delta, respectively (https://www.who.int/en/activities/tracking-SARS-CoV-2-variants/).

*Corresponding author, *E-mail address:* hf2340@cumc.columbia.edu

https://doi.org/10.1016/j.yamp.2021.06.006
2589-4080/21/

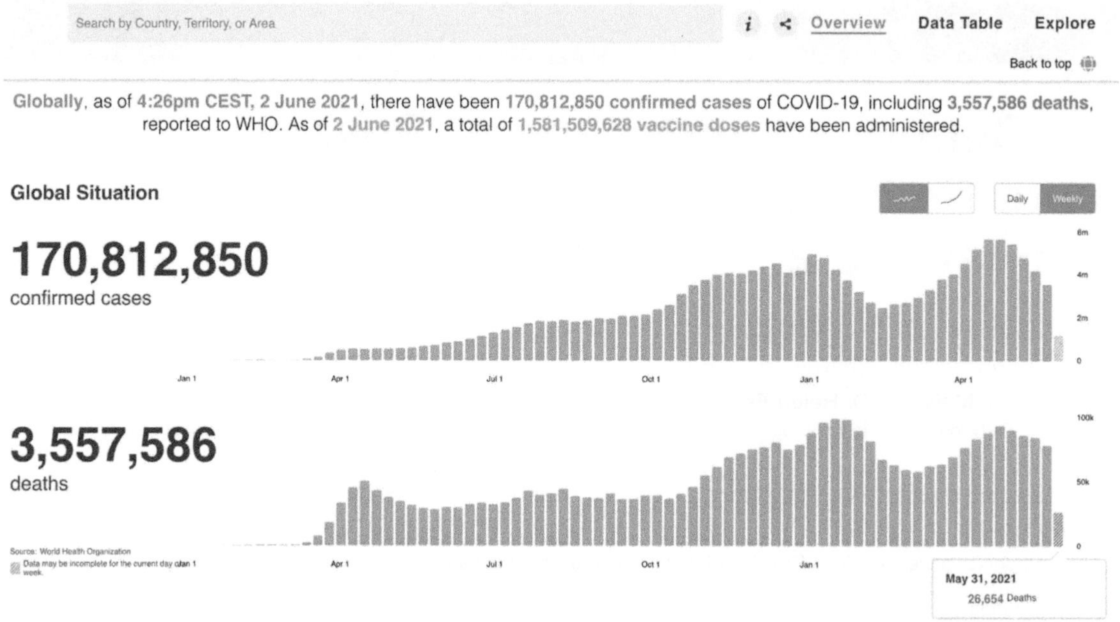

FIG. 1 Depicts the global pattern of COVID-19 infections and fatalities from April 2020 to April 2021. The waves represent variants of concern that emerge in different countries. (Source: World Health Organization.)

Some variants seem to have enhanced transmissibility or infectivity than the wild-type virus and other circulating strains. These acquired characteristics of SARS-CoV-2 have been responsible for the continued surge of cases and the increased fatality in different parts of the globe (Fig. 2). Additionally, early clinical trials have demonstrated reduced vaccine efficacy against novel strains compared with the original strain, most notable being the 501Y.V2 (B1.351) variant in South Africa. As several nations enter into a second wave of cases, reports of reinfection with the new circulating variants arise regularly, generating concern on the status of acquired immunity from prior exposure.

VARIANTS OF CONCERN IN RESOURCE-LIMITED SETTINGS

India and Brazil represent 2 important locations to examine given the recent surge in cases primarily owing to novel variants of concern. The B.1.617 variant first detected in India in October 2020 is characterized by L452R, D614G, and P681R substitutions within the spike protein domain. Three sublineages have been characterized, with B.1.617.2 being the predominant strain currently devastating India during its second wave. Based on the observed growth in sequenced cases, the B.1.617.2 variant is more transmissible than the B.1.1.7 variants [2,3]. An additional cause for concern as India battles this variant is that, despite high levels of seroprevalence, indicating prior infection, in regions such as Delhi (56%), Mumbai (≤75%), and Hyderabad (54%), the number of cases in these cities is once again surging [4]. This pattern is not at all unique to India.

In Manaus, Brazil, a variant with an E484K substitution was associated with a recent surge in cases despite a reported seroprevalence of 76% as of October 2020 [5]. An important caveat to seroprevalence studies is that detectable humoral immunity does not capture the entire scope of immunity, including T-cell reactivity. However, the estimated infection rate in Manaus is greater than the theoretic herd immunity threshold of 67% using a case reproduction number (R_0) of 3 [6]. The abrupt surge in hospitalizations that hit Manaus in January 2021 followed a period during which physical distancing requirements were eased (see ref. [5]). This surge that surprisingly included SARS-CoV-2 reinfection of individuals in addition to new individuals, was attributed to a novel strain containing an E484K substitution [7]. Reinfection in the city of Manaus has been associated with the P.1 lineage characterized by 10 unique spike protein mutations, including E484K and N501K [8]. In a Brazilian case of reinfection

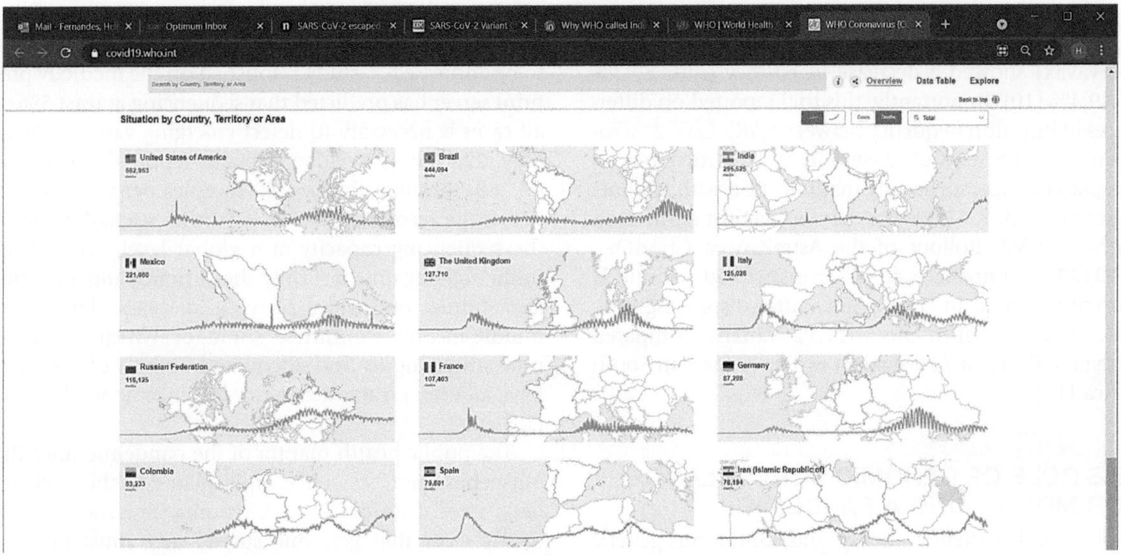

FIG. 2 Shows the global landscape of SARS-CoV-2 infections over time. The patterns of emergence, representing increased infectivity, are seen. (Source: World Health Organization.)

9 months after initial infection, the reinfecting virus carried all lineage-defining mutations of P.1, but 11 additional amino acid substitutions in the S-protein relative to the primary infecting virus.

Interestingly, the unique molecular signatures that characterize the novel strains seem to be responsible for the lack of protection in previously infected individuals. Variants with E484Q or E484K substitutions have been found to have reduced neutralization by protective antibodies, or are, in other words, able to escape optimal protection by humoral immunity. This has been demonstrated effectively by an international research collaboration led by the Africa Health Research Institute (Durban, South Africa). This team used in vitro live viral neutralization assays, with plasma from individuals infected during the country's first and second waves. They clearly demonstrated that convalescent plasma from individuals infected with the wild-type virus during the first wave was unable to neutralize the 501Y.V2 (B1.1.351) virus that was responsible for roughly 97% of cases during the second wave in South Africa [9].

SEROPREVALENCE AND EFFICACY OF VACCINES

Returning to the idea of herd immunity, the resurgence in Brazil and India despite a seroprevalance of greater than 70% causes us to reconsider our current mathematical models for herd immunity. This model is represented by equation $R = (1 - p_c)(1 - p_I)R_0$, where R is the effective reproduction number, p_c, is the relative reduction in transmission owing to nonpharmaceutical measures, p_I is the proportion of immune individuals, and R_0 is the reproduction number in the absence of controls in a fully susceptible population. In this model, herd immunity is achieved when R is less than 1, hopefully indicating an end to future large outbreaks. If this model holds true, then the only way to explain the surges in Brazil and India is if current seroprevalance studies no longer accurately represent the proportion of immune individuals, or p_I, because seropositivity of an older strain would not represent immunity to a novel variant of concern. The other potential explanation would be if the R_0 of these variants were greater than that of the prior circulating strains. Potentially, both of these situations may be true. Whatever the explanation, given the dynamic nature of the virus, genomic surveillance is key to understanding the variant landscape of the infecting virus.

Notably, we have not yet raised the question of whether current SARS-CoV-2 vaccines are effective against novel strains, or whether they affect p_c in the way they have increased p_c for early strains. Preliminary results from clinical trials suggest that the vaccines developed for the wild-type virus may have a decreased efficacy against variants of concern. So far, in South Africa, at least 2 clinical trials during the second wave reported a decrease in vaccine efficacy against the 501Y.V2 strain. The NVX-CoV2373 subunit vaccine (Novavax) showed a decrease in efficacy from 89.3% to 49.4% [10]. Importantly, this trial reported no differences in infection frequency between SARS-CoV-2–seropositive and SARS-CoV-2–seronegative participants in the placebo arm, suggesting that infection with variants other than 501Y.V2 does not protect against reinfection with 501Y.V2. Rollout of the AstraZeneca ChAdOx1 AZD1222 chimpanzee adenovirus-vectored vaccine is currently paused in South Africa after displaying only 10% efficacy against the 501Y.V2 variant, compared with an efficacy of 75% against earlier variants in South Africa [11].

THE ROLE OF GENOMIC SURVEILLANCE FOR MONITORING A PANDEMIC

Representative, quality, timely, and continuous genetic surveillance of SARS-CoV-2 is critical to the COVID-19 outbreak response. In addition to acquiring information on the infectivity and virulence of the virus, quick identification genomic alterations helps to elucidate the molecular mechanisms that allow variants of concern to evade vaccine-induced immunity and/or targeted therapy. Sequencing can also potentially alert us to variants that may eventually render current diagnostic tests ineffective.

Currently, there is a lack of capacity for genomic surveillance globally. Rapid progress is occurring in scaling up genomic surveillance. However, the level of surveillance has not reached the necessary breadth to track and manage the pandemic. Large numbers of samples were sequenced in the UK, the United States, Australia, and Iceland and data were shared promptly. However, as of May 22, 2021, the United States has shared 11.7 sequences per 1000 cases and currently ranks 25th in the number of genomic sequences shared to the online genome repository GISAID compared with the UK with 85.1 sequences shared per 1000 cases and 16 days to deposition [12]. Since November 2020, the US Centers for Disease Control and Prevention have accepted SARS-CoV-2 samples from state health departments and other public health agencies for sequencing and further necessary characterization in a program called the National SARS-CoV-2 Strain Surveillance System (see ref. [1]). Although this program continues to grow there is additional work to be done, especially because the United States has the highest number of reported cases. The lack of capacity for testing alone, in the United States does not explain the deficiency in sequencing. There is an enormous virus-sequencing capacity, but funding, coordination, and systemic problems in sharing samples and data are hurdles that need to be addressed. A study published on the medRxiv preprint server has predicted that sequencing at least 5% of all cases is necessary to detect emerging variants. As of May 22, the last 7-day average reported cases was 27,789, meaning that at 750 samples per week we are below the recommended 5%. Further strengthening of the sequencing capacity at a global level would help in the fight against not only the current pandemic, but also future outbreaks of viral diseases. Low- and middle-income countries, some of which are even now struggling to find adequate numbers of vaccines, have an even greater deficiency in genomic surveillance [13].

The public health mantra of the pandemic since the outset has been "test, trace, and isolate." As the phylogenetic tree of SARS-CoV-2 blossoms, it is now abundantly clear that genomic surveillance must buttress our testing. Otherwise, we may be unsuccessful in tackling this to the best of our capacity. Perhaps the greatest aspect of human creativity is the ability to do highly impactful work with limited resources, making the best of what we have available. With diagnostic stewardship, it is possible to scale up genomic surveillance worldwide, although we will need to be strategic about how the scarce genomic sequencing resources are used and shared globally. In areas where this infrastructure is limited, genomic surveillance still can and must be done, although it will need to be much more targeted. For example, in resource-limited settings, genomic surveillance may be limited to only patients who present with reinfections. This approach can then be broadened to entire geographic areas that develop surges in infection despite having reached herd immunity, or regions with unexpectedly high rates of transmission. It is also important to correlate variant and lineage details with epidemiologic data to inform public health decisions. We have entered a new era in the COVID-19 pandemic. However, it may also be a promising turning point in pandemic preparedness.

REFERENCES

[1] Genomic surveillance for SARS-CoV-2 variants – CDC. 2021. Available at: https://www.cdc.gov/coronavirus/2019-ncov/cases-updates/variant-surveillance.html. Accessed May 21, 2021.

[2] SAGE 89 minutes: coronavirus (COVID-19) response, 13 May 2021. In: Eighty-ninth SAGE meeting on COVID-19. 2021. Available at: https://www.gov.uk/government/publications/sage-89-minutes-coronavirus-covid-19-

response-13-may-2021/sage-89-minutes-coronavirus-covid-19-response-13-may-2021 2021. Accessed May 26, 2021.

[3] Narang D. COVID-19: the second wave may not be the last – but which one will be? Science, the Wire. 2021. Available at: https://science.thewire.in/health/covid-19-the-second-wave-may-not-be-the-last-but-which-one-will-be/. Accessed May 24, 2021.

[4] Hyderabad SARS-CoV-2 serosurvey – Ministry of Science and Technology, Govt. of India, Council of Scientific and Industrial Research, Centre for Cellular and Molecular Biology. Available at: https://www.ccmb.res.in/press-covrg/Hyderabad_SARS_CoV2_serosuvey.pdf. Accessed May 26, 2021.

[5] Sabino EC, Buss LF, Carvalho MPS, et al. Resurgence of COVID-19 in Manaus, Brazil, despite high seroprevalence. Lancet 2021;397(10273):452–5.

[6] Fontanet A, Cauchemez S. COVID-19 herd immunity: where are we? Nat Rev Immunol 2020;20(10):583–4.

[7] Nonaka CKV, Franco MM, Gräf T, et al. Genomic evidence of SARS-CoV-2 reinfection involving E484K spike mutation, Brazil. Emerg Infect Dis 2021;27(5):1522–4.

[8] Faria NR, Claro IM, Candido D, et al. Genomic characterisation of an emergent SARS-CoV-2 lineage in Manaus: preliminary findings. 2021. Virological.Org.

[9] Cele S, Gazy I, Jackson L, et al. Escape of SARS-CoV-2 501Y.V2 from neutralization by convalescent plasma. Nature 2021;593(7857):142–6.

[10] Shinde V, Bhikha S, Hoosain Z, et al, 2019nCoV-501 Study Group. Efficacy of NVX-CoV2373 Covid-19 vaccine against the B.1.351 variant. N Engl J Med 2021; 384(20):1899–909.

[11] Madhi SA, Baillie V, Cutland CL, et al, NGS-SA Group, Wits-VIDA COVID Group. Efficacy of the ChAdOx1 nCoV-19 Covid-19 vaccine against the B.1.351 variant. N Engl J Med 2021;384(20):1885–98.

[12] Global sequencing coverage, COVID-19 CoV genetics, enabled by data from GISAID. Available at: https://cov-idcg.org/?tab=global_sequencing. Accessed May 23, 2021.

[13] Cyranoski D. Alarming COVID variants show vital role of genomic surveillance. Nature 2021;589(7842):337–8.